Quality of Life Outcomes in Clinical Trials and Health-Care Evaluation

STATISTICS IN PRACTICE

Advisory Editor

Stephen Senn
University of Glasgow, UK

Founding Editor

Vic Barnett
Nottingham Trent University, UK

Statistics in Practice is an important international series of texts which provide detailed coverage of statistical concepts, methods and worked case studies in specific fields of investigation and study.

With sound motivation and many worked practical examples, the books show in down-to-earth terms how to select and use an appropriate range of statistical techniques in a particular practical field within each title's special topic area.

The books provide statistical support for professionals and research workers across a range of employment fields and research environments. Subject areas covered include medicine and pharmaceutics; industry, finance and commerce; public services; the earth and environmental sciences, and so on.

The books also provide support to students studying statistical courses applied to the above areas. The demand for graduates to be equipped for the work environment has led to such courses becoming increasingly prevalent at universities and colleges.

It is our aim to present judiciously chosen and well-written workbooks to meet every-day practical needs. Feedback of views from readers will be most valuable to monitor the success of this aim.

A complete list of titles in this series appears at the end of the volume.

Quality of Life Outcomes in Clinical Trials and Health-Care Evaluation

A Practical Guide to Analysis and Interpretation

Stephen J. Walters

School of Health and Related Research, University of Sheffield, UK

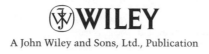

A John Wiley and Sons, Ltd., Publication

Library of Congress Cataloguing-in-Publication Data

Walters, Stephen John.
  Quality of life outcomes in clinical trials and health-care evaluation : a practical guide to analysis and interpretation / Stephen Walters.
    p. ; cm.
  Includes bibliographical references and index.
  ISBN 978-0-470-75382-8 (cloth)
  1. Clinical trials. 2. Quality of life. 3. Outcome assessment (Medical care) I. Title.
  [DNLM: 1. Cross-Sectional Studies. 2. Randomized Controlled Trials as Topic. 3. Outcome Assessment (Health Care) 4. Quality of Life. 5. Research Design. WA 950 W235q 2009]
  R853.C55W35 2009
  610.72′4 – dc22

2009024883

A catalogue record for this book is available from the British Library.

ISBN: 978-0-470-75382-8

Set in 10/12pt Times Roman by Laserwords Pvt Ltd, Chennai, India
Printed and bound in Great Britain by CPI Antony Rowe, Chippenham, Wiltshire

Contents

Preface

Quality of life (QoL) outcomes or person/patient reported outcome measures (PROMs) are now frequently being used in randomized controlled trials (RCTs) and observational studies. This book aims to be a practical guide to the design, analysis and interpretation of studies that use such outcomes. Since there are numerous QoL instruments now available, it emphasizes that, for busy and time-constrained researchers, it is easier to use an 'off-the-shelf' QoL instrument than to design your own. This book gives practical guidance on how to choose between the various instruments.

QoL outcomes tend to generate data with discrete, bounded and skewed distributions. Hence, many investigators are concerned about the appropriateness of using standard statistical methods to analyse QoL data and want guidance on what methods to use. This book provides such practical guidance, based on the author's extensive experience. Other texts, on the analysis of QoL outcomes, concentrate mainly on clinical trials and ignore other frequently used study designs such as cross-sectional surveys and non-randomized health-care evaluations. Again this book rectifies this and provides practical guidance on the analysis of QoL outcomes from such observational designs. It presents simple conventional methods to tackle these problems (such as linear regression), before addressing more advanced approaches, including ordinal regression and computer-intensive methods (such as the bootstrap).

The book is illustrated throughout with real-life case studies and worked examples from RCTs and other observational studies, taken from the author's own experience of designing and analysing studies with QoL outcomes. Each analysis technique is carefully explained and the mathematics, as far as possible, is kept to a minimum. Hopefully, it is written in a style suitable for statisticians and clinicians alike!

The practical guidance provided by this book will be of use to professionals working in and/or managing clinical trials, in academic, government and industrial settings, particularly medical statisticians, clinicians and trial co-ordinators. Its practical approach will appeal to applied statisticians and biomedical researchers, in particular those in the biopharmaceutical industry, medical and public health organizations. Graduate students of medical statistics will also find much of benefit, as will graduate students of the medical and health sciences who have to analyse QoL data for their dissertations and projects.

Most of the book is written at an intermediate level for readers who are going to collect and analyse their own QoL data. It is expected that readers will be familiar with basic statistical concepts such as hypothesis testing (P-values), confidence intervals, simple statistical tests (e.g. the t-test and chi-square test) and simple linear regression. The more advanced topics, in the later chapters, such as marginal generalized linear models for longitudinal data, will require a more thorough statistical knowledge, but are explained in as simple a way as possible with examples.

Stephen J. Walters
Sheffield, UK

1

Introduction

Summary

Quality of life (QoL) is a complex concept with multiple dimensions. This book will assume a wide definition for this concept. It will describe the design, assessment, analysis and interpretation of single- and multi-item, subjective measurement scales. These measurement scales all have the common feature of using a standardized approach to assessing a person's perception of their own health by using numerical scoring systems, and may include one or several dimensions of QoL. This chapter will provide a brief history of QoL assessment; describe the different types of QoL assessment tools available and give reasons why it is important to measure QoL.

1.1 What is quality of life?

Quality of life (QoL) is a complex concept with multiple aspects. These aspects (usually referred to as domains or dimensions) can include: cognitive functioning; emotional functioning; psychological well-being; general health; physical functioning; physical symptoms and toxicity; role functioning; sexual functioning; social well-being and functioning; and spiritual/existential issues (see Figure 1.1). This book will assume a wide definition for this concept. It will describe the design, assessment, analysis and interpretation of single- and multi-item, subjective measurement scales. This broad definition will include scales or instruments that ask general questions, such as 'In general, how would you rate your health now?', and more specific questions on particular symptoms and side effects, such as 'During the past week have you felt nauseated?'. These measurement scales all have the common feature of using a standardized approach to assessing a person's perception of their own health by using numerical scoring systems, and may include one or several dimensions of QoL.

Quality of Life Outcomes in Clinical Trials and Health-Care Evaluation   Stephen J. Walters
© 2009 John Wiley & Sons, Ltd

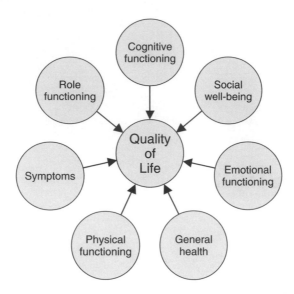

Figure 1.1   Examples of QoL domains.

1.2   Terminology

Researchers have used a variety of names to describe QoL measurement scales. Some prefer to use the term *health-related quality of life* (HRQoL or HRQL), to stress that we are only concerned with health aspects. Others have used the terms *health status* and *self-reported health*. The United States Food and Drug Administration (FDA) has adopted the term *patient-reported outcome (PRO)* in its guidance to the pharmaceutical industry for supporting labelling claims for medical product development (FDA, 2006). However, not all people who complete such outcomes are ill and patients, and hence PRO could legitimately stand for *person-reported outcome*. Mostly, we shall assume that the QoL instrument or outcome is self-reported, by the person whose experience we are interested in, but it could be completed by another person or proxy. The term *health outcome assessment* has been put forward as an alternative which avoids specifying the respondent. This book will follow convention and use the now well-established term *quality of life*.

1.3   History

The World Health Organisation (WHO, 1948) declared health to be 'A state of complete physical and mental social well-being, and not merely the absence of disease and infirmity'. This definition was one of the first to emphasize other facets of health, such as physical, mental and social, in connection with disease and infirmity.

The Karnofsky Performance Scale (Karnofsky and Burchenal, 1949) was one of the first instruments to undertake a wider assessment of patients' functional impairment apart from clinical and physiological examination. It involves health-care staff assessing patients, using a simple single-item 11-point scale ranging from 0 for 'dead' to 100

Table 1.1   The Karnofsky Performance Scale.

Description	Score
Normal; no complaints; no evidence of disease	100
Able to carry on normal activity; minor signs and symptoms of disease	90
Normal activity with effort; some signs and symptoms of disease	80
Cares for self; unable to carry on normal activity or do work	70
Requires occasional assistance, but is able to care for most personal needs	60
Requires considerable assistance and frequent medical care	50
Disabled; requires special care and assistance	40
Severely disabled; hospitalization indicated although death not imminent	30
Very sick; hospitalization necessary; requires active support treatment	20
Moribund; fatal processes progressing rapidly	10
Dead	0

for 'Normal' (see Table 1.1). It can be used to compare effectiveness of different therapies and to assess the prognosis in individual patients.

This led to the development of the next generation of questionnaires which focused on broader aspects of QoL, such as emotional well-being, social functioning, impact of illness, perceived distress and life satisfaction. These included the Nottingham Health Profile (NHP, Hunt *et al.*, 1980, 1981) and the Sickness Impact Profile (SIP, Deyo *et al.*, 1982). Again, I shall describe the NHP and SIP as QoL scales although their developers neither designed them nor claimed them as QoL scales.

Newer instruments such as the Medical Outcomes Study (MOS) Short Form (SF)-36 (Ware and Sherbourne, 1992) now place more emphasis on the subjective aspects of QoL, such as emotional, role, social and cognitive functioning. The SF-36 is the most commonly used QoL measure in the world today. It contains 36 questions measuring health across eight dimensions: Physical Functioning (PF); Role-Physical (role limitations due to physical health, RP); Social Functioning (SF); Vitality (VT); Bodily Pain (BP); Mental Health (MH); Role-Emotional (role limitations due to emotional problems, RE); and General Health (GH).

Quality of life was introduced by the MEDLINE (Medical Literature Analysis and Retrieval System Online) international literature database of life sciences and biomedical information as a heading in 1975, and accepted as a concept by Index Medicus in 1977. Since then there has been a rapid expansion of interest in the topic, with an exponential increase in the number of citations of QoL in the medical literature (see Figure 1.2).

In 1991, the first edition of a new international, multidisciplinary journal devoted to the rapid communication of original research, theoretical articles and methodological reports related to the field of QoL in all the health sciences was published, entitled *Quality of Life Research*. The February 2004 issue was largely devoted to the publication of abstracts from the first meeting of the International Society for Quality of Life Research (ISOQOL), held in Brussels. ISOQOL's mission is the scientific study of QoL relevant to health and health care. The Society promotes the rigorous investigation of health-related QoL measurement from conceptualization to application and practice. ISOQOL fosters the worldwide exchange of information through scientific publications, international conferences, educational outreach, and collaborative support for QoL initiatives.

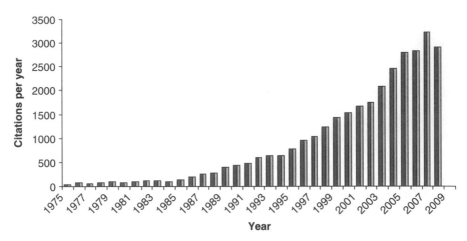

Figure 1.2 MEDLINE database 'quality of life' focused subject heading citations, 1975–2008.

1.4   Types of quality of life measures

The SF-36 is an example of a QoL instrument that is intended for general use, irrespective of the illness or condition of the patient. Such instruments are often termed *generic* measures and may often be applicable to healthy people too and hence used in population surveys. Figure 1.3 shows the distribution of the eight main dimensions of the SF-36 from a general population survey of United Kingdom residents (Brazier *et al.*, 1992). The SF-36 dimensions are scored on a 0 to 100 ('good health') scale. Figure 1.3 shows that the SF-36 outcome, in common with many other QoL scales, generates data with a discrete, bounded and skewed distribution. Figure 1.4 shows how physical functioning in the general population (Walters *et al.*, 2001a) declines rapidly with increasing age.

The SF-36 is also an example of a *profile* QoL measure since it generates eight separate scores for each dimension of health (Figure 1.3). Other generic profile instruments include the SIP and NHP (see Section 1.3). Conversely, some other QoL measures generate a single summary score or *single index*, which combines the different dimensions of health into a single number. An example of a single index QoL outcome is the EuroQol or EQ-5D as it is now named (EuroQol Group, 1990).

Generic instruments are intended to cover a wide range of conditions and have the advantage that the scores from patients with various diseases may be compared against each other and against the general population. For example, Figure 1.5 compares the mean SF-36 dimension scores of a group of patients six months after acute myocardial infarction (AMI) with an age and sex matched general population sample (Lacey and Walters, 2003). The AMI sample has lower QoL on all eight dimensions of the SF-36 than the general population sample. On the other hand, generic instruments may fail to focus on the issues of particular concern to patients with disease, and may often lack the sensitivity to detect differences that arise as a consequence of treatments that are compared in clinical trials. This has led to the development of *condition-* or *disease-specific* questionnaires. Disease-specific QoL measurement scales are comprehensively reviewed by Bowling (2001, 2004). Examples of disease-specific QoL questionnaires include the

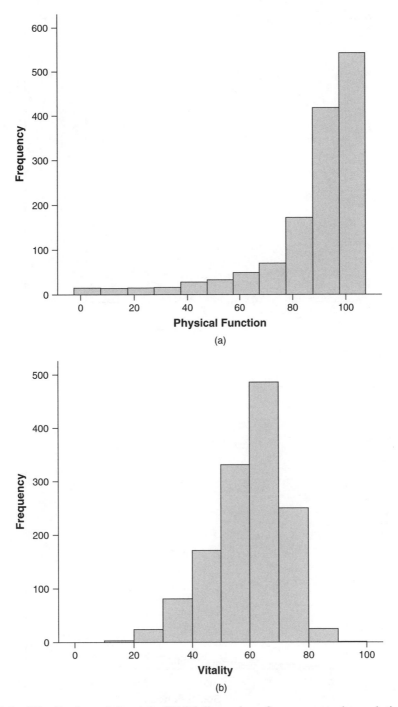

Figure 1.3 Distribution of the eight SF-36 dimensions from a general population survey (*n* = 1372); a score of 100 indicates 'good health' (data from Brazier *et al.*, 1992).

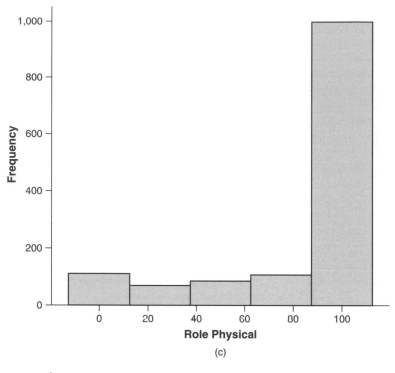

(c)

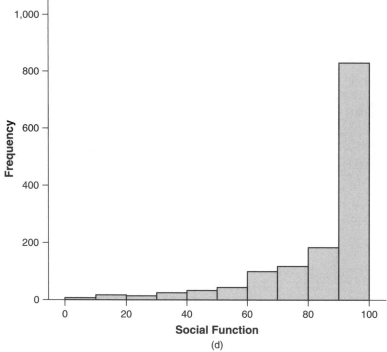

(d)

Figure 1.3   (*Continued*)

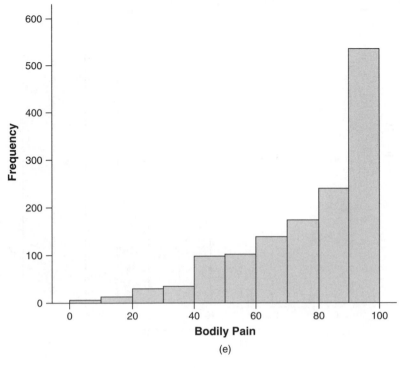

Bodily Pain

(e)

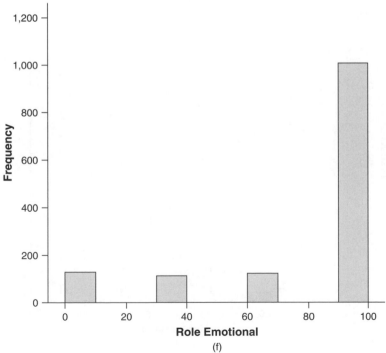

Role Emotional

(f)

Figure 1.3   (*Continued*)

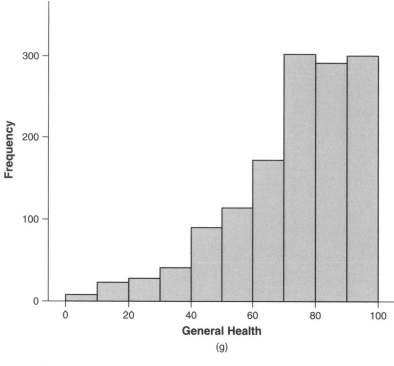

(g)

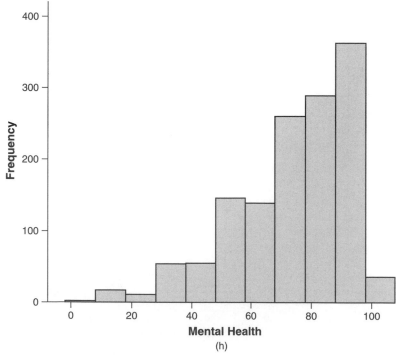

(h)

Figure 1.3   (*Continued*)

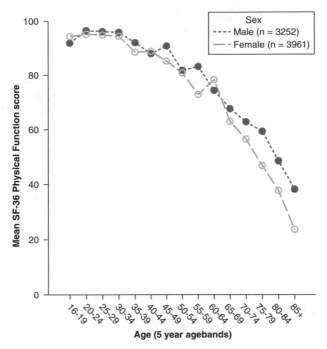

Figure 1.4   Mean SF-36 Physical Functioning age profile by sex (data from Walters *et al.*, 2001a).

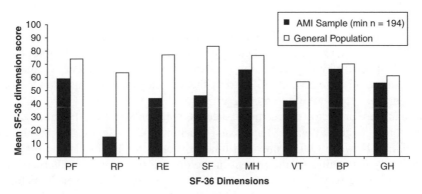

Figure 1.5   Profile of mean SF-36 scores for an acute myocardial infarction sample (six weeks after infarction) compared with an age and sex matched general population sample (data from Lacey and Walters, 2003).

cancer-specific 30-item European Organisation for Research and Treatment of Cancer (EORTC) QLC-30 questionnaire (Aaronson *et al.*, 1993) and the cancer-specific 30-item Rotterdam Symptom Checklist (RSCL, de Haes *et al.*, 1990).

The instruments described above claim to measure general QoL, and usually include at least one question about overall QoL or health. Sometimes investigators may wish to explore particular aspects or concepts in greater depth. There are also instruments for specific aspects of QoL. These specific aspects may include anxiety and depression, physical functioning, pain and fatigue. Examples of instruments which evaluate specific aspects of QoL are: the Hospital Anxiety and Depression Scale (HADS, Zigmond and Snaith, 1983) and the Beck Depression Inventory (BDI, Beck *et al.*, 1961) instruments for measuring anxiety and depression; the McGill Pain Questionnaire (MPQ, Melzack, 1975) for the measurement of pain; the Multidimensional Fatigue Inventory (MFI, Smets *et al.*, 1995) for assessing fatigue and the Barthel Index (Mahoney and Barthel, 1965) for assessing disability and functioning.

1.5   Why measure quality of life?

There are several reasons why we should measure quality of life in both a research setting and in routine clinical practice. The use of QoL assessment in routine clinical practice may make communication with patients easier and help find out information about the range of problems that affect patients. Medicine and health care have traditionally tended to focus on symptom relief as the main outcome measure. QoL assessment may help improve symptom relief, care or rehabilitation for an individual patient. Using QoL instruments may reveal other issues that are equally or more important to patients than just symptom relief. The patient's self-assessment of their own QoL may differ substantially from the judgement of other health-care staff. Individual patient preferences may also differ from those of other patients. Therefore it is important to measure QoL from the patient's perspective, using a self-completed questionnaire to establish their views and preferences. Cured patients and long-term survivors may have ongoing problems long after their treatment is successfully completed. These ongoing problems may be overlooked, so again it important to measure QoL long term and to look for late problems of psychosocial adaptation.

QoL assessments may be included in research studies such as randomized controlled trials (RCTs). The main reason is to compare the study treatments with respect to those aspects of QoL that may be affected by the treatment. These treatment comparisons will include both the positive benefits from trials that are expected to improve QoL, and any negative changes, from toxicity and side effects of treatment.

QoL can be a predictor of treatment success, and hence pre-treatment assessment of QoL may have prognostic value. Fayers and Machin (2007) suggest that the direction of the association between QoL scores and treatment outcome is not clear. Do QoL scores reflect an early perception by the patient of the disease progression? Alternatively, does QoL status in some way influence the course of the disease? Whatever the nature of the association, it is important to assess QoL and use it when making medical decisions for individual patients.

QoL assessment can also be used to make decisions on treatments at a population level, rather than an individual patient level. QoL outcomes can be used in economic evaluations alongside clinical trials to asses the clinical and cost-effectiveness of new health technologies.

There is an ongoing thoughtful discussion about the meaning of QoL, and about what should be measured. In the face of this debate, it is still important to measure quality of life as well as clinical and process-based outcomes. This is because 'All of the these [QoL] concepts reflect issues that are of fundamental importance to patients' well-being. They are all worth investigating and quantifying' (Fayers and Machin, 2007).

1.6   Further reading

The two books by Bowling extensively describe the numerous QoL instruments now available (Bowling 2001, 2004). The book by Fayers and Machin (2007) covers all aspects of QoL assessment, analysis and interpretation. Fairclough (2002) goes into more detail about the statistical analysis of QoL data in RCTs with a strong emphasis on imputation methods for missing data and the modelling of longitudinal data. The book edited by Fayers and Hays (2005) covers a variety of topics in its 27 chapters with contributions from 31 authors and provides an overview of QoL assessment, analysis and interpretation.

2

Measuring quality of life

Summary

This chapter describes the principles of measurement scales and introduces the methods for developing and validating new questionnaires. Psychometric methods lead to scales that are based upon items reflecting a patient's level of QoL. The clinimetric approach makes use of composite scales that may include symptoms and side effects. The remainder of the chapter provides an overview of the stages of developing and validating new questionnaires and the principles that are involved.

2.1   Introduction

Questionnaires for assessing QoL usually contain multiple questions or items, although rarely a few may attempt to rely upon a single global question to assess overall QoL. For example, 'Overall, what has your quality of life been like over the last week?'. Some QoL questionnaires are designed so that all items are combined together to produce an overall score. Most instruments attempt to group the items into separate 'scales' corresponding to different dimensions of QoL. This chapter explores the relationship between items and scales and introduces the concepts underlying QoL scales and their measurement.

2.2   Principles of measurement scales

2.2.1   Scales and items

Most QoL instruments consist of many questions or items. These items are usually combined to generate a dimension or domain score. Figure 2.1 shows this process graphically. Some of these items may aim to measure a relatively simple aspect of QoL, such as physical symptoms like nausea, vomiting or constipation. For these relatively simple aspects of QoL a single question or item may be sufficient to measure the underlying dimension.

Quality of Life Outcomes in Clinical Trials and Health-Care Evaluation   Stephen J. Walters
© 2009 John Wiley & Sons, Ltd

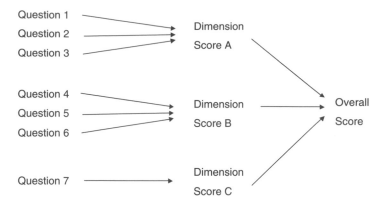

Figure 2.1   Items and scales.

For example, the EORTC QLQ-C30 questionnaire (Aaronson *et al.*, 1993), measures the symptom of constipation with the single question, 'During the past week, have you been constipated?'. The question has four possible response options: not at all; a little; quite a bit; very much.

The more complex psychological dimensions of QoL such as anxiety and depression are usually more vaguely defined in a subject's understanding of QoL. These dimensions are typically measured by the use of several questions in multi-item scales. For example, the Hospital Anxiety and Depression scale (HADS) consists of 14 items, with seven items on the 'anxiety' aspect and the other seven items assessing 'depression' (Zigmond and Snaith, 1983).

2.2.2   Constructs and latent variables

Fayers and Machin (2007) describe QoL as a complex construct that cannot be adequately measured by a single global question. They suggest that QoL has a number of dimensions (see Figure 1.1), each of which should be thought of as an underlying 'construct'. These constructs are represented or measured by 'latent variables', which we measure by asking the subject one or, more typically, a number of separate questions. For this reason QoL instruments commonly contain multiple questions to assess the underlying latent variables.

Example: Hospital Anxiety and Depression Scale (Zigmond and Snaith, 1983)

The HADS questionnaire (see Appendix A) is a QoL instrument with a simple theoretical structure (see Figure 2.2). It assumes that there are two different and distinct constructs of 'anxiety' and 'depression', which are meaningful to patients and can be quantified. It is assumed that anxiety and depression cannot be adequately measured by a single question, such as 'How anxious are you today?' (not at all, a little, quite a bit, very much), and that multiple questions must be employed. The HADS consists of 14 items, with seven questions relating to anxiety and seven questions relating to depression.   □

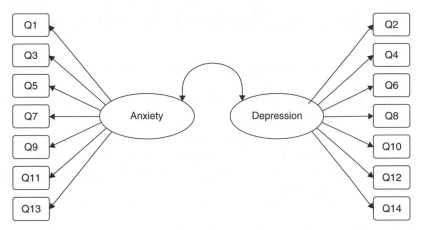

Figure 2.2   The theoretical structure of HADS. Reproduced with permission from *Fayers, P.M., Machin, D., Quality of Life: The Assessment, Analysis and Interpretation of Patient-reported Outcomes*. 2nd edition. John Wiley & Sons Ltd, Chichester. © 2007 John Wiley & Sons Ltd.

2.3   Indicator and causal variables

2.3.1   Indicator variables

Most items in personality tests, intelligence tests, educational attainment tests and other psychometric assessments reflect a level of ability or a state of mind. Such items do not alter or influence the latent construct that they measure. These items are *indicator variables* (Fayers and Machin, 2007). In common with most questionnaires that assess psychological aspects of QoL, the HADS items (see Appendix A) are mainly indicator variables. For example, 'During the past week, I feel tense or "wound up"'. The question has four possible response options: most of the time; a lot of the time; from time to time; not at all.

2.3.2   Causal variables

The symptoms (such as nausea, vomiting and constipation) assessed in QoL scales, such as the EORTC QLQ-C30 (Aaronson *et al.*, 1993) may cause a change in QoL. A patient who gets serious symptoms is likely to have their QoL affected by those symptoms. The reason for including symptoms in QoL instruments is principally that symptoms are believed to affect QoL. However, having a poor QoL does not imply that the patient has specific symptoms (such as nausea, vomiting and constipation). Typically, a single causal item may be enough to change the latent QoL variable. It is unnecessary, and usually rare, for each patient to suffer from all the symptoms in order to have a poor QoL. One serious symptom, such as extreme nausea, may be enough to reduce overall QoL.

Fayers and Machin (2007) caution that the above distinction between indicator and causal variables is not entirely clear-cut. Variables may frequently be partly indicator

---

Box 2.1 Identifying causal items (Fayers and Machin, 2007)

- "Thought test"
    - Consider a typical patient from the target population. For an item called, say, item X:
        - a) If the level of item X changes, is the patent's quality of life likely to change?

        - b) If the patient's quality of life improves (or deteriorates), do we expect this to be reflected by a change in item X?
    - If the answer to (a) is "yes" and (b) is "no", the item is likely to have a causal component.

---

and partly causal. For example, a patient may experience symptoms such as nausea and vomiting, become anxious and depressed, and then perceive and report the symptoms as being worse than they are. An initial causal variable has acquired indicator properties. So how can we identify causal variables? Fayers and Machin (2007) describe the *thought test* for identifying causal variables (see Box 2.1).

2.3.3 Why do we need to worry about the distinction between indicator and causal items?

Indicator variables assume that the observed responses to the items depend solely upon the level of the underlying latent variable. That is, if QoL is 'good', then this should be reflected in good or high levels of response on the various items. Furthermore, if the observed values of the items are correlated, then these correlations arise solely because of the effect of the latent variable. Causal variables are not correlated with each other through the different levels of QoL. They do not have correlations that arise through their parallel nature. Their correlations arise through an underlying variable – such as treatment, or stage or extent of disease. Thus causal variables may exhibit seemingly strange correlations that are nothing to do with changes in QoL. Causal items do not reflect QoL, they affect it. Therefore indicator and causal items behave in fundamentally different ways and this will have a considerable impact upon the design of QoL scales.

2.3.4 Single-item versus multi-item scales

Multi-item scales are commonly used to assess specific aspects of QoL. Responses from multiple items usually have several advantages over a score estimated from the responses to a single item in terms of reliability, precision, validity and scope (see Box 2.2).

2.4 The traditional psychometric model

The most common psychometric model is the *parallel tests* model. In this model each measurement item is a 'test' or question that reflects the level of the underlying construct or latent variable. Each item is distinct from the others, but is similar and comparable in all important respects. They differ only as a consequence of random error. These items

---

Box 2.2 Single-item versus multi-item scales

- *Reliability.* A reliable test is one that measures something in a consistent, repeatable and reproducible manner. Patient variability means that a single-item test is potentially unreliable since we only have one attempt to measure the QoL aspect we are interested in. Reliability is increased by including and averaging a number of 'parallel' items.

- *Precision.* Multi-item tests can have greater precision.

- *Validation.* The items of a multi-item scale can be compared against each other.

- *Scope.* QoL is a complex issue and not easily assessed by a single question.

Box 2.3 The traditional psychometric model – parallel tests

1. Each item is a test, which gives an unbiased estimate of the latent variable, with a random error term ε.

2. The error terms of the items are uncorrelated.

3. The error terms are uncorrelated with the latent variable.

4. The amount of influence from the latent variable to each item is assumed to be the same for all items.

5. Each item is assumed to have the same amount of error as any other item. The influence of extraneous factors is assumed to be equal for all items.

---

are then described as being parallel. The theory of parallel tests underpins the majority of QoL instruments which use simple summated (Likert) scales (see Box 2.3).

2.4.1   Psychometrics and QoL scales

The majority of QoL instruments have been designed on the principles of parallel tests and summated Likert scales. The related psychometric methods to a large extent assume that the scales contain solely indicator variables. The inter-item correlations that exist between causal variables can render these methods inapplicable (Fayers and Machin, 2007).

2.5   Item response theory

So-called modern psychometric theory largely centres on *item response theory* (IRT, Van der Linden and Hambleton, 1997). Items have varying 'difficulty'. It is assumed that patients will have different probabilities of responding positively to each item, according to their level of ability (that is, the level of the latent variable). Traditional methods focus upon averages; whereas IRT emphasizes the probabilities of responses. The design of scales using IRT methods is markedly different from traditional methods.

2.5.1   Traditional scales versus IRT

Traditional Likert summated scales assume items of broadly similar difficulty, with response categories to reflect severity or degree of response level. In contrast, IRT scales are based upon items of varying difficulty, and frequently each item will have only two response categories, such as 'yes' or 'no'. IRT models assume that the observed variables reflect the value of the latent variable, and that the item correlations arise solely by virtue of this relationship with the latent variable. Thus it is implicit that all items are indicator variables. The IRT model is inappropriate for symptoms and other causal variables (Fayers and Machin, 2007).

Example: A scale with items of varying difficulty – the SF-36 Physical Functioning dimension score

Question 3 of the SF-36 (see Appendix A) has 10 items of varying difficulty about activities that you might do during a typical day. The least difficult or 'easiest' item to answer, if the respondent has a good level of physical functioning, is the question on bathing and dressing oneself (question 3j). In general, most people with good physical functioning will not be limited at all in carrying out this daily activity. Conversely, the most difficult or 'hardest' item to answer, if the respondent has a poor level of physical functioning, is the question on vigorous activities (question 3a). The other eight items on the questionnaire appear to reflect levels of varying difficulty on the underlying latent physical functioning scale.   □

2.6   Clinimetric scales

Many clinical scales possess fundamentally different attributes from psychometric scales. Their development and validation should therefore proceed along separate paths. A 'good' and useful *clinimetric* scale may consist of items comprising a variety of symptoms and other clinical indices. It does not necessarily need to satisfy the same requirements that are demanded of other scales. Clinicians try to measure multiple attributes with a single index – for example, the Apgar Score (Apgar, 1953) for assessing the health of newborn babies or the Glasgow Coma Score (Teasdale and Jennett, 1974).

Example: The Glasgow Coma Score (Teasdale and Jennett, 1974)

The Glasgow Coma Scale (GCS) is a neurological scale which aims to give a reliable, objective way of recording the conscious state of a person, for initial as well as continuing assessment. The GCS was initially used to assess the level of consciousness after head injury, and it is now used by doctors as being applicable to all acute medical and trauma patients. In hospital it is also used in chronic patient monitoring in, for instance, intensive care. The scale combines three seemingly disparate symptoms related to the eye, verbal and motor responses. The lowest possible GCS score is 3 (deep coma or death), whilst the highest is 15 (fully awake person). Generally, comas are classified as: severe, with GCS ≤ 8; moderate, GCS 9–12; minor, GCS ≥ 13.   □

2.7   Measuring quality of life: Indicator or causal items

QoL instruments commonly contain both indicator and causal variables. Psychometric methods assume that all items are indicator variables. Clinimetric methods are more relevant for causal items. Fayers and Machin (2007) suggest that QoL instruments serve two different functions:

1. They alert the clinician to problems concerning symptoms and side effects.

2. They assess overall QoL and its aspects.

For the first purpose each symptom is usually reported separately, but if a multi-item scale is needed, then this is best constructed on clinimetric principles. For the second purpose, indicator variables are usually the most effective, chosen and validated using psychometric techniques.

2.8   Developing and testing questionnaires

Development of QoL instruments requires much painstakingly detailed work, patience, time and resources. The validation of a new QoL scale depends upon collecting and analysing data from samples of patients or others. Statistical and psychometric techniques can only confirm that a scale is valid in so far as it performs in the manner that is expected. Thus quantitative techniques presuppose that the scale has been carefully and sensibly designed. Therefore QoL scale development should follow rigorous pre-specified qualitative and quantitative procedures.

QoL instrument development, modification and validation usually occur in a non-linear fashion with a varying sequence of events, simultaneous processes or iterations. This iterative process is shown in Figure 2.3 and is discussed in detail below. One or more parts of the original process may be repeated in a new QoL instrument development, modification, or change in application of an existing instrument. This section describes the steps usually taken in the development of a QoL instrument.

2.8.1   Specify the research question and define the target population

The first stage when developing a QoL instrument is to clearly specify the research question. This should include specification of the objectives in measuring QoL, a working definition of what is meant by 'quality of life', the identification of the intended groups of respondents, and suggestions as to the concepts or dimensions of QoL that are to be assessed (Fayers and Machin, 2007).

Examples of the objectives are whether the new instrument is intended for comparison of treatment groups in randomized clinical trials, or for use in routine clinical practice for individual patient treatment and management. Possible definitions of QoL might place greater or lesser importance upon symptoms, psychological, spiritual or other aspects. Depending on the definition of the target population of respondents, there may be more or less prominence given to disease and treatment-related issues. All these factors will

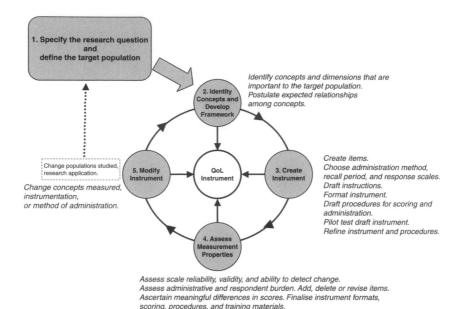

Figure 2.3 The QoL instrument development and modification process (adapted from FDA, 2006).

affect decisions about the dimensions of QoL to be assessed, the number of questions, length of the questionnaire and the scope and content of the questions.

Before identifying the concepts to be measured by the new QoL instrument, it is essential to define the target population. What is the range of diseases to be investigated? Are the symptoms and QoL issues the same for all disease subgroups? What is the range of treatments? For example, in cancer there can be a wide range of treatments, including chemotherapy, radiotherapy, hormone therapy and surgery. What is the severity range (advanced or early disease)? A QoL instrument should ensure that it is appropriate for the range of diseases and treatments to be investigated. As Fayers and Machin (2007) comment, the detailed specification of the intended target population is second in importance only to the specification of the research questions and the definition of QoL or of the aspects of QoL that are to be investigated.

2.8.2   Identify concepts

The second phase of developing a QoL instrument is to identify the concepts and dimensions that are important to the subjects (the intended target population) and the research application (both of which were defined in the previous step). This phase involves generating an extensive and exhaustive list of all QoL issues that are relevant to the dimensions of interest, by searching the literature, interviews with health-care professionals, discussions with patients and expert opinion.

Once the concepts have been identified, it is helpful to hypothesize the expected relationships among these concepts. This should include how individual items are associated with each other, how items are associated with each dimension, and how dimensions are associated with each other and the general concept of interest. A diagram of the expected relationships among the items and dimensions can help show these relationships. Figure 2.1 shows a general example of a conceptual framework where dimensions A, B and C each represent related but separate concepts. Items in this diagram are aggregated into dimensions. For dimension C a single item is sufficient to measure this aspect of QoL. In some measures, dimensions can be aggregated into an overall score.

Example: EORTC head and neck cancer-specific module (Bjordal *et al.*, 1994)

Literature searches:

46 relevant references were found. Hence 57 potential issues were identified. These were divided into five areas: pain-related, nutrition, dental status, other symptoms, and functional aspects.

Specialist interviews:

21 specialist nurses, oncologists and surgeons.

17 of the 57 issues identified in the literature search were regarded as being irrelevant, too rare, or too broad in scope.

59 new issues were also proposed; 11 were added, resulting in a provisional list of 43 issues.

Patient interviews:

6   of the issues that were felt by patients to be of low relevance or unimportant were deleted.

21 new symptom or problem issues and 5 new function issues were identified. The revised list covered 37 issues.   □

2.8.3   Create instrument

2.8.3.1   Item generation

Having identified all the relevant dimensions, items can be generated to reflect these dimensions. The first stage of item generation usually involves searches of relevant journals and bibliographic databases, to ensure that all the dimensions previously thought to be relevant are included. Any existing instruments that address the same or related areas of QoL assessment should be identified and reviewed. From these sources, a list of potential QoL items for inclusion in the questionnaire can be identified.

As before, there are several approaches to generating items: reviewing the literature (i.e. other questionnaires – this is a very incestuous business!); interviews with health-care professionals; interviews with patients; and expert opinion. There is always a certain amount of editing by instrument designers in order to limit the size of the questionnaire, remove ambiguity (see Box 2.4 on the wording of the questions) and to fit into a standard format. There is a trade-off between reliability, requiring more than one item per concept, and practicality, requiring the minimum number of items.

Box 2.4 Wording of questions

- Make questions and instructions brief and simple.
  For example, ill patients and the elderly may be confused by long, complicated sentences.

- Avoid small, unclear typefaces.
  Elderly patients may not have good eyesight.

- 'Not applicable' questions may result in missing or ambiguous answers.
  For example, 'Do you have difficulty going up stairs?' is not applicable to someone bedridden.

- Potentially embarrassing or offending questions should be avoided, put at the end, or made optional.
  For example, before a question about sex life, the FACT-G writes: 'If you prefer not to answer it, please check this box and go to the next section.'

- Avoid double negatives.
  For example, 'I don't feel less interest in sex (Yes/No)'.

- If two questions have similar wording, emphasize the differences, using underlining, bold, or italics.
  For example, questions 4 and 5 of the SF-36 are very similar apart from the underlined phrases 'as a result of your physical health' and 'as a result of any emotional problems'.

- Underlining and similar methods also draw attention to key words or phrases.
  For example, emphasize the time frame of questions, such as 'during the past 7 days'.

- Consider including both positively phrased and negatively phrased items.
  For example, the HADS includes 'I feel tense or "wound up"' and 'I can sit at ease and feel relaxed'.

2.8.3.2   Choice of administration or data collection method

Developers of QoL instruments should consider how the new QoL questionnaire is to be administered to the subjects. Possible modes of administration include: interview, paper-based self-administration, electronic, web-based, and interactive voice response formats. The majority of QoL instruments are designed to be self-completed paper-based questionnaires.

2.8.3.3   Choice of recall period

The development of the items for the QoL instrument should also consider the choice of recall period for the questions. The choice of recall period that is most suitable will depend on the purpose and intended use of the instrument, the characteristics of the disease or condition and the treatment to be tested. However, QoL instruments with items that require respondents to rely on memory, particularly if they must recall their

QoL over a long period of time or to average their response over a period of time, may have reduced accuracy and should be avoided. It is usually best to construct items that ask subjects to describe their current QoL status, rather than to ask them to compare their current state with an earlier period or attempt to average their experiences of over time. For example, the question 'How would you rate your overall quality of life today?' is to be preferred to 'Compared to one year ago, how would you rate your overall quality of life now?'.

2.8.3.4 Choice of response options

It is also important to make sure that the response options to the items are consistent with the purpose and intended use of the QoL instrument. Table 2.1 describes the types of response options that are typically used in QoL instruments.

Response choices are usually regarded as being suitable when:

- The wording used in the responses is clear and appropriate.

- Responses are appropriate for the intended target population.

- Responses offer a clear distinction between choices.

- Instructions to subjects for completing the questionnaire and selecting response options are adequate.

- Response options are appropriately ordered and appear to represent equal intervals.

- Response options avoid potential floor or ceiling effects.

- Response options do not bias the direction of responses.

2.8.3.5 Draft procedures for scoring of items and dimensions

For each item, numerical scores are generally assigned to each response category based on the most appropriate scale of measurement for the item (e.g. nominal, ordinal, interval or ratio scales – see Box 2.5).

The scoring systems in most questionnaires are often arbitrary and chosen for their simplicity. A common method involves 'adding the ticks', or for Likert scales, with n response options, simply assigning scores between 1 and n or between 0 and $n - 1$, for each response, and then adding the item response numbers to derive an overall score for the domain (e.g. the SF-36 and the HADs).

Example: Scoring the HADS (Zigmond and Snaith, 1983)

- The HAD scale consists of 14 items on two subscales (seven for anxiety and seven for depression).

- Ratings by subjects are made on four-point ordinal scales, which represent the degree of distress: 0 = not at all; 1 = occasionally; 2 = a lot of the time; 3 = most of the time.

- Items are summed on each of the seven-item anxiety and depression subscales to generate a score ranging from 0 to 21.

Table 2.1 Types of response options.

Type	Description	Example
Visual analogue scale (VAS)	A horizontal or vertical line of fixed length (usually 100 mm) with words that anchor the scale at the extreme ends and no words describing intermediate positions. Subjects are instructed to place a mark on the line corresponding to their perceived state.	• How would you rate your overall quality of life, today? Poor ——————————— Excellent
Anchored or categorized VAS	A VAS that has the horizontal or vertical line of fixed length (usually 100 mm) with words that anchor the scale at the extreme ends and words describing intermediate positions.	• How would you rate your overall quality of life, today? Poor Fair Good Very Good Excellent
Likert scale	An ordered set of discrete terms or statements from which subjects are asked to choose the response that best describes their state or experience.	• How would you rate your overall quality of life, today? ○ ○ ○ ○ ○ Poor Fair Good Very Good Excellent
Rating scale	A set of numerical categories from which subjects are asked to choose a category that best describes their state or experience. The ends of the rating scales are anchored with words but the intermediate categories do not have descriptive labels.	• How would you rate your overall quality of life, today? 0 1 2 3 5 Poor Excellent
Checklist	Checklists provide a simple choice between a limited set of response options such as Yes, No, and Don't know.	• Today would you rate your overall quality of life as good? ○ ○ ○ Yes No Do not Know
Binary format	The simplest checklist with only two responses options such as yes or no.	• Today would you rate your overall quality of life as good? ○ ○ Yes No

---

Box 2.5 Scoring/scaling – the theory

- It is important to bear in mind the distinction between ordinal, interval and ratio scales.

- Consider the following example:
  1) I lie awake most of the night

  2) I sleep badly at night

  3) I wake up occasionally at night

- An *ordinal* scale simply involves ranking statements e.g 3) > 2) > 1).

- An *interval* scale is where it is assumed that the intervals are equal. In this example this would mean that hte difference between 2) and 3) was equal to the difference between 1) and 2). An example is scales of temperature.

- A *ratio* scale is where it is possible to say that 3) is X times as bad as 1).

- High scores on each scale indicate the presence of problems.

- Non-cases ≤ 7; doubtful cases $= 8-10$; definite cases ≥ 11.   □

An alternative approach is to derive weights from a panel of 'experts', lay people or patients using some method of eliciting preferences, such as a visual analogue scaling or standard gamble. Whichever method is used, it is important to ask whether the scale has ordinal, interval or ratio properties since this has implications for the statistical analysis and interpretation.

2.8.3.6 Pilot or pre-test draft version of the questionnaire

Seemingly simple, lucid questions may present unanticipated problems. Therefore it is important that all questions are extensively tested before use by a pilot or 'pre-test' study. A pilot study will help to identify and solve potential problems with the new QoL instrument. For example, some questions may be ambiguous and not clearly phrased, with inappropriate response options which are not clearly laid out. Patients complete the provisional questionnaire, and are then debriefed using a pre-structured interview. The ideal debriefing interview will ask questions such as: Were any questions difficult to answer, confusing, or upsetting? Were all questions relevant, and were any important issues missed? Any other comments?

Example: Pre-testing – EORTC head and neck cancer module (Bjordal *et al* 1994)

Pre-testing of the EORTC head and neck module identified several items that were ambiguous, difficult or poorly worded. These items were rephrased. Some patients found positively worded functional items confusing: 'Have you been able to talk on the telephone? (Never, . . . , very often)' was reworded to 'Have you had any trouble talking on the telephone? (Not at all, . . . , very much)'.

Swallowing problems are common with head and neck cancer patients, and tubes are inserted for extreme swallowing difficulty. These patients may leave this question blank as 'not applicable'. Some report 'no problems' because they no longer need to swallow or report 'a lot of problems' because they cannot swallow.   □

2.8.4   Assess measurement properties

The next stage in developing a QoL questionnaire is to assess the measurement properties of the new instrument. New QoL instruments, in order to be useful, should satisfy the four basic properties of validity, reliability, responsiveness (ability to detect change) and interpretability (see Table 2.2).

Table 2.2   Assessment of the measurement properties of new QoL instruments.

Measurement property	Test	What is assessed
Validity	*Criterion (concurrent)*	Assessing the QoL instrument against the true value.
	Criterion (predictive)	Whether future outcomes can be predicted by current QoL scores.
	Content	Whether the items and response options are relevant measures of the dimension/concept.
	Content (face)	Are the items credible (e.g. asking elderly folk with bronchitis about vigorous activity)?
	Construct	Whether the relationships among items, dimensions and concepts conform to what is predicted by the conceptual framework for the QoL instrument.
Reliability	*Test–retest*	Stability of QoL scores over time when no change has occurred in the concept of interest.
	Internal consistency	Whether the items in a dimension are correlated with each other, as assessed by an internal consistency statistic (e.g. Cronbach's alpha).
	Inter-rater (interviewer)	Agreement between responses when the QoL instrument is administered by two or more different interviewers.

Table 2.2   (*Continued*)

Measurement property	Test	What is assessed
Responsiveness (ability to detect change)	*The extent to which an instrument is able to detect a clinically important change.*	Whether QoL scores are stable when there is no change in the subject, and the scores change in the predicted direction when there has been a notable change in the subject as evidenced by some effect size statistic. Ability to detect a change is always specific to a time interval.
Interpretability	*Smallest difference and/or change in QoL score that is considered clinically or practically important (the MID).*	Difference in mean QoL scores between treatment groups that provides convincing evidence of treatment benefit. Can be based on experience with the measure using a distribution-based approach, a clinical or non-clinical anchor, an empirical rule or a combination of approaches. The definition of an MID using a clinical anchor is called a minimum clinically important difference (MCID).
	Individual responder definition	Change in QoL score that would give clear evidence that an individual patient experienced a treatment benefit.

2.8.4.1   Reliability

Reliability is the stability, in QoL scores, between repeated administrations in a population who have not experienced any health change or change in QoL. This includes stability: over time (i.e. test–retest reliability); between raters or interviewers (i.e. inter-rater reliability); and between locations, such as hospital and home. Another form of reliability is *internal reliability* or *internal consistency reliability*. For scales which use multiple items to assess a particular dimension of QoL, all items should be consistent, meaning that they should all measure the same concept.

2.8.4.2   Validity

Validity is the extent to which an instrument measures what it is intended to measure. Validity is a difficult and some would say impossible thing to prove in the case of QoL

Box 2.6 Types of validity

Content	Item coverage and relevance
Criterion	Concurrent
	Predictive
Construct	Known-groups
	Convergent
	Discriminant

---

measurement, since there is no 'gold standard'. So how can you judge if a new QoL instrument measures what it is intended to measure? There are several types of validity (see Box 2.6), and confusingly a variety of terminology is used in the literature to define these different types. I shall describe the 'three Cs' of *content* validity, *criterion* validity and *construct* validity (Streiner and Norman, 2003).

Content validity looks to see if the items of an instrument are sensible and comprehensively cover the domain of interest. Face validity, which is often considered to be a form of content validity, assesses if the items in a QoL instrument appear on the face of it to cover the domain of interest clearly and unambiguously. The main distinction between the two types of content validity is that face validity concerns the critical review of the items of a new instrument after it has been constructed but before use, whereas item coverage and relevance are usually looked at during the instrument construction.

Criterion validity is the extent to which the new QoL scale has an association or correlation with external criteria such as other established instruments or measures (which are generally regarded as more accurate), or the true value (the *criterion variable*). Criterion validity is usually divided into two types: *concurrent* validity and *predictive* validity. With concurrent validity we are concerned with the correlation between the new QoL scale and the criterion variable, both of which are measured at the same time. When the new QoL measurement correlates with future values of the criterion variable or other outcomes, then we are concerned with predictive validity, that is, whether future outcomes or health status can be predicted by the current scores on the new QoL instrument.

Construct validity is the extent to which an instrument measures the construct or concept that it is designed to measure. This involves forming a theoretical model that describes the constructs being assessed and the expected relationships between these constructs. Data are then collected, and a judgement is made as to the extent to which these relationships are confirmed. If the results confirm prior expectations then the instrument may be valid.

Construct validity is usually divided into three types: *known-groups* validity; *convergent* validity; and *discriminant* validity. Known-groups validity is based simply on the assumption that certain specified groups of subjects may be expected to score differently from other groups, and the new instrument should be sensitive to these differences. A scale that cannot sensibly distinguish between groups with known differences is not likely to be useful. A more complex aspect of construct validity is convergent validity. Convergent validity shows that a postulated dimension of QoL correlates appreciably with those dimensions that theory suggests it should. Conversely, discriminant validity recognizes that some dimensions of QoL are expected to be relatively unrelated and that their correlations should be low. Convergent and discriminant validity are effectively the two opposite sides of the same coin and are usually considered together.

2.8.4.3 Responsiveness

Responsive is the extent to which an instrument is able to detect a clinically or practically important change in QoL status. That is, when the concept changes, the scores for the QoL instrument measuring that concept should change. This is the sensitivity of a measure to health change. Strictly speaking, it is a form of validity and hence again it is difficult to prove. It can be assessed by effect size statistics, that is, ratios of mean changes to standard deviations.

2.8.4.4 Interpretability

Many QoL instruments are able to detect mean changes or differences that are very small. Therefore it is important to consider whether such changes are meaningful. To help interpret the scores of QoL instruments it is important to identify (and specify) the smallest difference or change in QoL scores between individuals or groups that is clinically and practically important. This benchmark value is usually called the minimum important difference (MID). An MID is usually specific to the population under study. The FDA (2006) describes a variety of methods for determining MIDs (see Box 2.7).

There may be circumstances where it is more reasonable to characterize the meaningfulness of an individual's response to treatment rather than a group's average response. This leads to the definition of an *individual responder* to treatment. This individual response to treatment definition should be based upon pre-specified criteria. Examples include categorizing a patient as a responder based upon a pre-specified change from baseline in one or more scales, a change in score of certain size or greater (e.g. a 10-point change on a 100-point scale) or a percentage change from baseline. The definition of a responder should be backed by empirical evidence that such a change in QoL scores truly benefits individual patients.

Box 2.7 Methods for determining the minimum important difference

- Using a clinical or non-clinical anchor-based approach (mapping changes in QoL scores to clinically relevant and important changes in non-QoL measures of treatment outcome in the condition of interest).

- Mapping changes in QoL scores to other QoL scores to arrive at an MID that is appreciable to patients (e.g. when multi-item QoL scores are mapped to a single question asking the patient to rate their global impression of change since the start of treatment).

- Using a distribution-based approach (e.g. definition of the MID as 0.5 times the standard deviation of the QoL scores).

- Using an empirical rule (e.g. 8% of the theoretical or empirical range of scores).

The measurement properties of a new QoL instrument are typically assessed by field-testing on a large heterogeneous sample of patients (which is representative of the full range of intended responders). This field-testing may result in modifications to the instrument.

2.8.5   Modify instrument

When a QoL instrument is modified, additional validation studies may be needed to confirm the adequacy of the modified instrument's measurement properties. The FDA (2006) recommends additional validation of a modified QoL instrument when one or more of the following modifications occur.

1. An instrument that is developed and validated to measure one concept is used to measure a different concept.

2. An instrument developed for use in one population or condition is used in a different patient population or condition.

3. An instrument is altered in item content or format.

4. An instrument's data collection mode is altered.

5. An instrument developed in one language or culture is adapted or translated for use in another language or culture.

2.9   Further reading

Designing and developing new QoL instruments constitutes a complex and lengthy process. It is advisable not to develop your own instrument – unless you must. It is preferable to use an off-the-shelf QoL measure. If you do wish to develop a new QoL instrument, perhaps because no other measures are suitable, then be prepared for much hard work over a period of years. Fayers and Machin (2007) provide an overview of the process. The EORTC Quality of Life Study Group has developed and published comprehensive guidelines for the development of new QoL instruments, including Blazeby *et al.* (2002). These manuals are downloadable from the EORTC website http://groups.eortc.be/qol/documentation_manuals.htm. The next chapter will give practical guidelines, when designing a study, on how to choose between the many hundreds of QoL questionnaires now available.

3

Choosing a quality of life measure for your study

Summary

There are numerous QoL instruments now available. By far the easiest way to assess QoL is to use an 'off-the-shelf' instrument rather than designing your own. So how do you choose between the various QoL instruments? This fundamentally depends on the purpose of the study and then the appropriateness, acceptability, feasibility, validity, reliability, responsiveness, precision and interpretability of the instrument. This chapter describes these issues in detail. A 'belt-and-braces' approach is recommended for the assessment of QoL. That is, both a generic and condition-specific instrument should be used.

3.1 Introduction

The successful use of QoL outcomes in studies depends a great deal on the choice of appropriate instruments. There are many QoL instruments now available and the choice of a QoL instrument for a particular study should be made carefully. The choice of instrument will depend on the objectives of the study, the characteristics of the target population and the appropriateness, acceptability, feasibility, validity, reliability, responsiveness, precision and interpretability of the instrument. In this chapter we explore the issues in detail.

3.2 How to choose between instruments

The first step is to consider the aim or purpose of the intended study. Box 3.1 describes four different purposes for the intended study and the ideal properties of a QoL instrument for such a purpose.

Quality of Life Outcomes in Clinical Trials and Health-Care Evaluation   Stephen J. Walters
© 2009 John Wiley & Sons, Ltd

Box 3.1 Purpose of the intended study

1. *To describe the health of a population.* The chosen QoL instrument should have good discriminative properties (i.e. be sensitive to health differences) and generate a single index and/or profile of scores.

2. *To conduct a clinical trial.* Evaluative properties (responsive to health changes), single index (to assess overall effectiveness) and/or profile of scores.

3. *To conduct an economic evaluation alongside a clinical trial.* Evaluative properties; single index, explicitly incorporates preferences into the scoring.

4. *To use in routine clinical practice.* Acceptable and feasible to use, good evaluative properties (sensitive to health changes), incorporates domains that are important to the patient/clinician.

Box 3.2 Eight questions that need to be answered in relation to choosing a QoL measure for a study (from Fitzpatrick *et al*. 1998)

1. *Appropriateness.* Is the content of the QoL instrument appropriate to the questions which the study is intended to address?

2. *Acceptability.* Is the QoL instrument acceptable to patients?

3. *Feasibility.* Is the QoL instrument easy to administer and process?

4. *Validity.* Does the QoL instrument measure what it claims to measure?

5. *Reliability.* Does the QoL instrument produce results that are reproducible and internally consistent?

6. *Responsiveness.* Does the QoL instrument detect changes over time that matter to patients?

7. *Precision.* How precise are the scores of the QoL instrument?

8. *Interpretability.* How understandable are the scores of the QoL instrument?

The review by Fitzpatrick *et al*. (1998) identified eight questions or criteria that need to be addressed when choosing a QoL outcome measure for a clinical trial (see Box 3.2 and Figure 3.1 for more details). The majority of these criteria are applicable to most research study designs and not just clinical trials.

Let us assume that you have formed a shortlist of potential QoL instruments that appear to be suitable for the intended purpose of your study. The next steps are to review the instruments and to consider the eight criteria identified by Fitzpatrick *et al*. (1998) when choosing a QoL instrument for your study.

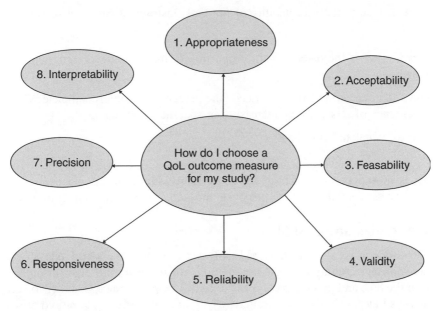

Figure 3.1   How do I choose a QoL outcome for my study? Eight questions to ask and answer.

3.3   Appropriateness

This requires careful consideration of the aims of the study, with particular reference to the QoL research questions. As discussed in the previous chapter, this consideration should include specification of the objectives in measuring QoL, a working definition of what is meant by 'quality of life', the identification of the intended groups of respondents, and suggestions as to the concepts or dimensions of QoL that are to be assessed.

For this reason, it is very difficult to give specific recommendations about what in general makes a QoL instrument appropriate to a study, because this is essentially a decision based on the concordance between the investigators' specific study research questions and the content of the instruments.

3.4   Acceptability

It is vital that the QoL instrument is acceptable to the study subjects. It is important to obtain high response rates to QoL instruments in order to make the results of studies more easily interpretable, more generalizable and less prone to bias from non-response. Fitzpatrick *et al.* (1998) state that pragmatically the best measure of acceptability of a QoL instrument in a clinical trial is the end result. That is, whether or not the trialists obtain data that are as complete as possible from the study patients. However, this can only be determined after the study has been carried out.

More realistically, the acceptability of the QoL instrument can be assessed in terms of:

(i) response rate – the percentage or proportion of the sample who returned the questionnaire;

(ii) item and dimension completion rate – the percentage of items completed (e.g. there is evidence of missing data increasing in specific subgroups);

(iii) time to complete instrument.

Other criteria being equal, then, you should choose the QoL instrument for your study that is most acceptable, that is, the instrument with the most evidence that its use is consistently associated with high response and item/dimension completion rates.

Example: Older adults study

The SF-36 is one of the most widely used QoL instruments in the world today. However, there was some uncertainty over the acceptability of using the SF-36 with older adults (aged 65 and over), and particular concerns over low response rates, inability to complete postal surveys independently, and questions which may be irrelevant to retired or severely impaired respondents. Walters et al. (2001a) report the results of study which aimed to establish whether the SF-36 could be successfully used in a large postal survey of community-dwelling older adults.

The overall response rate to the SF-36 was 82% (8117/9887). The response rate was above 80% for all age groups except that aged 85 and over, which achieved 69%. Individual item completion was high, being greater than 93% for all questions. Dimension completion (i.e. completion of all items in a dimension, allowing it to be calculated without interpolation) ranged from 86.4% to 97.7%. Dimension completion was lowest among those aged 85 or over, ranging from 83.3% to 94.4%. Based on these results, the authors concluded, that the SF-36 is an acceptable QoL instrument to use in postal surveys of older people living in the community.   □

3.5   Feasibility

When choosing a QoL instrument it is important to consider the impact upon staff and researchers in administering, collecting and processing the information from the QoL instrument. There may be additional staff effort and costs involved in personally administering the questionnaires over postal delivery. The length and complexity of a QoL instrument may mean that it requires additional staff time to assist and help explain how more complex questions are to be filled out by patients. So other criteria being equal then one should choose the QoL instrument for your study that is easiest to administer and process. Typically, the shorter, simpler instruments require less time and effort to process.

Example: Leg ulcer study

Walters et al. (1999) compared four generic QoL instruments – the MOS 36-item Short-Form Health Survey (SF-36), EuroQol (EQ-5D), the McGill Short Form Pain Questionnaire (SF-MPQ) and the Frenchay Activities Index (FAI) – in 233 people with venous leg ulcers. The mean time to complete all four instruments at initial assessment was 19.3 minutes (standard deviation 6.3). This was split into 10.8 (4.3), 1.6 (1.3), 3.6 (1.8) and 3.4 (1.7) minutes to complete the SF-36, EQ-5D, FAI and SF-MPQ, respectively.   □

Unfortunately, the time required to collect, process and analyse a QoL outcome measure is frequently not reported, so evidence on the feasibility of using the instrument may not be available. So a judgement on this aspect of an instrument may have to be made without evidence, but fortunately this is only one component of the burden on participants that will determine the overall feasibility of the study and therefore the value of its final results.

3.6   Validity

Validity, which was described in Chapter 2, is the extent to which an instrument measures what it is intended to measure. Validity is a difficult – some would say impossible – thing to prove in the case of QoL measurement since there is no 'gold standard' (i.e. criterion validity). So how can you judge whether a QoL instrument measures what it is intended to measure, and which QoL questionnaire is better and more valid for your study? Chapter 2 and Box 2.5 described three main types of validity – content, criterion and construct – and there different variations. There are several tests for the different types of validity.

3.6.1   Tests for criterion validity

Criterion validity is the extent to which the new QoL scale has an association or correlation with external criteria such as other established instruments or measures (which are generally regarded as more accurate), or the true value (the *criterion variable*). However, with QoL measures there is rarely, if ever, a perfect 'gold standard' measurement which exists to test the criterion validity of a new QoL instrument against. One exception may be when a longer version of the questionnaire can be used as the 'gold standard' to develop a shorter version of the same established instrument (Fitzpatrick *et al.*, 1998).

Example: Use of a longer version of an instrument to develop a shorter version

Ware *et al.* (1996) used regression methods to select and score 12 items from the MOS 36-item Short-Form Health Survey (SF-36) to reproduce the Physical Component Summary and Mental Component Summary scales in the general US population ($n = 2333$). The resulting 12-item short-form (SF-12) achieved multiple R^2 values of 0.911 and 0.918 in predictions of the SF-36 Physical Component Summary and SF-36 Mental Component Summary scores, respectively. Scoring algorithms from the general population used to score 12-item versions of the two components (Physical Component Summary and Mental Component Summary) achieved R^2 values of 0.905 with the SF-36 Physical Component Summary and 0.938 with SF-36 Mental Component Summary when cross-validated with the scores from the longer 36 items in the Medical Outcomes Study.   □

3.6.2   Tests for face and content validity

Face validity looks at whether a QoL instrument appears to be measuring what it purports to be measuring, while content validity looks in more detail at the items in the QoL instrument and whether or not these items comprehensively cover all aspects of the dimension of interest. There are no formal statistical tests for face and content validity. Tests for face and content validity largely involve a qualitative judgement of whether the items in the QoL instrument clearly reflect the intended QoL dimension of interest and whether or not these items cover most of the aspects of the QoL dimension of interest.

3.6.3   Tests for construct validity

Construct validity is the extent to which an instrument measures the *construct* or concept that it is designed to measure. This involves forming a theoretical model that describes the constructs being assessed and the expected relationships between these constructs. Data are then collected, and a judgement is made as to the extent to which these relationships are confirmed. If the results confirm prior expectations then the instrument may be valid.

Construct validity is usually divided into three types: *known-groups* validity, *convergent* validity and *discriminant* validity. Known-groups validity is based simply on the assumption that certain specified groups of subjects may be expected to score differently from other groups, and the new instrument should be sensitive to these differences. Convergent validity shows that a postulated dimension of QoL correlates appreciably with those dimensions that theory suggests it should. Conversely, discriminant validity recognizes that some dimensions of QoL are expected to be relatively unrelated and that their correlations should be low. Known-groups construct validity involves comparing the QoL scores between groups with obviously different health (e.g. patients with osteoarthritis with the general population, or patients with different severity of condition) and looking for differences. A valid QoL scale should show differences, in the expected direction, between these groups.

Example: Known-groups construct validity

In a study of 110 patients with osteoarthritis (OA) of the knee, Brazier *et al.* (1999) expected that patients with more severe OA (as assessed by their physician) would have poorer QoL than patients with mild or moderate disease. They used four instruments to assess QoL: the Western Ontario McMaster Osteoarthritis index (WOMAC); Health Assessment Questionnaire (HAQ); SF-36 and EQ-5D. Table 3.1 gives the mean QoL instrument score for each group, the mean difference and its associated confidence interval and *P*-value. In the paper the authors reported that:

> Mean score differences between patients with a clinical assessment of mild/moderate vs. severe disease were highly significant for all three dimensions of the WOMAC questionnaire and the HAQ at the 1% level. Six dimensions of the SF-36 also discriminated significantly between the patient groups in terms of severity. Results for the EQ were mixed, where differences between the EQ-5D index, but not the rating scale reached significance levels.

□

Table 3.1 Mean score differences between rheumatology clinic patients with mild/moderate and severe knee osteoarthritis (data from Brazier et al., 1999).

	Severity Mild/Moderate			Severe			Mean difference	95% CI		P-value[1]	Effect size[2]
	n	Mean	sd	n	Mean	sd		Lower	Upper		
WOMAC											
Pain	66	1.7	(0.8)	45	2.5	(0.7)	-0.8	-1.1	-0.5	0.001	-1.05
Stiffness	65	2.1	(0.9)	44	2.8	(0.8)	-0.7	-1.0	-0.4	0.001	-0.81
Physical Function	66	1.8	(0.9)	46	2.4	(0.6)	-0.7	-1.0	-0.4	0.001	-0.85
HAQ											
Disability Index	65	1.5	(0.8)	43	1.9	(0.4)	-0.4	-0.7	-0.2	0.001	-0.66
SF-36											
Physical Functioning	63	34.8	(24.0)	43	17.8	(16.4)	17.0	8.6	25.3	0.001	0.80
Social Functioning	65	60.5	(29.5)	44	42.2	(28.6)	18.3	7.1	29.6	0.002	0.63
Role Physical	64	18.4	(27.9)	41	3.0	(10.0)	15.3	6.3	24.3	0.001	0.67
Role Emotional	63	51.3	(43.9)	41	25.2	(39.3)	26.1	9.3	42.9	0.003	0.62
Bodily Pain	65	37.9	(19.9)	45	25.2	(17.1)	12.8	5.5	20.0	0.001	0.68
Mental Health	65	65.0	(19.7)	43	60.4	(21.9)	4.7	-3.3	12.7	0.250	0.23
Vitality	66	41.2	(19.3)	41	32.0	(19.2)	9.3	1.7	16.8	0.017	0.48
General Health	60	48.8	(21.8)	43	40.6	(25.1)	8.2	-1.0	17.4	0.081	0.35
EQ											
EQ-5D Index	64	51.3	(15.5)	43	38.1	(15.7)	13.2	7.1	19.3	0.001	0.85
EQ VAS Rating scale	65	60.0	(19.3)	41	54.7	(21.0)	5.3	-2.5	13.2	0.182	0.27

Scores for the SF-36 and EQ lie in the range 0–100, with high scores indicating good health. The range for the WOMAC is 0–4. The range for the HAQ is 0–3. For both these instruments, low scores indicate good health.

[1] P-value from two independent samples t-test.

[2] Effect size = (mean score of mild/moderate group) – (mean score of severe group) divided by the overall pooled standard deviation.

Convergent validity and *discriminant* validity involve looking at correlations between a QoL instrument and other QoL instruments that measure the same and different dimensions of QoL. This involves comparing the correlations with other instruments with overlapping constructs and assessing the extent to which they converge or diverge (if the constructs are not overlapping). This approach requires developers of instruments to hypothesize that an instrument that we wish to test should have stronger relationships with some variables and weaker relationships with others.

For example, a new measure of physical functioning should correlate more strongly with existing measures of physical functioning than with measures of emotional well-being. Basically the correlations are expected to be strongest with the most related constructs and weakest with other unrelated constructs. Statistical tests for convergent validity and discriminant validity involve calculating all the pairwise correlation coefficients between the scores on the different QoL scales. There are no agreed standards for how high correlations should be between a QoL instrument being assessed and other variables in order to establish convergent construct validity (Fitzpatrick *et al.*, 1998), although a correlation of 0.60 or more may be strong evidence in support of convergent construct validity.

Example: Convergent validity and discriminant validity

Walters *et al.* (1999) examined the construct validity of four instruments in measuring QoL in patients with venous leg ulcers: the MOS 36-item Short-Form Health Survey (SF-36); the EuroQol (EQ); the McGill Short Form Pain Questionnaire (SF-MPQ); and the Frenchay Activities Index (FAI). Table 3.2 shows some of the observed correlations. For example, the largest correlation, 0.72, was observed between the Physical Functioning dimension of the SF-36 and the FAI (another measure of physical functioning). Much lower correlations, ranging from 0.21 to 0.42, were observed between the Physical Functioning dimension of the SF-36 and the various pain dimensions of the SF-MPQ. The high correlations between the similar constructs supported the predictions of convergent validity, while the lower correlations between the other subscales supported the discriminant validity.   □

All these tests cannot prove a QoL instrument is valid; they can only provide support or otherwise for its validity. Other criteria being equal, then, you should choose a QoL instrument for your study which provides the most comprehensive evidence that it is valid for the purpose of your study and your intended target population.

3.7 Reliability

Reliability, which was described in Chapter 2, is the reproducibility or stability, in QoL scores, between repeated administrations in a population who have not experienced any health change or change in QoL. This includes stability: over time (i.e. test–retest reliability); between raters or interviewers (i.e. inter-rater reliability); and between locations, such as hospital and home. This is sometimes called *repeatability reliability* (Fayers and Machin, 2007). Another form of reliability is *internal reliability* or *internal consistency reliability*. For scales which use multiple items to assess a particular dimension of QoL, all items should be consistent, meaning that they should all measure the same concept.

Table 3.2 Correlations* between dimensions of health status measures at baseline (data from Walters *et al.* 1999).

	PF	RP	BP	GH	VT	SF	RE	MH	DSI	FAI	PRI(S)	PRI(A)	VAS Now	VAS Day	VAS Night
SF-36:															
PF	1.00														
RP	0.41	1.00													
BP	0.43	0.43	1.00												
GH	0.40	0.35	0.41	1.00											
VT	0.48	0.38	0.45	0.66	1.00										
SF	0.50	0.51	0.48	0.51	0.52	1.00									
RE	0.23	0.50	0.30	0.38	0.41	0.40	1.00								
MH	0.27	0.25	0.31	0.55	0.67	0.38	0.41	1.00							
EuroQol:															
DSI	0.67	0.43	0.64	0.55	0.66	0.54	0.36	0.54	1.00						
Frenchay:															
FAI	0.72	0.25	0.28	0.30	0.45	0.35	0.11	0.26	0.54	1.00					
SF-MPQ:															
PRI(S)	−0.27	−0.26	−0.53	−0.25	−0.32	−0.20	−0.31	−0.24	−0.54	−0.12	1.00				
PRI(A)	−0.26	−0.16	−0.43	−0.18	−0.29	−0.13	−0.30	−0.24	−0.48	−0.13	0.70	1.00			
VAS Now	−0.24	−0.21	−0.55	−0.22	−0.31	−0.19	−0.29	−0.27	−0.46	−0.20	0.55	0.45	1.00		
VAS Day	−0.21	−0.24	−0.57	−0.25	−0.34	−0.22	−0.29	−0.25	−0.47	−0.13	0.62	0.53	0.71	1.00	
VAS Night	−0.42	−0.37	−0.55	−0.36	−0.44	−0.32	−0.32	−0.30	−0.57	−0.34	0.57	0.40	0.62	0.62	1.00

*Pearson's product moment correlation coefficient.

Key to abbreviations: PF, Physical Functioning; RP, Role Physical; BP, Bodily Pain; GH, General Health; VT, Vitality; SF, Social Functioning; RE, Role Emotional; MH, Mental Health; DSI, EuroQol Derived Single Index; FAI, Frenchay Activities Index; PRI(S), Pain Rating Index (Sensory); PRI(A), Pain Rating Index (Affective); VAS Now, Visual Analogue Scale, amount of pain now; VAS Day, Visual Analogue Scale, amount of pain in the daytime; VAS Night, Visual Analogue Scale, amount of pain at night.

From a statistical perspective, both internal and repeatability reliability are assessed using similar statistical techniques.

3.7.1 Repeatability reliability

Repeatability reliability is based on looking at the relationship between repeated QoL measurements. The measurements are either repeated over time (*test–retest reliability*), by different observers (*inter-rater reliability*) or by different variants of the instruments (*equivalent forms reliability*). Repeatability reliability is usually assessed by the statistical techniques listed in Table 3.3. A fuller description of these techniques is given in Chapter 5.

Example: Estimating test–retest reliability

Table 3.4 shows the two-week test–retest reliability estimates for the eight SF-36 dimensions for a sample of ($n = 31$) patients with rheumatoid arthritis who reported that their arthritis and overall health had remained the same during this time (Ruta *et al.*, 1998). The authors used the ICC to assess test–retest reliability for SF-36 scales they regarded as continuous and kappa for scales with ordinal characteristics. The authors obtained reasonably high ICCs, greater than 0.76, for the Physical Functioning, Mental Health, Vitality and General Health scales, which they believed were 'sufficient for the scales to be used with individuals'. Kappa was calculated for the three remaining SF-36 scales (Social Functioning, Role Physical and Role Emotional). The values for kappa were low, less than 0.59, indicating 'poor test–retest reliability'.   □

3.7.2 Graphical methods for assessing reliability between two repeated measurements

As shown in Figure 3.2, Bland and Altman (1986) advocate graphically plotting the scores from the two administrations of the QoL instrument to assess reliability. Here the difference in scores between the two administrations (QoL measurement at time 1 minus

Table 3.3 Statistical techniques for assessing repeatability reliability for different types of QoL data.

Type of data	Statistical technique
Binary	Proportion of agreement Kappa (κ)
Ordered categorical	Weighted kappa (κ)
Continuous	Intra-class correlation coefficient (ICC) Mean QoL score differences between test and retest and the 95% confidence limit for this difference Plots of differences by mean score

Table 3.4 Two-week test–retest reliability estimates for the eight SF-36 subscales for a sample of ($n = 31$) patients with rheumatoid arthritis. Reproduced from Ruta, D.A., Hurst, N.P, Kind, P., Hunter, M., Stubbings, A., 'Measuring health status in British patients with rheumatoid arthritis: reliability, validity and responsiveness of the short form 36-item health survey (SF-36).' *British Journal of Rheumatology*, 1998, 37, 425–436, by permission of Oxford University Press.

SF-36 dimension	Mean difference (SD of difference)	Reliability
		ICC
Physical Functioning	−1.8 (12.2)	0.93
Pain	2.9 (16.9)	0.76
General Health	0.2 (10.7)	0.91
Vitality	−1.9 (12.8)	0.83
Mental Health	3.2 (12.1)	0.78
		Kappa
Social Functioning		0.26
Role Physical		0.37
Role Emotional		0.59

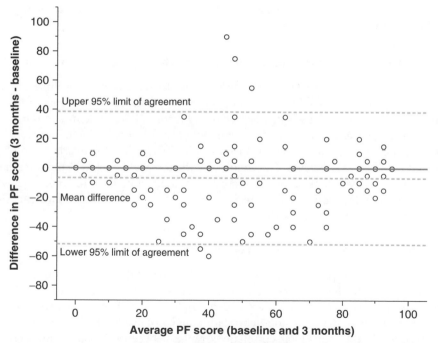

Figure 3.2 Plot of difference against average SF-36 Physical Functioning score in $n = 129$ leg ulcer patients who reported that their health was the same, plus the observed mean difference and 95% limits of agreement plot (data from Walters *et al.*, 1999).

QoL measurement at time 2) is plotted against their average. Three things are readily observable with this type of plot:

(i) the size of the differences between administrations;

(ii) the distribution of these differences about zero;

(iii) whether the differences are related to the size of the measurement (for this purpose the average of the two QoL scores acts as the best estimate of the true unknown value).

How well do the QoL scores on our two assessments agree? We could simply quote the mean difference and standard deviation of the differences (SD_{diff}). However, it is more useful to use these to construct a range of values which would be expected to cover the agreement between the methods for most subjects (Altman, 1991) and the 95% limits of agreement are defined as the mean difference $\pm 2SD_{Diff}$.

Figure 3.2 shows such a graph for 129 leg ulcer patients who reported that their overall health was the same at 3-month follow-up using the SF-36 Physical Functioning dimension (Walters *et al.*, 1999). In Figure 3.2, only 5 out of 129 (or 4 per cent) of the observations are outside the 95% limits of agreement. However, there is considerable variability in the difference in SF-36 Physical Functioning scores between baseline and 3-month follow-up, even though the mean difference is small, −6.6. The limits of agreement are wide, approximately 90 points, which is almost all the SF-36 Physical Functioning score range. This suggests that there is poor to moderate agreement between two administrations of the SF-36.

3.7.3   Internal reliability or internal consistency reliability

This is the degree of homogeneity between items in the same domain or dimension. It is the extent to which the individual items of a dimension appear to be tapping the same health domain or concept, that is, the degree of coherence between items and dimensions. Internal consistency can be measured in a number of different ways including: correlation between items and their own dimension score after correction for overlap; Cronbach's alpha; and reliability coefficients. The simplest of the three approaches to measure internal consistency is simply to look at the correlation of individual items to the scale as a whole, omitting that item. Fitzpatrick *et al.* (1998) suggest, as a rule of thumb, that items should correlate at least 0.20 with the scale.

Example: Internal consistency reliability

Table 3.5 shows the mean raw item scores, on the 1–3 scale, for the 10 questions that make up the SF-36 Physical Functioning dimension and the overall mean scale score (when the responses to the 10 items are added up). Table 3.6 shows the mean scale score if the item is deleted, the item–total correlation and Cronbach's alpha coefficient if the item is removed. The item–total correlations range between 0.57 and 0.83, suggesting that some of the items are potentially redundant from the Physical Functioning scale. The high values of Cronbach's alpha (0.92 or more) also suggest that some of the items could be removed from the Physical Functioning scale without any loss of internal consistency reliability. □

Table 3.5   Mean scores, standard deviations and sample sizes for the 10 items of the SF-36 Physical Functioning scale (data from Brazier *et al.*, 1992).

Item	Question	Label	Mean	SD	n
1.	Q3a	Vigorous activities	2.24	0.74	1514
2.	Q3b	Moderate activities	2.79	0.49	1514
3.	Q3c	Lifting or carrying	2.74	0.55	1514
4.	Q3d	Climbing several flights of stairs	2.59	0.65	1514
5.	Q3e	Climbing one flight of stairs	2.85	0.46	1514
6.	Q3f	Bending, kneeling or stooping	2.68	0.58	1514
7.	Q3g	Walking more than 1 mile	2.71	0.61	1514
8.	Q3h	Walking half a mile	2.82	0.50	1514
9.	Q3i	Walking 100 yards	2.90	0.38	1514
10.	Q3j	Bathing and dressing	2.92	0.35	1514

Statistics for	Mean	Variance	SD	Items
PF SCALE	27.25	18.09	4.25	10

Table 3.6   Internal consistency reliability of the 10-item SF-36 Physical Functioning scale (data from Brazier *et al.*, 1992).

Item	Scale mean if item deleted	Scale variance if item deleted	Corrected item–total correlation	Alpha if item deleted
Q3a	25.00	14.35	0.57	0.94
Q3b	24.45	14.77	0.81	0.92
Q3c	24.51	14.63	0.75	0.92
Q3d	24.65	13.98	0.77	0.92
Q3e	24.40	14.93	0.84	0.92
Q3f	24.57	14.48	0.74	0.92
Q3g	24.54	14.02	0.81	0.92
Q3h	24.42	14.66	0.83	0.92
Q3i	24.35	15.68	0.75	0.92
Q3j	24.32	16.16	0.66	0.93

Reliability coefficient for all 10 items, Cronbach's alpha = 0.93

A low correlation suggests an item does not belong to the dimension. A very high correlation suggests redundancy. Hence, a moderate correlation is required. For these reasons, it has been suggested that good internal consistency implies good retest reliability. Streiner and Norman (2003) emphasize that reliability cannot be seen as a fixed property of a particular QoL instrument. It should be borne in mind that any QoL measure will have a certain degree of reliability when applied to specific populations under particular conditions.

Two established and often quoted standards for acceptable values of the reliability coefficients of a QoL instrument are a minimum of 0.70 for use in research and a minimum of 0.90 for individual use in routine clinical practice (Streiner and Norman, 2003; Nunnally, 1978). The reasons for the lower minimum reliability standards for research are that in a research study, such as an RCT, the results and conclusions will typically be based on a mean QoL score averaged across many individuals. In these circumstances the sample size will in general tend to reduce the measurement error in comparison to the between-groups differences. Other criteria being equal, then, you should choose a QoL instrument for your study which provides evidence that it satisfies the minimum standards of reliability for the purpose of your study and your intended study population.

3.8   Responsiveness

Responsiveness is the extent to which an instrument is able to detect a clinically significant or practically important change. This is the ability of a measure to detect a health change. Strictly speaking, it is a form of validity and hence again it is difficult to prove. Fayers and Machin (2007) distinguish between the *sensitivity* and responsiveness of a QoL instrument. They define sensitivity as the ability of an instrument to detect differences between groups, for example between two groups in an RCT. They regard responsiveness as the ability of the QoL instrument to detect changes over time. Sensitivity can be assessed by cross-sectional studies, but responsiveness can only be assessed in longitudinal studies of subjects in whom a change in health is expected to occur.

Responsiveness and sensitivity can be assessed by *effect size* statistics, that is, ratios of mean changes or differences to standard deviations (see Table 3.7). Whether or not an instrument is likely to be responsive can also be examined by looking at the proportion of patients at the 'floor' and 'ceiling' of the measure to determine the extent to which a person can move on the scale if their QoL changes over time. Guyatt *et al.* (1993) emphasize the distinction between *discriminative* instruments intended to be particularly valid in distinguishing between respondents at a point in time, and *evaluative* instruments that need to be particularly sensitive to changes within individuals over time. Just as with reliability and validity, it should be noted that any estimates of responsiveness for a QoL measure are applicable to specific populations under particular conditions and should not be regarded as an inherent property of the instrument (Fitzpatrick *et al.*, 1998).

3.8.1   Floor and ceiling effects

One of the main limitations on the responsiveness of a QoL instrument is the range of responses for the scale. The actual form or wording of the questionnaire items may reduce the chance of further improvement or deterioration being recorded since they may preclude the reporting of most favourable or worst health states. A high percentage of subjects responding at the worst end of the response scale is referred to as a *floor effect*. Conversely, a high percentage of subjects responding at the optimal end of the response scale is called a *ceiling effect*.

Example: Floor and ceiling effects

Table 3.8 shows the mean SF-36 dimension scores and the percentages of subjects on the floor or ceiling of the scale for a sample of ($n = 233$) patients with rheumatoid arthritis (Ruta *et al.*, 1998). There is some suggestion of floor effects for the Physical Functioning,

Table 3.7 Statistical methods of evaluating responsiveness.

Method	Summary	Equation	Denominator
Paired t-test	Change score for instrument divided by standard error of the change score	$t = \dfrac{(\bar{x}_2 - \bar{x}_1)}{SE(x_2 - x_1)}$	SE of change
Relative efficiency/ relative validity of two scales.	Ratio of the squares of the statistics for the two scales	$\dfrac{t_{S1}^2}{t_{S2}^2}$	
Effect size	Change score for instrument divided by standard deviation of baseline measure of instrument	$\dfrac{\bar{x}_2 - \bar{x}_1}{SD(x_1)}$	SD of baseline (x_1)
Cross-sectional effect size	Change score for instrument divided by standard deviation of baseline measure of instrument	$\dfrac{\bar{x}_2 - \bar{x}_1}{SD(x_1)}$	Pooled SD (x)
Standardized response mean	Change score for instrument divided by standard deviation of change score	$\dfrac{\bar{x}_2 - \bar{x}_1}{SD(x_2 - x_1)}$	SD of change
Modified standard response mean	Change score for instrument divided by standard deviation of change score individuals otherwise identified as stable	$\dfrac{\bar{x}_2 - \bar{x}_1}{SD(x^*)}$	SD of change for individuals otherwise identified as stable.
Ceiling and floor effects	Proportion/percentage of sample at floor or ceiling	$100\dfrac{x_{\text{Floor}}}{N}$	$N =$ No. in sample

Role Physical, Role Emotional and Social Functioning dimensions which all had 10% or more of subjects scoring 0 on the dimension. There is some suggestion of ceiling effects for the Role Physical, Social Functioning and Role Emotional dimensions which all had 15% or more of subjects scoring 100 on the dimension.   □

Example: Effect sizes

Walters *et al.* (1999) evaluated the cross-sectional sensitivity of four QoL instruments in 233 patients with venous leg ulcers. The four different tools used were: the MOS

Table 3.8 Mean SF-36 dimension scores and the percentages of subjects on the floor or ceiling of the scale for a sample of ($n = 233$) patients with rheumatoid arthritis. Reproduced from Ruta, D.A., Hurst, N.P, Kind, P., Hunter, M., Stubbings, A., 'Measuring health status in British patients with rheumatoid arthritis: reliability, validity and responsiveness of the short form 36-item health survey (SF-36).' *British Journal of Rheumatology*, 1998, 37, 425–436, by permission of Oxford University Press.

SF-36 dimension	Mean (SD)	% Floor (scoring 0)	% Ceiling (scoring 100)
Physical Functioning	31 (29)	22	0
Role Physical	25 (38)	59	15
Bodily Pain	37 (23)	6	1.7
General Health	44 (23)	0.9	0.4
Vitality	39 (24)	4	0
Social Functioning	54 (42)	11	19
Role Emotional	59 (42)	29	45
Mental Health	69 (20)	0.4	3

36-Item Short-Form Health Survey (SF-36); the EuroQol (EQ); the McGill Short Form Pain Questionnaire (SF-MPQ); and the Frenchay Activities Index (FAI). Table 3.9 shows the effect sizes for patients in relation to age, mobility, leg ulcer size, current ulcer duration and maximum ulcer duration. Mean score differences between patients under and over 75 years of age were highly significant for three dimensions of the SF-36 (PF, GH, MH) and the FAI. For the SF-MPQ and the EQ DSI, all of the effect sizes were less than 0.20. Five dimensions of the SF-36 (PF, RP, BP, VT, SF), the DSI, FAI and VAS Night scale of the SF-MPQ produced significant differences in relation to patients' ability to walk freely and unaided. Small effect sizes across all four instruments were found in relation to initial leg ulcer size. Only the PF, MH, FAI and VAS Night dimensions showed evidence of statistical significance. Similarly, small effect sizes were observed in relation to current ulcer duration and maximum ulcer duration.

Walters *et al.* (1999) also looked at the longitudinal responsiveness of the four QoL instruments. Patients were assessed at enrolment and after 3 months. At the 3-month follow-up, the initial leg ulcers of 39 patients were known to have healed. Table 3.10 shows the standardized response mean (SRM) effect sizes from baseline to 3-month follow-up by leg ulcer healed status. For most dimensions (PF, RP, GH, VT, SF, RE, DSI, FAI, PRI(A)) health status had deteriorated by the 3-month follow-up, as indicated by the negative mean change/SRM. However, there was no evidence of a differential 'health change' between the healed and not healed groups except for two dimensions of the SF-MPQ (PRI(S) and VAS Now). On these two dimensions there was more improvement in the ulcer-related pain in those patients whose ulcer had healed. The authors concluded that 'only the SF-MPQ appears sensitive enough to detect a difference in HRQoL between those patients whose leg ulcer had healed or not'.   □

The measure with the largest effect size for a given change would be regarded as the 'best'. As with construct validity, it is necessary to establish a change has occurred, for example, before and after a successful operation. The following benchmarks for effect size statistics have now conventionally been accepted in the QoL literature. An effect size of 0.30–0.50 is regarded as 'small', 0.50–0.80 as 'moderate', 0.80 and above as

Table 3.9 Effect sizes[1] for patients in relation to age[2], mobility[3], leg ulcer size[4], current ulcer duration[5] and maximum ulcer duration[6] (data from Walters et al., 1999).

Health Status measure	Age[2]		Mobility[3]		Initial ulcer size[4]		Current ulcer duration[5]		Maximum ulcer duration[6]	
	Effect size	P	Effect size	P	Effect size	P	Effect size	P	Effect size	P-value[7]
SF-36:										
PF	0.44	0.001	1.18	0.001	0.25	0.06	-0.10	0.44	-0.16	0.21
RP	0.08	0.56	0.46	0.001	-0.14	0.31	-0.11	0.41	0.08	0.55
BP	-0.21	0.12	0.45	0.001	0.12	0.36	-0.03	0.82	0.04	0.78
GH	-0.36	0.006	0.21	0.11	-0.09	0.53	-0.33	0.01	0.05	0.69
VT	-0.14	0.28	0.37	0.005	-0.15	0.27	-0.11	0.39	-0.05	0.68
SF	-0.04	0.76	0.46	0.001	-0.06	0.64	-0.06	0.66	-0.06	0.65
RE	-0.18	0.18	0.16	0.21	0.05	0.71	0.19	0.16	0.25	0.06
MH	-0.39	0.002	0.09	0.51	-0.31	0.02	-0.30	0.02	0.03	0.80
EuroQol:										
DSI	-0.09	0.48	0.78	0.001	0.12	0.39	-0.24	0.07	-0.04	0.76
Frenchay:										
FAI	0.40	0.002	0.94	0.001	0.35	0.009	0.01	0.93	-0.16	0.24
SF–MPQ:										
PRI(S)	0.11	0.40	-0.15	0.27	-0.17	0.22	0.07	0.62	-0.24	0.06
PRI(A)	0.14	0.30	-0.13	0.32	-0.14	0.30	-0.06	0.64	-0.32	0.02
VAS Now	-0.02	0.90	-0.28	0.37	-0.14	0.32	0.07	0.59	-0.05	0.72
VAS Day	0.15	0.26	-0.21	0.12	-0.30	0.03	0.09	0.51	-0.21	0.10
VAS Night	0.00	0.98	-0.48	0.001	-0.22	0.11	0.06	0.67	0.01	0.94

[1]Effect size = mean score group 1 minus mean score group 2, divided by the pooled standard deviation.
[2]The cut-off value for the groups is the median age (i.e. ≤75 years; >75 years).
[3]The cut-off value for the groups is being able to walk freely or having to walk with an aid/chair/bed bound.
[4]The cut-off value for the groups is the median initial leg ulcer size (i.e. ≤5.61 cm²; >5.61 cm²).
[5]The cut-off value for the groups is the median current leg ulcer duration (i.e. ≤7 months; >7 months).
[6]The cut-off value for the groups is the median maximum leg ulcer duration (i.e. ≤7 years; >7 years).
[7]The P-values are from two-sample t-test comparing mean scores in each group. An effect size of 0.20 is regarded as small, one of 0.50 as moderate, and one of 0.80 or greater as large.

Table 3.10 Responsiveness of instruments as indicated by standardised response mean (SRM)* at 3-month follow-up by leg ulcer healed status at 3 months (data from Walters *et al.*, 1999).

	Leg ulcer healed at 3 months							
	Not healed				Healed			
	n	Mean Change	SD change	SRM	n	Mean Change	SD change	SRM
SF-36								
Physical Functioning	163	−5.3	22.9	−0.23	37	−1.6	27.0	−0.06
Role Physical	162	−11.3	43.4	−0.26	36	−12.5	39.9	−0.31
Bodily Pain	162	2.4	27.2	0.09	37	−3.3	35.3	−0.09
General Health	161	−8.4	18.7	−0.45	36	−7.3	16.5	−0.44
Vitality	160	−6.8	21.7	−0.31	36	−5.8	17.5	−0.33
Social Functioning	163	−6.6	28.2	−0.23	35	−8.9	28.7	−0.31
Role Emotion	161	−6.8	49.6	−0.14	35	−18.1	48.7	−0.37
Mental Health	162	−1.2	20.1	−0.06	36	0.0	21.1	0.00
EQ-5D								
EQ Single Index	161	−1.7	16.2	−0.10	37	−4.2	20.2	−0.21
SF-MPQ								
PRI(S)	154	1.7	7.9	0.21	35	4.8	7.9	0.60
PRI(A)	158	0.3	3.4	0.08	35	1.1	3.7	0.30
VAS Now	160	0.3	3.3	0.09	37	1.9	3.0	0.63
VAS Day	160	1.2	3.2	0.37	36	2.2	3.2	0.68
VAS Night	160	1.4	3.7	0.38	37	2.6	3.4	0.76

*The SRM is the mean change in score from initial assessment to 3-month follow-up, divided by the standard deviation of the change in scores. A negative SRM indicates that health-related quality of life has deteriorated from initial assessment to 3-month follow-up. An SRM of 0.20 is regarded as small, one of 0.50 as moderate, and one of 0.80 or greater as large.

'large' (Cohen, 1988; Kazis *et al.*, 1989). The most responsive instruments should have the largest effect size indices. Other criteria being equal, then, you should choose the most responsive instrument for your study, that is, the instrument which provides evidence that it generates the largest effect size indices for the purpose of your study and your intended study population.

3.9   Precision

Here we are interested in how precise are the scores of the QoL instrument and how the scores distinguish between difference levels of health and illness. One of the main influences on the precision of an instrument is the format of the response categories to the questions. Table 2.1 described the different types of response categories, ranging from a 'yes' or 'no' binary response category to a 100-point Visual Analogue Scale. Binary response categories have the advantage of simplicity but they may not allow respondents to report the degrees of difficulty or severity that they experience and consider important to distinguish (Fitzpatrick *et al.*, 1998). So other factors being equal, more items, each with a wider range of categories, will produce a greater theoretical range of values and scores for a QoL scale.

Many QoL instruments use Likert format response categories where degrees of agreement with a statement are given progressively lower (or higher) values – for example, poor = 1; fair = 2; good = 3; very good = 4; excellent = 5. The direction of such values is entirely arbitrary and can be reversed so that greater agreement is given a high numerical value. There are basically two different methods of scoring multi-item QoL measures with such Likert scale responses. One simple method is just to add up or take the average score of all the items for a dimension. Each item is given equal importance or weight in the scoring of the dimension or scale. This is sometimes referred to as the method of *summated ratings* or *Likert summated scales* (Fayers and Machin, 2007). Many commonly used QoL measures such as the HAD, SF-36 and EORTC QLQ-C30 use this simple method of scoring.

An alternative but more complex method of scoring multi-item QoL measures is to give each item or response a different weight or level of importance. The EQ-5D (see Appendix A), for example, has five items, each with a three-point Likert scale response of: no problems; some problems; cannot do activity. This generates 243 different possible combinations of responses or health states. Each of these 243 combinations of responses has been given a different value or weight to reflect the relative severity of the health state. This results in scale with a range of −0.59 to 1.00, with a score of 1.00 indicating 'full health' (Dolan *et al.*, 1995). Figure 3.3 shows a histogram of the distribution of the EQ-5D scores for a sample of 241 patients aged 20–64 with low back pain (Thomas *et al.*, 2006). The wide range of scores is readily apparent from the graph.

Many QoL measures, such as the SF-36 and EORTC QLQ C30, recode the numerical values so that the items are expressed as percentages or proportions of the total scale score. For example (see Figure 3.4), the Role Emotional dimension of the SF-36 consists of three questions each with a binary response option. There are only four possible combinations of responses to the three questions which would produce different scores or responses of 3, 4, 5 or 6. Instead of scoring the responses 3, 4, 5, or 6 or 1, 2, 3, or 4 the scores are transformed into percentages of a total: 0%, 33.3%, 66.7%, 100%. Although this approach produces a theoretical range of values between 0 and 100, the

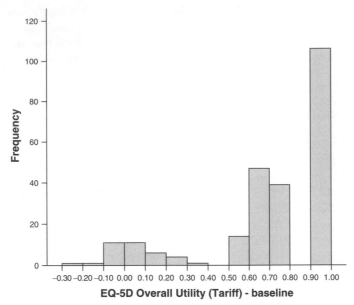

Figure 3.3   Histogram of EQ-5D utility scores for a sample of 241 patients aged 20–64 with low back pain (data from Thomas *et al.*, 2006).

During the <u>past 4 weeks</u>, have you had any of the following problems with your work or other regular daily activities <u>as a result of any emotional problems</u> (such as feeling depressed or anxious)?

(circle one number on each line)

	YES	NO
a. Cut down on the **amount of time** you spent on work or other activities	1	2
b. **Accomplished less** than you would like	1	2
c. Didn't do work or other activities as **carefully** as usual	1	2

Figure 3.4   The three items for the Role Emotional dimension of the SF-36.

simple and limited basis from which the values have been derived means that actually only four different values are possible. Figure 3.5 clearly shows that the actual range of possible values for the SF-36 Role Emotional dimension is small and the dimension does not have a high level of precision.

So when choosing a QoL measure for your study it is important to look at the format of the response categories to the questions and how these questions are scaled and combined to generate a dimension score. Other criteria being equal, then, you should choose the QoL instrument for your study which has the most precision, that is, the instrument that

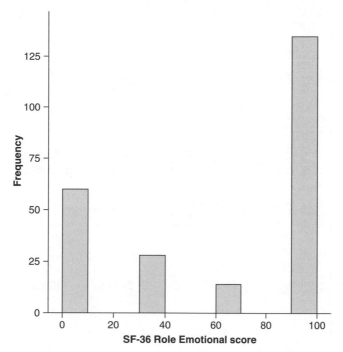

Figure 3.5 Histogram of SF-36 Role Emotional scores for a sample of 237 patients aged 20–64 with low back pain (data from Thomas *et al.*, 2006).

generates the greatest range of actual possible values for the purpose of your study and your intended target population.

3.10   Interpretability

Interpretability is concerned with how understandable the scores from a QoL instrument are. For example, what does a score of 70 mean on a 100-point QoL scale, compared to a score of 80? Chapter 2 discussed the issue of how to interpret QoL scores. Many QoL instruments are able to detect mean changes or differences that are very small. Therefore it is important to consider whether such changes are meaningful. To help interpret the scores of QoL instruments it is important to identify (and specify) the smallest difference or change in QoL scores between individuals or groups that is clinically and practically important. This benchmark value is usually called the minimum important difference (MID). An MID is usually specific to the population under study. The FDA (2006) describes four methods for determining minimum important difference (see Box 2.7).

Example: MID of the SF-6D and EQ-5D utility measures

Walters and Brazier (2005) used distribution and anchor-based methods to determine and compare the MID for the SF-6D and EQ-5D from eight longitudinal studies in 11 patient groups that used both instruments. The SF-6D is scored on a 0.29 to 1.00 scale and the EQ-5D on a −0.59 to 1.00 scale, with a score of 1.00 on both indicating 'full health'.

Table 3.11 MIDs, SRMs, half a standard deviation and effect size for those who reported some change at follow-up (data from Walters and Brazier, 2005).

Study/patient group		Period of time between assessments	Some change n*	MID	0.5SD	8% of empirical range
Leg ulcer I	*SF-6D*	Baseline to 3 months	44	0.03	0.07	0.05
	EQ-5D		44	0.14	0.16	0.13
Leg ulcer II	*SF-6D*	Baseline to 12 months	37	0.06	0.05	0.06
	EQ-5D		37	0.11	0.15	0.13
Back pain	*SF-6D*	Baseline to 12 months	63	0.10	0.05	0.05
	EQ-5D		63	0.08	0.15	0.13
Early rheumatoid arthritis (RA) patients	*SF-6D*	Baseline to 12 months	99	0.04	0.06	0.05
	EQ-5D		99	0.13	0.15	0.11
Limb reconstruction	*SF-6D*	Baseline to 12 months	27	0.04	0.06	0.05
	EQ-5D		27	0.05	0.16	0.10
Irritable bowel syndrome (IBS) patients	*SF-6D*	Baseline to 6 months	55	0.02	0.07	0.04
	EQ-5D		55	0.07	0.14	0.09
IBS controls	*SF-6D*	Baseline to 6 months	25	0.03	0.08	0.04
	EQ-5D		25	0.04	0.16	0.08
Acute myocardial infarction (AMI) patients	*SF-6D*	Baseline to 12 months	72	0.06	0.04	0.03
	EQ-5D		72	0.09	0.11	0.11
Osteoarthritis (OA) of the knee	*SF-6D*	Baseline to 6 months	55	0.04	0.05	0.03
	EQ-5D		55	0.12	0.17	0.11
Patients with chronic obstructive pulmonary disease (COPD I)	*SF-6D*	Baseline to 12 months	25	0.01	0.05	0.03
	EQ-5D		25	0.00	0.12	0.08
COPD II	*SF-6D*	Baseline to 6 months	30	0.04	0.05	0.04
	EQ-5D		30	−0.01	0.15	0.07

*No. of patients with valid baseline and follow-up SF-6D and EQ-5D score and who reported some change on the follow-up global change score.

Patients were followed for a period of time, then asked, using question 2 of the SF-36 as the anchor, if their general health is much better (5), somewhat better (4), stayed the same (3), somewhat worse (2) or much worse (1) compared to the last time they were assessed. They considered patients whose global rating score was 4 or 2 as having experienced some change equivalent to the MID.

Table 3.11 shows the MIDs, SRMs, half a standard deviation and effect size for those who reported some change at follow-up for the 11 data sets. From the 11 reviewed studies the MID for the SF-6D ranged from 0.011 to 0.097 (mean 0.041). The corresponding SRMs ranged from 0.12 to 0.87 (mean 0.39) and were mainly in the 'small to moderate' range using Cohen's criteria, supporting the MID results. The mean MID for the EQ-5D was 0.074 (range -0.011 to 0.140). The mean MID for the EQ-5D was almost double that of the mean MID for the SF-6D. The authors concluded that: 'Further empirical work is required to see whether or not this holds true for other utility measures, patient groups and populations.'   □

Other criteria being equal, then, you should choose a QoL instrument for your study which provides meaningful and interpretable scores. Ideally, the MID for the QoL measure for your intended target population will already have been defined.

3.11   Finding quality of life instruments

There are a number of books providing wide-ranging reviews of both generic and disease-specific QoL instruments. Examples include Bowling (2001, 2004) and McDowell and Newell (1996).

The Patient-Reported Outcome and Quality of life Instruments Database (PRO-QOLID) is available through the Internet at http://www.proqolid.org/. The PROQOLID database aims to:

  (i) provide an overview of existing QoL instruments;

 (ii) provide relevant and updated information on QoL instruments;

(iii) facilitate access to the instruments and their developers;

(iv) facilitate the choice of an appropriate QoL instrument.

The information on the PROQOLID website is structured in two levels. The first level is available to all visitors to the website at no charge. For each instrument in the database, you will find basic information (e.g. author, objective, mode of administration, original language, existing translations, pathology and number of items). The second more advanced level, which is accessible to subscribers only on payment of a fee, presents a greater degree of practical information on the instruments and, when available, includes the review copy of the instrument, its translations and the user manual.

4

Design and sample size issues: How many subjects do I need for my study?

Summary

This chapter will describe how sample sizes may be estimated for a variety of different study designs using QoL outcomes. The study designs will include two-group clinical trials, cross-over trials, cross-sectional surveys and reliability studies. The method of statistical analysis to be used with the subsequently collected QoL data needs to be specified, as do the significance/confidence level and power. The consequences of comparing more than two groups or simultaneously investigating several QoL outcomes are discussed.

4.1 Introduction

Quality of life measures are becoming more frequently used in clinical trials and health services research, both as primary and secondary endpoints. Investigators are now asking statisticians for advice on how to plan and analyse studies using QoL measures, which includes questions on sample size. Sample size calculations are now mandatory for many research protocols and are required to justify the size of clinical trials in papers before they will be accepted by journals.

Thus, when an investigator is designing a study to compare the outcomes of an intervention, an essential step is the calculation of sample sizes that will allow a reasonable chance (power) of detecting a predetermined difference (effect size) in the outcome variable, at a given level of statistical significance. Sample size is critically dependent on the purpose of the study, the outcome measure and how it is summarized, the proposed effect size and the method of calculating the test statistic.

Quality of Life Outcomes in Clinical Trials and Health-Care Evaluation   Stephen J. Walters
© 2009 John Wiley & Sons, Ltd

Whatever type of study design is used, the problem of sample size must be faced. In principle, there are no major differences between planning a study using QoL outcomes and those using conventional clinical outcomes. Pocock (1983) outlines five key questions regarding calculating sample sizes for clinical trials:

1. What is the main purpose of the trial?

2. What is the principal measure of patient outcome?

3. How will the data be analysed to detect a treatment difference?

4. What type of results does one anticipate with standard treatment?

5. How small a treatment difference is it important to detect and with what degree of certainty?

Thus, after deciding on the purpose of the study and the principle or primary outcome measure, the investigator must decide how the data are to be analysed to detect a treatment difference. We must also identify the smallest treatment difference that is of such clinical value that it would be very undesirable to fail to detect it. Given answers to all of the five questions above, we can then calculate a sample size.

4.2   Significance tests, P-values and power

The traditional approach to sample size determination for clinical trials is by consideration of significance or hypothesis tests. Suppose we are planning a two-group randomized controlled trial (RCT) to assess the efficacy or superiority of a new test (T) versus a control (C) treatment, and the main outcome is a continuous QoL measure, which is Normally distributed. We set up a null hypothesis (H_0) that the two population mean QoL scores, for the Test and Control treatments, μ_T and μ_C are equal, that is, $H_0 : \mu_T - \mu_C = 0$. After we have conducted the trial and collected some QoL outcome data, we carry out a significance test, such as the two independent samples t-test (see Chapter 7), to test this hypothesis. We calculate the observed difference in mean QoL scores between the test (observed mean, $\bar{x}_T$) and control (mean, $\bar{x}_C$) groups, $\bar{x}_T - \bar{x}_C = \bar{d}$. This significance test results in a P-value, which is the probability of getting the observed result, $\bar{d}$, or a more extreme one, if the null hypothesis H_0 (of no treatment difference) is true, by chance. If the P-value obtained from the trial data is less than or equal to α, then one rejects the null hypothesis and concludes that there is a statistically significant difference in QoL outcomes between the treatments. The value we take for α is arbitrary, but conventionally it is either 0.05 or 0.01. On the other hand, if the P-value is greater than α, we do not reject the null hypothesis.

Even when the null hypothesis, of no treatment effect or difference in QoL scores between the groups, is true there is still a risk of making a mistake and rejecting it. To reject the null hypothesis when it is actually true is to make a false positive or Type I error. Clearly, the associated probability of rejecting the null hypothesis when it is true is α. The quantity α is variously termed the test size, significance level or probability of a Type I (false positive) error.

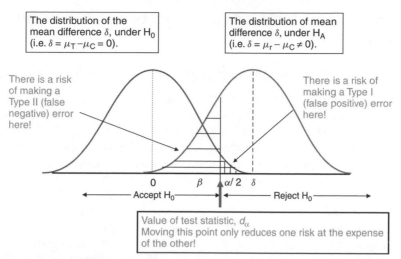

Figure 4.1   Distribution of the mean difference δ under the null and alternative hypotheses. Reproduced with permission from Campbell, M.J., Machin, D., Walters, S.J., *Medical Statistics: A Text Book for the Health Sciences*. 4th edition. John Wiley & Sons Ltd, Chichester. © 2007 John Wiley & Sons Ltd.

The left-hand curve in Figure 4.1 shows the expected distribution of the observed treatment difference $\bar{d}$ under the null hypothesis $H_0 : \delta = \mu_T - \mu_C = 0$ centred at zero. If $\bar{d}$ is greater than some critical value d_α which is determined so that the shaded area to right of d_α is equal to α, then H_0 is rejected.

The clinical trial could yield an observed difference $\bar{d}$ that could lead to a *P*-value above α, even though the null hypothesis is not true, that is, μ_T is indeed not equal to μ_C and there is a treatment difference. In such a situation, we then accept (or, more correctly, fail to reject) the null hypothesis although it is actually truly false. This is called a Type II (false negative) error and the probability of this is denoted by β.

The probability of a Type II error is based on the assumption that the null hypothesis is not true, that is $\delta = \mu_T - \mu_C \neq 0$. There are clearly many possible values of δ in this instance and each would imply a different alternative hypothesis, H_A, and a different value for the probability β.

The power is defined as one minus the probability of a Type II error, that is, power $= 1 - \beta$. The power is the probability of obtaining a statistically significant *P*-value if the null hypothesis is truly false. The right-hand curve of Figure 4.1 illustrates the distribution of $\bar{d}$ under the alternative hypothesis H_A, centred around the expected difference in means, $\delta = \mu_T - \mu_C$.

Conventionally a minimum power of 0.80 $(1 - \beta)$ or 80% is required in a trial. So the Type I error, α (of 0.05), is less than the Type II error, β (of 0.20). Why this difference in error rates? The simple answer is that researchers are innately conservative. They would prefer to accept an established treatment against the evidence that a new treatment is better, rather than risk going over to a new treatment, with all its possible attendant problems such as long-term side effects, and different procedures.

4.3   Sample sizes for comparison of two independent groups

4.3.1   Normally distributed continuous data – comparing two means

Suppose we are planning a two-group RCT to assess the efficacy or superiority of a new test (T) versus a control (C) treatment, and the main outcome is a continuous QoL measure. If the QoL outcome is assumed to be continuous and plausibly sampled from a Normal distribution, then the best summary statistic for the data is the sample mean, and the mean difference in QoL scores between the two groups is an appropriate comparative summary measure. The usual hypothesis test for a difference in location or shift in mean population parameters between two independent samples is the two-sample t-test (Campbell et al., 2007). See Chapter 7 for more details on the t-test.

For two independent groups with continuous and Normally distributed data, the effect size is the expected mean value of the test outcome, μ_T, minus the expected mean value of the control outcome, μ_C, that is, $\delta = \mu_T - \mu_C$. If this difference is then divided by the standard deviation of the outcomes, σ, then Δ_{Normal} is the *standardized effect size index*,

$$\Delta_{Normal} = \frac{\mu_T - \mu_C}{\sigma} = \frac{\delta}{\sigma}, \tag{4.1}$$

where μ_T and μ_C are the expected group outcome variable means under the null and alternative hypotheses and σ is the outcome variable standard deviation (assumed to be the same under the null and alternative hypotheses).

In a two-group study comparing mean QoL between the two groups, the number of subjects per group n for a two-sided significance level α and power $1 - \beta$ is given by

$$n_{Normal} = \frac{2[z_{1-\alpha/2} + z_{1-\beta}]^2}{\Delta_{Normal}^2}, \tag{4.2}$$

where $z_{1-\alpha/2}$ and $z_{1-\beta}$ are the appropriate values from the standard Normal distribution for the $100(1 - \alpha/2)$ and $100(1 - \beta)$ percentiles, respectively. Table 4.1 shows some typical percentage points for the standard Normal distribution.

For the commonly occurring situation of $\alpha = 0.05$ (two-sided) and $\beta = 0.2$, $z_{1-\alpha/2} = 1.96$ and $z_{1-\beta} = 0.8416$, and equation (4.2) simplifies to:

$$n_{Normal} = \frac{16}{\Delta_{Normal}^2}. \tag{4.3}$$

Example calculations

Suppose we are planning a two-group RCT, in men aged 50–74, to see if a daily exercise regime for a year will lead to improved QoL compared to a control group. The primary outcome will be the Physical Functioning (PF) dimension of the SF-36 at 12-month follow-up. We know from published data on the SF-36 QoL measure that at this age men have a mean score on the PF dimension of 66.4, with a standard deviation of 29.5 (Walters et al., 2001a). Figure 4.2 shows a histogram of the SF-36 PF dimension from

Table 4.1   Percentage points of the Normal distribution for α and $1 - \beta$.

α 2-sided	α 1-sided	$1 - \beta$	Z
0.001	0.0005	0.9995	3.2905
0.005	0.0025	0.9975	2.8070
0.010	0.0050	0.9950	2.5758
0.020	0.0100	0.9900	2.3263
0.025	0.0125	0.9875	2.2414
0.050	0.0250	0.9750	1.9600
0.100	0.0500	0.9500	1.6449
0.200	0.1000	0.9000	1.2816
0.300	0.1500	0.8500	1.0364
0.400	0.2000	0.8000	0.8416
0.500	0.2500	0.7500	0.6745
0.600	0.3000	0.7000	0.5244
0.700	0.3500	0.6500	0.3853
0.800	0.4000	0.6000	0.2533

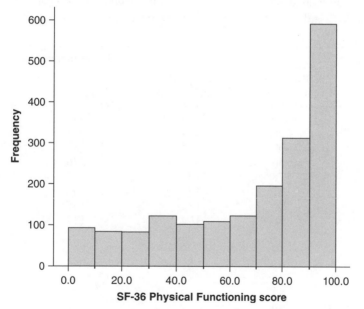

Figure 4.2   Histogram of SF-36 Physical Functioning dimension for 1817 men aged 50–74 (data from Walters *et al.*, 2001a).

a general population survey. Clearly the PF dimension has a skewed distribution in this sample. Let us assume that the PF data are Normally distributed in our population of men aged 50–74.   □

Suppose that the effect of the daily exercise regime on Physical Functioning will be considered important if it increases the PF dimension of the SF-36 by at least 10 points.

We want a high probability of detecting such a difference, so we set the power to be 0.90 (90%) and choose a 5% significance level.

For sample size calculations we usually round up the standard deviation, to reflect our uncertainty about the variability of the outcome. So $\sigma = 30.0$ (rounded up from 29.5), $\delta = 10.0$, $\alpha = 0.05$ and $\beta = 0.10$. Using equation (4.1), this results in a standardized effect size Δ_{Normal} of $10.0/30.0 = 0.33$. Using Table 4.1, With $\alpha = 0.05$ (two-sided) and $\beta = 0.10$, the appropriate z values, $z_{1-\alpha/2}$ and $z_{1-\beta}$, from the standard Normal distribution (Table 4.1) are 1.96 and 1.2816, respectively. So equation (4.2) becomes

$$n_{Normal} = \frac{2[1.96 + 1.2816]^2}{0.33^2} = 193.$$

This gives an approximate sample size of 193 men in each group (386 in total).

Using Table 4.2 with a standardized effect size of $\Delta_{Normal} = 0.30$ and 5% significance and 90% power gives an n per group of 172 and with $\Delta_{Normal} = 0.35$ gives an n per group of 234.

Table 4.2 Sample size n per group required for a comparison of two group means, μ_1 and μ_2, with common standard deviation, σ, with a *standardized effect size*, $\Delta = (\mu_2 - \mu_1)/\sigma$, with 80% and 90% power and 1% ($\alpha = 0.01$) and 5% ($\alpha - 0.05$) two-sided significance.

| Standardized | 5% significance | | 1% significance | |
Effect Size Δ	80% power Sample size	90% power Sample size	80% power Sample size	90% power Sample size
0.10	1600	2100	2350	3000
0.15	698	934	1045	1334
0.20	400	525	588	750
0.25	256	336	376	480
0.30	178	234	262	334
0.35	131	172	192	245
0.40	100	132	147	188
0.45	80	104	117	149
0.50	64	84	94	120
0.55	53	70	78	100
0.60	45	59	66	84
0.65	38	50	56	72
0.70	33	43	48	62
0.75	29	38	42	54
0.80	25	33	37	47
0.85	23	30	33	42
0.90	20	26	30	38
0.95	18	24	27	34
1.00	16	21	24	30

$\Delta = (\mu_2 - \mu_1)/\sigma$.
The cells in the table give the number of patients required in each treatment arm.

Example: Pre-study power and sample size calculation – the Community Postnatal Support Worker (CPSW) study

Morrell *et al.* (2000) undertook a two-group RCT in new mothers to assess the effectiveness of additional postnatal support provided by trained community postnatal support workers compared to usual care provided by community midwives. The primary endpoint was the General Health (GH) domain of the SF-36 at 6 weeks postnatally The GH domain of the SF-36 is scored on a 0 (poor) to 100 (good) health scale (Ware *et al.*,1993).

The developers of the SF-36 suggested that a 5-point difference (i.e. $\delta = 5.0$) in GH scores is the smallest difference in scores which could be considered 'clinically and socially relevant' (Ware *et al.*, 1993). A previous survey of the general population in the United Kingdom, using the SF-36, gave an estimated variability or standard deviation for the GH domain of 20 points (i.e. $\sigma = 20$) in women of child-bearing age, that is, women aged 16–45 (Brazier *et al.*, 1992). The standardized effect size, $\Delta_{Normal} = \delta/\sigma$ is 5/20 or 0.25.

Using Table 4.2, or equation (4.2), with an anticipated Δ_{Normal} of 0.25 (planned difference of 5 points in mean GH scores between the groups assuming a standard deviation of 20) and 90% power and 5% (two-sided) level of significance, estimates that we need 336 women per group (672 in total). □

4.3.2 Transformations

If the QoL outcome data is continuous but has a skewed distribution, it may be transformed using a logarithmic transformation. The transformed variable may have a more symmetric distribution that gives a better approximation to the Normal form. The problem is that certain QoL measures, for example the SF-36, are scored on 0–100 scales and the natural logarithm of 0 does not exist. We can get around this problem by adding 0.5 to all the QoL scores, so the scale now ranges from 0.5 to 100.5. Unfortunately, log-transforming the general population data, for the SF-36 PF dimension in Figure 4.2, did not make the distribution of the data more symmetric (see Figure 4.3).

The use of transformations, such as the natural logarithm, frequently does not make the transformed QoL data follow a more symmetric distribution. Therefore QoL data are usually not analysed on a transformed scale, since the use of transformations distorts QoL scales and make interpretation of treatment effects difficult (Fayers and Machin, 2007; Walters *et al.*, 2001b). So as an alternative we can use a non-parametric method to estimate sample sizes to compare two groups with continuous QoL outcome data.

4.3.3 Comparing two groups with continuous data using non-parametric methods

If the QoL outcome is assumed to be continuous and plausibly not sampled from a Normal distribution then the most popular (but not necessarily the most efficient) non-parametric test for comparing two independent samples is the two-sample *Mann–Whitney U*-test or the equivalent *Wilcoxon* rank sum test (Campbell *et al.*, 2007). Again, more details of this test are given in Chapter 7.

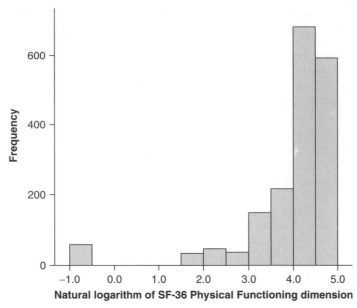

Figure 4.3 Histogram of the natural logarithm of the SF-36 Physical Functioning dimension for 1817 men aged 50–74 (data from Walters *et al.*, 2001a).

Suppose we have two independent random samples of subjects with QoL outcomes $X_1, X_2, \ldots, X_m$ and $Y_1, Y_2, \ldots, Y_n$ of size m and n respectively, and we want to test the hypothesis that the two samples have come from the same population against the alternative that the Y observations tend to be larger than the X observations. As a test statistic we can use the Mann–Whitney (MW) statistic U, given by

$$U = \#(Y_j > X_i), \qquad i = 1, \ldots, m; \; j = 1, \ldots, n,$$

which is a count of the number of times the Y_j are greater than the X_i. The magnitude of U has a meaning, because U/nm is an estimate of the probability that an observation drawn at random from population Y would exceed an observation drawn at random from population X.

Noether (1987) derived a sample size formula for the MW test, using an effect size, p_{Noether}, that makes no assumptions about the distribution of the data set (except that it is continuous), that can be used whenever the sampling distribution of the test statistic U can be closely approximated by the Normal distribution, an approximation that is usually quite good except for very small n. Noether's formula is

$$n_{\text{Non - normal}} = \frac{[z_{1-\alpha/2} + z_{1-\beta}]^2}{6(p_{\text{Noether}} - 0.5)^2}. \tag{4.4}$$

Hence to determine the sample size, we have to decide on a value for the 'effect size' p_{Noether} or the equivalent statistic $\Pr(Y > X)$. We could just decide *a priori* on a value for p_{Noether} and use this. However, unlike the effect size Δ_{Normal}, which can be interpreted as a difference of Δ standard deviations on the QoL scale, a meaningful and easily interpretable value of the effect size p_{Noether} is difficult to specify in advance. Post hoc there are several ways of estimating p_{Noether}. One way is simply to use the empirical estimate, $p_{\text{Noether}} = U/nm$. Unfortunately, this can only be estimated after we have collected the data or by computer simulation (see Walters and Campbell, 2005). We can make progress if we assume that $X \sim N(\mu_X, \sigma_X^2)$ and $Y \sim N(\mu_Y, \sigma_Y^2)$; then an estimate of $\Pr(Y > X)$ using the sample estimates of the mean and variance $(\hat{\mu}_X, \hat{\sigma}_X^2, \hat{\mu}_Y, \hat{\sigma}_Y^2)$ is given by

$$p_{\text{Noether}} = \Pr(Y > X) = \Phi\left(\frac{\hat{\mu}_Y - \hat{\mu}_X}{(\hat{\sigma}_Y^2 + \hat{\sigma}_X^2)^{1/2}}\right) \tag{4.5}$$

(Simonoff *et al.*, 1986), where Φ is the Normal cumulative distribution function.

If we assume that the QoL outcome is Normally distributed then equation (4.5) allows the calculation of two comparable 'effect sizes' p_{Noether} and Δ_{Normal}, thus enabling the two methods of sample size estimation to be directly contrasted. If the QoL outcome is not Normally distributed then we cannot use equation (4.5) to calculate comparable effect sizes and must rely on the empirical estimates of $p_{\text{Noether}} = U/nm$ calculated post hoc from the data. Alternatively, under certain assumptions, we can use computer simulation or bootstrap methods to estimate p_{Noether} (Walters and Campbell, 2005).

Example calculations

Suppose, as before, that we are planning a two-group RCT, in men aged 50–74, to see if a daily exercise regime for a year will lead to improved QoL compared to a control group. The primary outcome will be the PF dimension of the SF-36 at 12-month follow-up.

We believe the PF dimension of the SF-36 to be continuous, but not Normally distributed (see Figure 4.2) and are intending to compare SF-36 PF scores at 12 months in the two groups with a Mann–Whitney U-test. Therefore Noether's method will be appropriate. As before, if we assume a mean difference of 10.0 (i.e. $\hat{\mu}_X - \hat{\mu}_Y = 10.0$) and a standard deviation of 30.0 (i.e. $\hat{\sigma}_X - \hat{\sigma}_Y = 30.0$) for the SF-36 PF dimension, then using equation (4.5) leads to an effect size $p_{\text{Noether}} = \text{Prob}(Y > X)$ of 0.63. Substituting $p_{\text{Noether}} = 0.63$ in equation (4.4) with a two-sided 5% significance level and 90% power (or using Table 4.3) gives the estimated number of subjects per group as 104.   □

The two methods have given different sample size estimates $n_{\text{Normal}} = 193$ and $n_{\text{non-Normal}} = 104$. The two methods can be regarded as equivalent when the two distributions have the same shape and equal variances. When the two distributions are Normally distributed with equal variances, the MW test will require about 5% more observations than the two-sample t-test to provide the same power against the same alternative. For non-Normal populations, especially those with long tails, as in our example, the MW test may not require as many observations as the two-sample t-test (Elashoff, 1999).

4.3.4   Dichotomous categorical data – comparing two proportions

If the continuous QoL outcomes are condensed into a binary or dichotomous categorical scale, then an appropriate summary measure of the outcome data will usually be the sample rate or proportion. When comparing two groups or a single group over time, appropriate comparative summary measures may include the difference in rates or proportions, the relative risk or the odds ratio.

Table 4.3 Sample size n per group required for a comparison of two groups with non-Normally distributed continuous data, with an effect size $p_{Noether} = \Pr(Y > X)$ with 80% and 90% power and 1% ($\alpha = 0.01$) and 5% ($\alpha = 0.05$) two-sided significance.

Effect size $p_{Noether} = \Pr(Y > X)$	5% significance		1% significance	
	80% power Sample size	90% power Sample size	80% power Sample size	90% power Sample size
0.51	13082	17512	19465	24799
0.52	3271	4378	4867	6200
0.53	1454	1946	2163	2756
0.54	818	1095	1217	1550
0.55	524	701	779	992
0.56	364	487	541	689
0.57	267	358	398	507
0.58	205	274	305	388
0.59	162	217	241	307
0.60	131	176	195	248
0.61	109	145	161	205
0.62	91	122	136	173
0.63	78	104	116	147
0.64	67	90	100	127
0.65	59	78	87	111
0.70	33	44	49	62
0.75	21	29	32	40
0.80	15	20	22	28
0.85	11	15	16	21
0.90	9	11	13	16
0.95	7	9	10	13
1.00	6	8	8	10

The effect size $p_{Noether} = \Pr(Y > X)$ is an estimate of the probability that an observation drawn at random from population Y would exceed an observation drawn at random from population X.
The cells in the table give the number of patients required in each treatment arm.

The statistical hypothesis test used to compare two independent groups when the outcome is binary is the Pearson chi-squared test for a 2×2 contingency table (Campbell et al., 2007). In this situation, the anticipated effect size is $\delta_{Binary} = (\pi_T - \pi_C)$, where π_T and π_C are the proportions in the two treatment groups. In a two-group study comparing differences in rates or proportions between the groups, the number of subjects per group, n_{Binary}, for a two-sided significance level α and power $1 - \beta$ is given by

$$n_{Binary} = \frac{(z_{1-\alpha/2} + z_{1-\beta})^2 [\pi_T(1 - \pi_T) + \pi_C(1 - \pi_C)]}{(\pi_T - \pi_C)^2}. \tag{4.6}$$

Table 4.4 uses equation (4.6) to show the sample sizes per group for comparing two proportions with 80% power and 5% two-sided significance. Alternatively, the same difference between treatments may be expressed through the odds ratio (OR), which is

Table 4.4 Sample size n per group required for a given response rate in the control group (π_1) and the effect size anticipated ($\delta = \pi_2 - \pi_1$) with 80% power ($1 - \beta = 0.80$) and 5% ($\alpha = 0.05$) two-sided significance.

π_2	π_1 0.05	0.10	0.15	0.20	0.25	0.30	0.35	0.40	0.45	0.50	0.55	0.60	0.65	0.70	0.75	0.80	0.85	0.90
0.10	435																	
0.15	141	686																
0.20	76	199	906															
0.25	49	100	250	1094														
0.30	36	62	121	294	1251													
0.35	27	43	73	138	329	1377												
0.40	22	32	49	82	152	356	1471											
0.45	18	25	36	54	89	163	376	1534										
0.50	15	20	27	39	58	93	170	388	1565									
0.55	12	16	22	29	41	61	96	173	392	1565								
0.60	11	14	17	23	31	42	62	97	173	388	1534							
0.65	9	11	14	18	24	31	43	62	96	170	376	1471						
0.70	8	10	12	15	19	24	31	42	61	93	163	356	1377					
0.75	7	8	10	12	15	19	24	31	41	58	89	152	329	1251				
0.80	6	7	8	10	12	15	18	23	29	39	54	82	138	294	1094			
0.85	5	6	7	8	10	12	14	17	22	27	36	49	73	121	250	906		
0.90	4	5	6	7	8	10	11	14	16	20	25	32	43	62	100	199	686	
0.95	4	4	5	6	7	8	9	11	12	15	18	22	27	36	49	76	141	435
1.00	3	4	4	5	6	6	7	8	10	11	13	15	18	22	27	35	48	74

The cells in the table give the number of patients required in each treatment arm.

defined as

$$\text{OR}_{\text{Binary}} = \frac{\frac{\pi_T}{1-\pi_T}}{\frac{\pi_C}{1-\pi_C}} = \frac{\pi_T(1-\pi_C)}{\pi_C(1-\pi_T)}. \tag{4.7}$$

This formulation leads to an alternative for equation (4.6) for the sample size. Thus,

$$n_{\text{OR}} = \frac{2(z_{1-\alpha/2} + z_{1-\beta})^2/(\log \text{OR}_{\text{Binary}})^2}{\bar{\pi}(1-\bar{\pi})}, \tag{4.8}$$

where $\bar{\pi} = (\pi_T + \pi_C)/2$.

Equations (4.6) and (4.8) are quite dissimilar, but Julious and Campbell (1996) show that for all practical purposes they give very similar sample sizes, with divergent results only occurring for relative large (or small) $\text{OR}_{\text{Binary}}$.

Example calculations

Figure 4.2 indicates that approximately 50% of men aged 50–74 in the general population scored 75 or more on the PF dimension of the SF-36. Let us assume that a score of 75 or more can be regarded as 'good physical functioning' and a score of less than 75 regarded as 'poor physical functioning'. Suppose, as before, that we are planning a two-group RCT, men aged 50–74, to see if a daily exercise regime for a year will lead to improved QoL compared to a control group. The primary outcome this time will be binary and it will be the proportion of men who score 75 or more on the PF dimension of the SF-36 at 12-month follow-up. Let us assume that 50% of men in the control group will have good physical functioning. Suppose it is anticipated that this may improve to 60% having good physical functioning in the treatment group (following a daily exercise regime for a year). The anticipated treatment effect is thus $\delta_{\text{Binary}} = (\pi_T - \pi_C) = 0.60 - 0.50 = 0.10$. Using this effect size in equation (4.6) with a two-sided 5% significance level and 80% power gives the estimated number of subjects $n_{\text{Binary}} = 388$ per group.

Alternatively, this anticipated treatment effect can be expressed (using equation (4.7)) as $\text{OR}_{\text{Binary}} = (0.60/0.40)/(0.5/0.5) = 1.5$. Using this in equation (4.8) with $\bar{\pi} = (0.60 + 0.50)/2 = 0.55$ gives a sample size per group of $n_{\text{OR}} = 386$ patients. As we indicated previously, there is usually only a small and inconsequential difference between the calculations from the alternative formulae. □

4.3.5   Ordered categorical (ordinal) data

If the QoL outcomes are measured on an ordinal scale, then the statistical hypothesis test used (to compare two independent groups) is the Mann–Whitney U-test with allowance for ties or a chi-squared test for trend (Campbell et al., 2007). Whitehead (1993) derived a sample size formula for ordinal data using the odds ratio as an effect size. The odds ratio ($\text{OR}_{\text{Ordinal}}$) is defined as the odds of a subject being in a given category or lower in one group compared with the odds of a subject being in a given category or lower in the other group.

Suppose that we have two groups, treatment (T) and control (C), and the QoL outcome measure of interest Y has k ordered categories $y_i, i = 1, 2, \ldots, k$. Let p_{iT} be the probability of being in category i in group T and C_{iT} be the expected cumulative probability of being in category i or less in group T (i.e. $C_{iT} = \Pr(Y \le y_i)$). For category i, where $i = 1, \ldots, k-1$, the $OR_{Ordinal}$ is given by

$$OR_{Ordinal,i} = \frac{\dfrac{C_{iT}}{(1 - C_{iT})}}{\dfrac{C_{iC}}{(1 - C_{iC})}}. \tag{4.9}$$

The assumption of proportional odds specifies that the $OR_{Ordinali}$ will be the same for all categories $i = 1, \ldots, k-1$, and is equal to $OR_{Ordinal}$. This is the proportional odds assumption which underlies the proportional odds model and hence the derivation of the formulae.

Whitehead's method can be regarded as a 'non-parametric' approach as the derivation of the sample size formulae and analysis of data are based on the Mann-Whitney U-test, although it still relies on the assumption of a constant odds ratio for the data. Whitehead's method also assumes a relatively small log odds ratio and a large sample size, which will often be the case in QoL studies where dramatic effects are unlikely. The number of subjects per group for a two-sided significance level α and power $1 - \beta$ is given by

$$n_{Ordinal} = \frac{6[(z_{1-\alpha/2} + z_{1-\beta})^2 / (\log OR_{Ordinal})^2]}{\left[1 - \sum_{i-1}^{k} \bar{\pi}_i^3\right]}. \tag{4.10}$$

Here $\bar{\pi}_i$ is the average proportion of subjects anticipated in category i, that is, $\bar{\pi}_i = (\pi_{iT} + \pi_{iC})/2$.

Example calculations

Suppose the SF-36 PF data set of Figure 4.2 is recoded into a four-category ordinal variable. The four new physical functioning categories are (0–24, 25–49, 50–74 and 75–100). Table 4.5 shows the proportions in each category and the cumulative proportions.

Suppose (as before) that we are planning a two-group study to compare QoL (using a four-category ordinal physical function scale as the primary outcome) between the groups. We believe that the mean difference in QoL scores between the two groups is

Table 4.5   Anticipated cumulative proportions in test and control group.

Physical Functioning category		Control Group π_{iC}	Cumulative Proportion C_{iC}	Test Group π_{iT}	Cumulative Proportion C_{iT}	$\bar{\pi}_i$
1	0–24	0.122	0.122	0.085	0.085	0.1034
2	25–49	0.144	0.266	0.110	0.194	0.1269
3	50–74	0.236	0.502	0.207	0.402	0.2216
4	75–100	0.498	1.0	0.598	1.0	0.5482
		1.0		1.0		

not an appropriate comparative summary measure. However, the odds of a patient in the invention group having a QoL score in a given category or below compared to the odds for a patient in the control group are felt to be an appropriate comparative summary measure.

Let us assume that 50% of men in the control group will have good physical functioning (a score of 75 or more). Suppose it is anticipated that this may improve to 60% having good physical functioning in the treatment group (following a daily exercise regime for a year. Using equation (4.9)

$$OR_{Ordinal,i} = \frac{\dfrac{0.5}{(1-0.5)}}{\dfrac{0.6}{(1-0.6)}} = \frac{1.00}{1.5} = 0.67$$

leads to $OR_{Ordinal} = 0.67$ which is the reciprocal of OR_{Binary}.

If we assume proportions of patients of 0.122, 0.144, 0.236, and 0.498 respectively in the four physical function categories (0–24, 25–49, 50–74 and 75–100) in the control group, the cumulative proportions C_{iC} in category i for the control treatment C ($i =$ 1 to 4) are 0.122, 0.266, 0.502, and 1.000. Then, for a given constant $OR_{Ordinal} = 0.67$, the anticipated cumulative proportions (C_{iT}) for each category of treatment T are given by:

$$C_{iT} = \frac{OR_{Ordinal}C_{iC}}{OR_{Ordinal}C_{iC} + (1 - C_{iC})} \qquad i = 1, \ldots, k - 1.$$

After calculating the cumulative proportions (C_{iT}), the anticipated proportions falling in each treatment category, π_{iT} can be determined from the difference in successive C_{iT}. Finally, the combined mean ($\bar{\pi}_i$) of the proportions of treatments C and T for each category is calculated.

Using equation (4.10) with this OR and $\bar{\pi}_i$ with a two-sided 5% significance level and 80% power gives the estimated number of subjects per group as 347. Utilizing the ordinal nature of the four-category Physical Functioning outcome has resulted in a smaller estimated sample size than treating the scale as a binary outcome which gave the estimated number of subjects as $n_{Binary} = 388$ per group. □

If the number of categories is large it is difficult to postulate the proportion of subjects who would fall in a given category. Both Whitehead (1993) and Julious *et al.* (1995) point out that there is little increase in power (and hence saving in the number of subjects recruited) to be gained by increasing the number of categories beyond five. Categories that are equally likely to occur lead to the greatest efficiency.

Julious and Campbell (1996) show that, with two categories only, the method given by Whitehead is approximately equivalent to equation (4.6) for the binary case, even though at first sight the equations are very dissimilar. They state that the practical importance of this is to give the choice of two alternative measures of differences between groups: differences in proportions or odds ratios.

4.4   Choice of sample size method with quality of life outcomes

It is important to make maximum use of the information available from other related studies or extrapolation from other unrelated studies. The more precise the information, the better we can design the trial. I would recommend that researchers planning a study with QoL measures as the primary outcome pay careful attention to any evidence on the validity and frequency distribution of the QoL measures and its dimensions.

The frequency distribution of QoL dimension scores from previous studies should be assessed to see what methods should be used for sample size calculations and analysis. If the QoL outcome has a limited number of discrete values (say, less than seven categories) and/or the proportion of cases at the upper/lower bound (top or bottom category) is high (i.e. more than 50%), then I would recommend using Whitehead's method, $n_{Ordinal}$ (equation 4.10), to estimate the required sample size. In this case the alternative hypothesis of a simple location shift model (difference in mean QoL scores) is questionable and the proportional odds model will provide a suitable alternative with such bounded discrete outcomes.

If the QoL outcome has a larger number of discrete values (say, seven or more categories), most of which are occupied and the proportion of cases at the upper or bounds (i.e. scoring 0 or 100, in the case of the SF-36) is low then the location shift model (difference in mean QoL) is a useful working hypothesis. I would therefore recommend using n_{Normal} (equation (4.2)) or $n_{non-Normal}$ (4.4) to estimate the required sample size.

Computer simulation (Walters and Campbell, 2005) has suggested that if the distributions of the QoL dimensions are reasonably symmetric, and the proportion of patients at each bound is low, then under the location shift alternative hypothesis, the t-test appears to be slightly more powerful than the MW test at detecting differences in means. Therefore if the distribution of the QoL outcomes is symmetric or expected to be reasonably symmetric and the proportion of patients at the upper or lower bounds is low then equation (4.2) could be used for sample size calculations and analysis. The use of parametric methods for analysis (i.e. t-test) also enables the relatively easy estimation of confidence intervals, which is regarded as good statistical practice (Altman et al., 2000).

If the distribution of the QoL outcome is expected to be skewed then the MW test appears to be more powerful at detecting a location shift (difference in means) than the t-test. So in these circumstances the MW test is preferable to the t-test and Noether's method (equation (4.4)) and could be used for sample size calculations and analysis. However, using Noether's method for sample size estimation requires the effect size to be defined in terms of $Pr(Y > X)$, which is difficult to quantify and interpret.

If the QoL data have a symmetric distribution the mean and median will tend to coincide so either measure is a suitable summary measure of location. If the QoL data have an asymmetric distribution, then conventional statistical advice would suggest that the median is the preferred summary statistic (Altman et al., 2000). However, a case when the mean and mean difference might be preferred (even for skewed QoL outcome data) as a summary measure is when health-care providers are deciding whether to offer a new treatment or not to their population. The mean (along with the sample size) provides information about the total QoL benefit (and total cost) from treating all patients, which is needed as the basis for health-care policy decisions (Thompson and Barber, 2000). We cannot estimate the total QoL benefit (or cost) from the sample median.

If the sample size is 'sufficiently large' then the central limit theorem (CLT) guarantees that the sample means will be approximately Normally distributed. Thus, if the investigator is planning a large study and the sample mean is an appropriate summary measure of the QoL outcome, then pragmatically there is no need to worry about the distribution of the QoL outcome and we can use conventional methods (equations (4.1) and (4.2)) to calculate sample sizes. Although the Normal distribution is strictly only the limiting form of the sampling distribution of the sample mean as the sample size n increases to infinity, it provides a remarkably good approximation to the sampling distribution even when n is small and the distribution of the data is far from Normal. Generally, if n is greater than 25, these approximations will be good. However, if the underlying distribution is symmetric, unimodal and continuous a value of n as small as 4 can yield a very adequate approximation (Hogg and Tanis, 1988).

If a reliable pilot or historical data set of QoL data is readily available (to estimate the shape of the distribution) then bootstrap computer simulation (Walters and Campbell, 2005) may provide a more accurate and reliable sample size estimate.

4.5   Paired data

The previous sections have described sample size calculations for the comparison of two groups. These calculations have assumed that the QoL outcome data for one group are independent of the data in the other group. However, a common situation is when the data are paired in some way and so the assumption of independence no longer holds. Paired data arise in several ways: for example, subjects may have their QoL assessed before and after an intervention; treatments in a cross-over trial are evaluated on the same patient; or subjects with a disease may be matched with controls, by age, sex and area of residence, in a case–control study.

The purpose of this section is to describe methods for calculating sample sizes for studies which yield paired data. Two situations are described where the QoL outcomes are either continuous or binary.

4.5.1   Paired continuous data – comparison of means

For sample size calculations for continuous QoL outcome data we have to specify the anticipated difference, δ, in mean QoL scores for two occasions in a cross-over trial or the mean difference between the case and the corresponding matched control. In addition, we must specify, as in the two independent group case described earlier, the standard deviation of the data, $\sigma_{\text{Difference}}$. The standardized effect size is now defined as $\Delta = \delta / \sigma_{\text{Difference}}$.

Note that $\sigma_{\text{Difference}}$ is the anticipated standard deviation of the QoL outcome measured on the two occasions, or the difference between the QoL measurement on the case and the matched control. Thus $\sigma_{\text{Difference}}$ is the anticipated standard deviation of the N differences, in QoL scores, between the paired observations. It is not the standard deviation of the first QoL measurement, nor of the second QoL measurement, nor of the case values, nor of the corresponding control values.

The number of pairs, $N_{\text{Pairs\_means}}$, required to detect an anticipated standardized difference Δ, at a significance level α and power $1 - \beta$ is

$$N_{\text{Pairs\_means}} = \frac{(z_{1-\alpha/2} + z_{1-\beta})^2}{\Delta^2} + \frac{z_{1-\alpha/2}^2}{2}. \qquad (4.11)$$

A simple formula for the calculation of the number of paired observations required for a two-sided significance level of 5% and a power of 80% is

$$N_{\text{Pairs\_means}} = 2 + \frac{8}{\Delta^2}. \qquad (4.12)$$

Machin et al. (1997) point out that there is a relationship between the standard deviation for each subject group σ and the standard deviation of the difference $\sigma_{\text{Difference}}$. The relationship is:

$$\sigma_{\text{Difference}} = \sigma\sqrt{2(1 - \rho)}, \qquad (4.13)$$

where ρ is the correlation coefficient between the QoL values for the case and their controls.

Example calculations

Suppose, as in the previous example, that we are planning an exercise trial in men aged 50–74 to see if a daily exercise regime for a year will lead to improved physical functioning. However, this time we will use a cross-over design rather than two parallel groups. The subjects will be randomized to either the daily exercise (test) group or control group for the first 6 months. After this they will swap groups and receive the other treatment, daily exercise or control, for another 6 months. We are interested in the changes each man experiences in physical functioning on the test treatment compared to the control treatment.

We know from published data on the SF-36 QoL measure that at this age men have a mean score on the Physical Functioning dimension of 66.4, with a standard deviation of 29.5 (Walters et al., 2001a). This is an estimate of σ, but we require an estimate of $\sigma_{\text{Difference}}$. If we assume a correlation, ρ, of 0.60 between the QoL values on test and control treatments, then using equation (4.13) gives

$$\sigma_{\text{Difference}} = 29.5\sqrt{2(1 - \rho)} = 26.$$

Suppose the effect of the daily exercise regime on physical functioning will be considered important if it increases the PF dimension score of the SF-36 by at least 10 points. We want a high probability of detecting such a difference, so we set the power to be 0.9 (90%) and choose a 5% (two-sided) significance level. The standardized effect size is $\Delta = 10/26 = 0.38$. Using equation (4.11) gives an approximate total sample size of 77, i.e. 77 pairs of observations:

$$N_{\text{Pairs\_means}} = \frac{(1.96 + 1.2816)^2}{0.38^2} + \frac{1.96^2}{2} = 77. \qquad \square$$

Example: Pre-study power and sample size calculation for paired outcomes – the Health Status of Gypsies and Travellers in England study

Parry et al. (2007) undertook a matched case-control study to compare the QoL of Gypsies and Travellers with a control sample matched by age and sex. The primary outcome was the EQ-5D health utility measure. The EQ-5D is scored on a -0.59 (poor) to 1.00 (good) health scale (EuroQol Group, 1990). Sample size was calculated using data from a pilot study which suggested a difference of 0.14 (standard deviation 0.48) in EQ-5D scores between Gypsies and Travellers and a comparison group of poor White inner-city dwellers.

Using equation (4.11), with an anticipated standardized effect size of $\Delta = 0.10/0.48 = 0.21$ (planned difference, δ, of 0.10 points in mean EQ-5D scores between the Gypsies and Travellers and their age- and sex-matched comparison group assuming a standard deviation, $\sigma_{Difference}$, of 0.48) and 90% power and 5% (two-sided level) of significance, estimates that we need 250 Gypsies or Travellers paired with age- and sex-matched controls.   □

4.5.2   Paired binary data – comparison of proportions

Suppose we wish to design a cross-over trial in which patients' QoL is assessed on a binary categorical scale as 'good' or poor' on each of two treatments, test and control. We can summarize the results of such a trial in the format of Table 4.6. Thus the four possible combinations of pairs of responses are (Good, Good), (Good, Poor) (Poor, Good) and (Poor, Poor).

The usual test for analysing data in the form of Table 4.6 is McNemar's test (Campbell et al., 2007). The McNemar test for such paired data counts the number of N_{Pairs_binary} that are either (Good, Poor), denoted by s, or (Poor, Good), denoted by t. The data are often summarized using the odds ratio (OR), calculated as $\psi = s/t$. For a cross-over trial, ψ is a measure of how much more likely it is that a patient will have good QoL on treatment T and poor QoL on treatment C as opposed to good QoL on C and poor QoL on T.

In order to calculate the required sample size, we need to specify the anticipated proportion of discordant pairs, $\pi_{Discordant} = (s + t)N_{Pairs\_binary}$, and the odds ratio $\psi = s/t$.

Alternatively, an investigator may find difficulty in anticipating the values of s and t, but may be able to specify π_T and π_C, the marginal probabilities of response

Table 4.6   Notation for 2 × 2 cross-over trial.

Response to treatment T	Response to treatment C			
	Good QoL	Poor QoL	Total	Anticipated proportion
Good QoL	r	s	$r + s$	π_T
Poor QoL	t	u	$t + u$	$1 - \pi_T$
Total	$r + t$	$s + u$	N_{Pairs_binary}	
Anticipated proportion	π_C	$1 - \pi_C$		

to the test and control treatments. In this case we estimate the anticipated values with $sN_{Pairs\_binary} = \pi_T(1 - \pi_C)$ and $tN_{Pairs\_binary} = \pi_C(1 - \pi_T)$, and from these obtain the anticipated values for $\pi_{Discordant}$ and ψ. This calculation assumes that the response to treatment T is independent of the response to treatment C in each subject, which may not necessarily be the case.

The sample size required, here the total number of pairs, N_{Pairs_binary}, to be observed for a given anticipated proportion of discordant pairs $\pi_{Discordant}$ and anticipated odds ratio ψ, at significance level α and power $1 - \beta$, is given by

$$N_{Pairs\_binary} = \frac{\{z_{1-\alpha/2}(\psi + 1) + z_{1-\beta}\sqrt{(\psi + 1)^2 - (\psi - 1)^2\pi_{Discordant}}\}^2}{(\psi - 1)^2\pi_{Discordant}}. \tag{4.14}$$

Example calculations

Suppose we are unable to specify $\pi_{Discordant}$ but we believe that 50% of men on the control treatment will have good physical functioning and that this will increase to 60% having good physical functioning on the test treatment.

Here $\pi_C = 0.50$ and $\pi_T = 0.60$. Assuming independence of response for each subject, one anticipates therefore, that

$$s/N_{Pairs\_binary} = \pi_T(1 - \pi_C) = 0.60 \times (1 - 0.5) = 0.3,$$

$$t/N_{Pairs\_binary} = \pi_C(1 - \pi_T) = 0.5 \times (1 - 0.6) = 0.2.$$

These give $\pi_{Discordant} = 0.30 + 0.2 = 0.5$ and $\psi = 0.3/0.2 = 1.5$. Using equation (4.14) with $\alpha = 0.05$ and $1 - \beta = 0.80$ gives $N_{Pairs\_binary} = 390$.   □

4.6   Equivalence/non-inferiority studies

The classic RCT seeks to prove that a new treatment is *superior* to an existing one, and a successful conclusion is one in which such proof is demonstrated. In recent years, however, there has been an increasing interest in trials whose objective is to show that some new therapy is *no worse* as regards some outcome, such as QoL, than an existing treatment.

From the QoL point of view, we may wish to show that the new treatment is *equivalent* to the standard treatment with respect to QoL outcomes. However, it is important to be clear that failure to find a statistically significant difference between the treatment groups after completing the trial and analysing the QoL outcome data does not mean the two treatments are equivalent. It usually means the trial was too small or inadequately powered to detect the (small) actual difference, in QoL, between the two treatments. Indeed, with a finite number of subjects, one can never prove that two groups are exactly equivalent (Fayers and Machin, 2007).

However, having conducted a study to compare groups, one can calculate the summary QoL (such as the mean QoL) at a key stage for each group, and a $100(1 - \alpha)\%$ confidence interval (CI) for the true difference, δ, between the groups. This CI covers the true difference with a given probability or confidence, $1 - \alpha$.

At the design stage of an equivalence study, we need to specify α and also a limit, ε (>0), which is termed the *range of equivalence* between the QoL measure in the two groups. We set this so that if we ultimately observe an actual difference no greater than ε then we would accept that the two groups are essentially equivalent. We also need to specify the power, $1 - \beta$, of the test that the upper confidence limit (UL) for δ, calculated once the study is completed, will not exceed this pre-specified value ε.

Earlier when comparing two population means, μ_T and μ_C, for the test and control groups respectively we implied a null hypothesis, $H_0 : \mu_T = \mu_C$ (of no treatment difference), against an alternative hypothesis, $H_A : \mu_T \neq \mu_C$, (of treatment difference). Thus in a conventional test of significance we seek to test $\delta = \mu_T - \mu_C = 0$. In testing for equivalence, this is changed to testing for $\mu_T = \mu_C + \varepsilon$ (no treatment equivalence) against the alternative one-sided hypothesis $\mu_T < \mu_C + \varepsilon$ (treatment equivalence). These considerations lead to a $100(1 - \alpha)\%$ CI for $\delta = \mu_T - \mu_C$ of

$$\text{LL to (Difference} + z_{1-\alpha} \times \text{SE(difference))]}. \tag{4.15}$$

Here the value of LL (the lower confidence limit) depends on the context but not on the data (Machin *et al.*, 1997). Note that since this is a so-called one-sided CI it uses $z_{1-\alpha}$ and not $z_{1-\alpha/2}$.

The sample size formulae given previously have given us the number of subjects n per group, in a study for a two-sided test with significance level α and power $1 - \beta$. In this section on equivalence studies the sample size calculations use a one-sided significance level of 5% and a power of 80%, thus from Table 4.1, $z_{1-\alpha} = 1.6449$ and $z_{1-\beta} = 0.8416$.

4.6.1   Continuous data – comparing the equivalence of two means

When the two mean QoL scores are compared, the lower limit of the confidence interval for equation (4.15) is $LL = -\infty$ (minus infinity). The sample size per group, $n_{\text{Equivalence\_Means}}$, required for a comparison of means for two groups of equal size and anticipated to have the same population mean, μ, and standard deviation, σ, is

$$n_{\text{Equivalence\_Means}} = \frac{2(z_{1-\alpha} + z_{1-\beta})^2}{\Delta^2}, \tag{4.16}$$

where $\Delta = \varepsilon/\sigma$ can be thought of as the standardized effect size.

Example calculations

Suppose we are planning a two-group RCT, in patients with the lung condition chronic obstructive pulmonary disease (COPD) to compare a new community-based physiotherapy rehabilitation programme with the usual standard hospital-based physiotherapy rehabilitation programme.

Both rehabilitation programmes will last 2 months and the primary outcome will be the PF dimension of the SF-36 assessed immediately post rehabilitation (2-month follow-up). The study wants to show that a community-based physiotherapy rehabilitation programme is equivalent to the standard hospital-based physiotherapy rehabilitation programme with respect to QoL outcomes.

Published data on the SF-36 QoL measure in 124 COPD patients reported a mean score on the PF dimension of 29.0, with a standard deviation of 25.0 (Harper *et al.*, 1997). Suppose that the hospital- and community-based rehabilitation programmes will be considered equivalent if the difference in mean SF-36 PF scores post rehabilitation between the groups is less than five points. We want a high probability or power of 80% that the upper confidence limit for the true population difference in mean QoL between the groups, once the study is completed, will not exceed this pre-specified value of five points.

So $\sigma = 25.0$, $\varepsilon = 5.0$, $\alpha = 0.05$ (one-sided) and $\beta = 0.20$. Using equation (4.1), this results in a standardized effect size Δ of $5.0/25.0 = 0.20$. Using Table 4.1, With $\alpha = 0.05$ (one-sided) and $\beta = 0.20$, the appropriate z-values, $z_{1-\alpha}$ and $z_{1-\beta}$, from the standard Normal distribution (Table 4.1) are 1.64449 and 0.8416, respectively. So equation (4.16) becomes

$$n_{Equivalence\_Means} = \frac{2(1.6449 + 0.8416)^2}{0.20^2} = 310.$$

This gives an approximate sample size of 310 COPD patients in each group (620 in total).   □

4.6.2   Binary data – comparing the equivalence of two proportions

We assume that the QoL outcome of the trial has been dichotomized into a binary outcome as the proportion of patients with good or poor QoL. After testing for the equivalence of treatments, we would wish to assume that the proportions with 'good QoL' are for all practical purposes equal, although we might have evidence that they do in fact differ by a small amount. For this the purposes of comparison $LL = -1$ in equation (4.15), as that is the maximum possible difference in the proportion of responses in the two groups.

The sample size per group, $n_{Binary\_Equivalence}$, required for a comparison of proportions from two groups of equal size and expected to have the same population proportion π is:

$$n_{Binary\_Equivalence} = \frac{2\pi(1 - \pi)(z_{1-\alpha} + z_{1-\beta})^2}{\varepsilon^2}. \tag{4.17}$$

4.7   Unknown standard deviation and effect size

In practice the standard deviation of the QoL outcome will rarely be known in advance, although sometimes the investigator will be able to make use of an estimate of the standard deviation from previous data which is felt to be reasonably accurate. If no estimate is available there are several possible approaches. One way is to start the trial and use the data for the first patients to estimate the standard deviation and then the sample size needed. An alternative approach would be to estimate the standard deviation by a relatively small pilot investigation and then use this value. Another possibility is to specify the difference of interest directly in terms of the unknown standard deviation. All these solutions involve some degree of subjectivity.

As a rule of thumb, Norman et al. (2003) suggested that the value of half a standard deviation (0.5 SD) can serve as a default value for important patient-perceived change on QoL measures used with patients with chronic diseases. A fairly common situation when designing a clinical trial with a QoL outcome is that there is little evidence, for the proposed trial population, about how a QoL instrument will perform and what a clinically important treatment effect is. Therefore, in these circumstances, the sample size could be estimated based on an anticipated treatment difference of 0.5 SD.

4.7.1   Tips on obtaining the standard deviation

Often papers only give an estimate of the treatment effect, $\bar{d}$, plus its associated 95% CI. We need the standard deviation for the individual treatment groups (which we assume is the same for both groups). Let UL be upper limit and LL the lower limit of the 95% CI. Then we can use the fact that the width of the CI for the treatment difference, UL – LL, is about 4 standard errors (4 SE). We can also use the fact that the $SE(\bar{d}) = (\sqrt{2}SD)/\sqrt{n}$ (Machin *et al.*, 1997).

Example calculations

Suppose that we are planning a two-group RCT, in patients requiring total knee replacement (TKR) surgery, to compare a new artificial knee joint with an existing standard joint. The primary outcome measure will be the WOMAC pain dimension scores 12 weeks post surgery (Bellamy, 1988). The WOMAC pain dimension is scored on a 0 (no pain) to 20 (high pain) scale. Mitchell *et al.* (2005) describe the results of an RCT to assess the effectiveness of pre- and post-operative physiotherapy at home for unilateral TKR compared to usual care. They report the mean difference in WOMAC pain score at 12 weeks post surgery, between the intervention and control groups, as 0.5 (95% CI: −1.0 to 2.0) for 106 TKR patients.

The width of the CI is $2.0 - (-1.0) = 3.0$, which is four standard errors. So one standard error is $3.0/4 = 0.75$. The standard deviation is $(SE \times \sqrt{n})/\sqrt{2}$, that is, $(0.75 \times \sqrt{106})/\sqrt{2} = 5.8$. This value can then be used in equation (4.2) to calculate the required sample size.   □

4.8   Cluster randomized controlled trials

A cluster randomized controlled trial (cRCT) is one in which groups of patients (not individuals) are randomized. It is common in trials in primary care or general practice where patients under one general practitioner or in one practice all get randomized to the same treatment. To accommodate the clustering effect the sample size obtained assuming an individually randomized design, n_{random}, should be inflated by a design effect (DE):

$$n_{cluster} = \{1 + (k - 1)\rho_{intra}\} \times n_{random}, \tag{4.18}$$

where k is the average cluster size and ρ_{intra} is the intra-class or intra-cluster correlation (as described in Chapter 3).

The sample size depends on how closely the subjects in a cluster are related. This relationship is measured by the *intra-cluster correlation* coefficient (ICC), ρ_{intra}. If individuals within the same cluster are no more likely to have similar QoL outcomes than individuals in different clusters then the ICC will be 0. Conversely, if all individuals in the same cluster are identical with respect to their QoL outcomes, then ICC = 1. The higher the ICC (the closer it is to 1) the greater the number of subjects required. In the context of cluster-based evaluations, the ICC will usually assume small positive values (Ukoumunne *et al.*, 1999) less than 0.05.

Example calculations

Suppose when planning the exercise trial in men aged 50–74, to see if a daily exercise regime for a year will lead to improved QoL compared to a control group, we decide that, due to potential contamination effects, individual patient randomization is not appropriate. We therefore decide to randomize GP practices to receive the intervention or control intervention. We know from published data that the average cluster size (number of men aged 50–74) at a practice is about 300 and that the intra-cluster correlation is 0.01.

For an average cluster size, k, of 300 men aged 50–74 per GP practice and $\rho_{Intra} = 0.01$, we obtain to a design effect of

$$DE = 1 + ((300 - 1) \times 0.01) = 3.99,$$

and

$$n_{cluster} = 3.99 \times 193 = 771 \text{ per group (1542 in total)}.$$

The original calculation, ignoring the clustering, based on a standardized difference, Δ_{Normal}, of 0.33 gave an approximate total sample size of 386, i.e. $n_{random} = 193$ in each group. With an average cluster size of 300, this implies $1542/300 = 5.1$ or approximately 6 GP practices must be recruited (3 randomized to the intervention and 3 to the control treatment).   □

4.9   Non-response

Some allowance may be made for a proportion of subjects who withdraw or are lost to study during the course of an investigation. If a proportion, θ, are lost so that the outcome variables are not recorded, then the final analysis will be based on $1 - \theta$ times the number of subjects entering the study. To ensure an adequate sample size at the end of the study it would be necessary to start with a single sample size n', given by

$$n' = \frac{n}{1 - \theta},   \tag{4.19}$$

where n is the sample size determined by the methods given earlier in this chapter.

Example calculations

Suppose in the first example of the exercise trial in men aged 50–74 we assume that 20% (i.e. $\theta = 0.20$) of the subjects are going to withdraw from the study before the 1-year follow-up. The original calculation-based standardized difference, Δ_{Normal}, of 0.33 gave an approximate total sample size of 386, i.e. 193 in each group. So to ensure an adequate sample size at the end of the study it would be necessary to start with a sample of $386/(1 - 0.2) = 484$ men (242 per group).   □

4.10   Unequal groups

It is usually optimal, when comparing two groups, to have equal numbers in each group. But sometimes the number available in one group may be restricted. In this case the power can be increased to a limited extent by having more in the other group.

If one group contains m subjects and the other rm, then the study is approximately equivalent to a study with **n** in each group where (Armitage *et al.*, 2002)

$$\frac{2}{n} = \frac{1}{m} + \frac{1}{rm},$$ (4.20)

that is,

$$m = \frac{(r+1)n}{2r},$$ (4.21)

where r is the allocation ratio. This expression is derived by setting equal the expressions for the standard error of the difference between two means used in a two sample t-test, and is exact for a continuous variable and an approximate for the comparison of two proportions.

So, to plan a study with unequal sized groups, we first calculate n as if we were using equal groups and then calculate the modified group sample sizes m and hence rm.

Example calculations

In the exercise trial in men aged 50–74, originally 193 men were going to be recruited in each group. Suppose that it is easier to recruit twice as many men in the control group. So how many men could be needed if there were two men recruited into the control group for every one in the intervention group?

Using equation (4.21), with $r = 2$,

$$m = \frac{(r+1)n}{2r} = \frac{(2+1)193}{2 \times 2} = 145$$

That is, 145 men are needed in the intervention group and $(2 \times 145) = 290$ men in the control group, giving a combined sample size of 435.   □

Example: Pre-study power and sample size calculation with unequal allocation – acupuncture study

Thomas *et al.* (2006) undertook a two-group RCT in primary care patients with persistent non-specific low back pain to assess the effectiveness of a short course of traditional acupuncture compared to usual care provided by GPs. The primary endpoint was the bodily pain (BP) domain of the SF-36 at 12 months. The BP domain of the SF-36 is scored on a 0 to 100 (no pain) health scale (Ware *et al.*, 1993). A mean difference of 10 points between the groups was considered to be clinically important. On the basis of a pilot study they estimated the standard deviation of the BP scale to be 20.0.

Using Table 4.2 or equation (4.2), with an anticipated standardized effect size, Δ_{Normal}, of 0.50 (planned difference of 10 points in mean BP scores between the groups, assuming a standard deviation of 20) and 90% power and 5% (two-sided) level of significance, estimates that we need 84 patients per group (168 in total).

In order for effects between acupuncturists to be tested, the researchers decided on a 2:1 randomization to the acupuncture group compared to the control group. Using equation (4.21), with $r = 2$,

$$m = \frac{(r+1)n}{2r} = \frac{(2+1)84}{2 \times 2} = 63.$$

That is, 63 men are required in the control group and $(2 \times 63) = 126$ men in the acupuncture group, giving a combined sample size of 189. Allowing for 20% drop-out, the study eventually recruited and randomized 241 patients (160 randomized to acupuncture and 81 allocated to usual management). □

4.11   Multiple outcomes/endpoints

We have based the calculations above on the assumption that there is a single identifiable endpoint, or QoL outcome, upon which treatment comparisons are based (in our case the PF dimension of the SF-36). Sometimes there is more than one endpoint of interest; QoL outcomes are multi-dimensional (e.g. the SF-36 has ten dimensions including PF). If one of these dimensions is regarded as more important than the others, it can be designated as the primary endpoint and the sample size estimates calculated accordingly. The remainder should be consigned to exploratory analyses or descriptions only (Fayers and Machin, 2007).

A problem arises when these outcome measures are all regarded as equally important. One approach is to repeat the sample size estimates for each outcome measure in turn and then select the largest number as the sample size required to answer all the questions of interest. Here, it is essential to note the relationship between significance tests and power, as it is well recognized that P-values become distorted if many endpoints are each tested for significance, and adjustments should be made.

To guard against false statistical significance as a consequence of multiple hypothesis testing, it is a sensible precaution to examine the consequences of replacing the significance level α in the various equations by a significance level adjusted using the Bonferroni correction. The Bonferroni correction is

$$\alpha_{\text{Bonferroni}} = \alpha/h, \tag{4.22}$$

where h is the number of outcomes or hypothesis tests to be performed. Such a correction will clearly lead to larger sample sizes. The Bonferroni approach to adjusting for multiple comparisons tends to be conservative as it assumes that all the different endpoints are uncorrelated (Altman *et al.*, 2000). In the case of QoL outcomes there is likely to be a strong correlation between the different dimensions. This conservativeness implies that using criterion (4.22) will lead to failure to reject the null hypothesis on too many occasions. Fairclough (2002) gives a more comprehensive discussion of multiple endpoints and suggests several alternative methods to the simple Bonferroni approach when analysing QoL outcomes, including: limiting the number of hypothesis tests; using summary measures and statistics; and global multivariate hypothesis tests.

There is no general consensus on what procedure to adopt to allow for multiple comparisons. Altman *et al.* (2000) recommend reporting unadjusted P-values and confidence limits with a suitable note of caution with respect to interpretation. As Perneger (1998) concludes: 'Simply describing what tests of significance have been performed, and why, is generally the best way of dealing with multiple comparisons.'

Pragmatically, I do not like to use multivariate global hypothesis tests, since the interpretation of the results of such tests is difficult. I prefer using a set of univariate test statistics since they are much easier to implement and report. Throughout this book, I will favour a combination of Fayers and Machin's (2007) and Altman *et al.* (2000)

approaches to multiple comparisons/endpoints. My favoured approach is to identify the main study QoL endpoints in advance, limit the number of confirmatory hypothesis tests to these outcomes, and report unadjusted P-values and confidence limits with a suitable note of caution with respect to interpretation.

4.12   Three or more groups

Most clinical trials involve a simple comparison between two interventions or treatments. When there are more than two treatments the situation is much more complicated. This is because there is no longer one clear alternative hypothesis. Thus for example, with three groups, A, B and C, although the null hypothesis is that the population mean QoL scores are all equal, there are several potential alternative hypotheses. These include one which suggests that two of the group means are equal but differ from the third, and one that the group means are ordered in some way. The researchers may simply wish to compare the mean QoL outcomes of all three groups, leading to three pairwise comparisons (of treatment A vs. B, B vs. C, and A vs. C), but the three comparisons may not all be equally important.

One problem arising at the time of analysis is that such situations may lead to multiple significance tests, resulting in misleading P-values. Various solutions have been proposed, each resulting in different analysis strategies and therefore different design and sample size considerations.

One strategy that is commonly proposed is to carry out an analysis of variance (ANOVA) or similar global test, with pairwise or other comparisons of mean QoL scores between the groups only being made if the global ANOVA test is significant. Day and Graham (1989) describe a simple nomogram that can be used to determine sample size (and power) for comparing two (three, four or five) treatment groups, by ANOVA, in a clinical trial at two levels of statistical significance (1% and 5%). An alternative strategy is to use conventional significance tests but combined with an adjusted significance level obtained from the Bonferroni correction.

However, the simplest strategy to adopt is to regard a three-treatment comparison as little different from carrying out three independent trials (of treatment A vs. B, B vs. C, and A vs. C) and to use conventional significance tests without adjustment (Machin et al., 1997). The sample size is then estimated as if three independent comparisons are to be made, and for each treatment group we simply take the maximum of these as the sample size required.

4.13   What if we are doing a survey, not a clinical trial?

4.13.1   Sample sizes for surveys

As part of an epidemiological survey we may want to estimate the mean QoL in a particular population. For example, we may wish to estimate the mean QoL of patients treated in hospital for end-stage renal (kidney) failure. We are likely to want to know how many renal failure patients we need to survey in order estimate their QoL with a reasonable degree of precision.

The true population mean QoL, μ, can only be determined by surveying the entire population. However, an unbiased estimate of the mean QoL can be provided by selecting a sample from the population by simple random sampling. The size of the random sample for the survey is determined by three factors:

1. How precise should the mean QoL estimate be? For example, within ±5 points of the true population mean QoL.

2. The probability that the estimate is close to the population parameter we are trying to estimate. For example, we often strive for 95% confidence that the interval we have obtained contains the actual population mean QoL.

3. We need some idea of the variability or standard deviation of the QoL outcome in the population under study.

With this information we can then calculate the required sample size for the survey.

4.13.2 Confidence intervals for estimating the mean QoL of a population

If μ is the true population mean QoL and n is the number of subjects sampled, then $\bar{x}$ is the sample estimate of μ based on the n subjects. When estimating the population mean QoL, the precision or standard error (SE) of the sample mean estimate is

$$SE(\bar{x}) = \frac{\sigma}{\sqrt{n}},$$ (4.23)

where σ is the population standard deviation of the QoL outcome.

The $100(1-\alpha)\%$ CI for the mean QoL, in the population is calculated as

$$\bar{x} - \left(z_{1-\alpha/2} \times \frac{\sigma}{\sqrt{n}}\right) \text{ to } \bar{x} + \left(z_{1-\alpha/2} \times \frac{\sigma}{\sqrt{n}}\right),$$ (4.24)

where $z_{1-\alpha/2}$ is the $100(1-\alpha/2)$ percentile from the standard Normal distribution. Thus, for a 95% CI, $z_{1-\alpha/2} = 1.96$ (see Table 4.1) and the formula simplifies to

$$\bar{x} \pm \left(1.96 \times \frac{\sigma}{\sqrt{n}}\right).$$ (4.25)

We can use the CI formula to determine the required number of patients to survey to estimate the mean QoL of a particular population. The *upper limit* of the 95% CI (UL) is given by:

$$UL = \bar{x} + \left(1.96 \times \frac{\sigma}{\sqrt{n}}\right).$$ (4.26)

Rearranging to get n on the left-hand side gives

$$n = \frac{\sigma^2}{\left[\frac{UL - \bar{x}}{1.96}\right]^2}.$$ (4.27)

If we let $UL - \bar{x} = \omega$, then

$$n = \frac{\sigma^2}{[\omega/1.96]^2}. \tag{4.28}$$

Thus ω is the margin of error or precision within which we would like to estimate the population mean QoL. Hence to calculate n from equation (4.28) we need to specify, ω and an estimate of the standard deviation (SD), σ. However, at the planning stage we will not have any data to estimate σ and will have to use an informed guess or anticipated value for it. Note that n is the number of responders to the survey. We may have to survey more patients to allow for non-response.

Example calculations

Suppose that we are planning a study to estimate the mean QoL of patients treated in hospital for end-stage renal failure. We are going to use the SF-36 QoL measure, and the main outcome, for the purposes of sample size calculation, will be the General Health dimension of this instrument. GH is scored on a 0 (poor) to 100 (good health) scale.

We know from published data on the SF-36 QoL measure that the mean score on the GH dimension, from a general population survey of 1372 adults aged 16–74 is 72.3 with a standard deviation of 20.7 (Brazier et al., 1992). So how many renal failure patients do we need to survey in order estimate their mean general health (as measured by the SF-36) with a reasonable degree of precision?

We need to specify how precise we require the mean GH estimate to be. Suppose we wish to be within ±3 points of the true population mean. So the margin of error or precision within which we would like to estimate the population mean GH is ±3 points, that is, $\omega = 3$.

Using equation (4.28) with $\sigma = 21$ and $\omega = 3$ gives an estimated sample size for the survey of $n = 189$ renal patients. Note than $n = 189$ is the number of responders to the survey. We may have to survey more patients to allow for non-response. Therefore, assuming a 50% response rate to the survey we will have to send out $189/0.5 = 378$ questionnaires.   □

4.13.3   Confidence intervals for a proportion

If a continuous QoL outcome is condensed into a binary or dichotomous categorical scale, then an appropriate summary measure of the outcome data will usually be the sample rate or proportion. Let us assume that a continuous QoL scale is dichotomized into 'good' and 'poor' QoL. If π is the true population proportion with good QoL and n is the number of subjects sampled, then p is the sample estimate of this true value π, based on the n subjects. If x is the observed number of subjects with good QoL in a sample size of n then the estimated proportion who have the feature is $p = x/n$. The standard error of p is

$$SE(p) = \sqrt{\frac{\pi(1 - \pi)}{n}}. \tag{4.29}$$

The $100(1 - \alpha)\%$ CI for the proportion in the population is calculated as

$$p - [z_{1-\alpha/2} \times SE(p)] \text{ to } p + [z_{1-\alpha/2} \times SE(p)]. \tag{4.30}$$

Thus, for a 95% CI, $z_{1-\alpha/2} = 1.96$ and the formula simplifies to

$$p \pm \left[1.96 \times \sqrt{\frac{\pi(1-\pi)}{n}} \right]. \tag{4.31}$$

We can use the CI formula to determine the required number of patients to survey to estimate the prevalence of subjects with 'good' QoL in a population. The upper limit (UL) of the 95% CI is given by:

$$UL = p + 1.96\sqrt{\frac{\pi(1-\pi)}{n}}. \tag{4.32}$$

Rearranging to get n on the left-hand side gives

$$n = \frac{\pi(1-\pi)}{\left[\frac{UL-\pi}{1.96}\right]^2}. \tag{4.33}$$

If we let $UL - \pi = \omega$, then

$$n = \frac{\pi(1-\pi)}{[\omega/1.96]^2}. \tag{4.34}$$

Thus ω is the margin of error or precision within which we would like to estimate the population prevalence of good QoL, π. Hence, to calculate n from equation (4.34) we need to specify ω and an estimate of π. However, at the planning stage we will not have any data to estimate π and will have to use an informed guess or anticipated value for it. If we denote this anticipated value as π_{Plan} then Table 4.7 shows the number of subjects that need to be sampled for various levels of precision. Note that n is the number of responders to the survey. We may have to survey more subjects to allow for non-response. This traditional method is adequate in many circumstances, but is based on an approximation. It should not be used for very low or very high observed proportions. The restriction on the use of the traditional method is usually given as a requirement that neither r nor $n - r$ is less than 5.

Example calculations

Suppose we are planning a study to estimate the proportion of patients treated in hospital for end-stage renal failure who have good QoL. We are going to use the SF-36 QoL measure, and the main outcome, for the purposes of sample size calculation, will be the GH dimension of this instrument, scored on a 0 (poor) to 100 (good health) scale.

We know from published data on the SF-36 QoL measure that the mean score on the GH dimension, from a general population survey of 1372 adults aged 16–74, is 72.3 with a standard deviation of 20.7 (Brazier et al., 1992). A GH score of 72 or more will be classified as 'good' QoL (i.e. better than average for the general population) and a GH score less than 72 as 'poor' QoL.

Table 4.7 Sample size m required to estimate the anticipated prevalence of good QoL (π_{Plan}) with upper and lower confidence limits of ±0.01, ±0.02, ±0.05, ±0.06, or ±0.10 away from the anticipated value.

| π_{Plan} | Required precision, ω, for the upper and lower confidence limits for the anticipated prevalence π_{Plan} | | | | |
	±0.01	±0.02	±0.05	±0.06	±0.10
0.05	1825	457	73		
0.10	3458	865	139	97	35
0.15	4899	1225	196	137	49
0.20	6147	1537	246	171	62
0.25	7203	1801	289	201	73
0.30	8068	2017	323	225	81
0.35	8740	2185	350	243	88
0.40	9220	2305	369	257	93
0.45	9508	2377	381	265	96
0.50	9604	2401	385	267	97
0.55	9508	2377	381	265	96
0.60	9220	2305	369	257	93
0.65	8740	2185	350	243	88
0.70	8068	2017	323	225	81
0.75	7203	1801	289	201	73
0.80	6147	1537	246	171	62
0.85	4899	1225	196	137	49
0.90	3458	865	139	97	35
0.95	1825	457	73		

So how many renal failure patients do we need to survey in order estimate the prevalence of good QoL (as measured by the GH dimension of SF-36) with a reasonable degree of precision?

We need to specify how precise we require the estimated prevalence of good QoL to be. Suppose we wish to be within $\pm10\%$ of the estimate. So the margin of error or precision within which we would like to estimate the population mean GH is $\pm10\%$ points, that is, $\omega = 0.10$. We also need to have an informed guess or anticipated value for prevalence of good QoL, π_{Plan}. If we assume half or 50% of renal patients will have good QoL, then $\pi_{Plan} = 0.50$.

Using, Table 4.7 or equation (4.34) with $\pi_{Plan} = 0.50$ and $\omega = 0.10$ gives an estimated sample size for the survey of $n = 97$ renal patients. That is, with 97 patients we should be able to estimate the true population prevalence, of good QoL, in renal patients within $\pm10\%$, assuming a true value of 50%, with 95% confidence (i.e. 95% confidence limits ranging from 40% to 60%). Note than $n = 97$ is the number of responders to the survey. We may have to survey more patients to allow for non-response. Therefore, assuming a 50% response rate to the survey, we will have to send out $97/0.5 = 194$ questionnaires.   □

4.14 Sample sizes for reliability and method comparison studies

Suppose that we wish to assess the reliability or repeatability of a QoL instrument in a population to see if the scale produces reproducible and consistent results when used on the same subject while the subject's QoL has not changed. This repeated reliability is based upon the analysis of the correlations between the repeated measurements, where the measurements are repeated over time. For continuous QoL data, the intra-class correlation coefficient (ICC) measures the strength of agreement between repeated QoL measurements (see Chapter 3).

Sample size estimation for studies to assess the reliability of a QoL instrument depends on both the minimum acceptable level of reliability, ρ_{Min}, and the true reliability, ρ_1. A reliability coefficient of 0.90 is often recommended if measurements are to be used for evaluating individual patients, although most QoL instruments fail to obtain such levels. For discriminating between groups of patients in a clinical trial it is usually recommended that the reliability of an instrument should exceed 0.70 (Fayers and Machin, 2007).

Walter *et al.* (1998) developed a method to estimate the required number of subjects, n, for a reliability study where reliability is measured using the ICC. Table 4.8 shows the estimates of sample size n, for $\alpha = 0.05$, $\beta = 0.20$ and various values of ρ_{Min} and ρ_1 based on $r = 2$ repeated assessments.

Example calculations

Suppose we wish to assess the test–retest reliability of a new QoL instrument that is being developed for use in clinical trials. Subjects will complete the new QoL questionnaire twice a short time (say, one week) apart. If it is desirable to show that the reliability of the new QoL instrument is above 0.70 (i.e. $\rho_{Min} = 0.70$) with an anticipated true reliability ρ_1, of 0.8, then Table 4.8 (with $\rho_{Min} = 0.70$ and $\rho_1 = 0.8$) shows that two repeated measurements on 118 subjects are required. □

Table 4.8 Estimates of sample size n, for $\alpha = 0.05$, $\beta = 0.20$ and various values of ρ_{Min}, ρ_1 based on $r = 2$ repeated assessments (based upon Walter *et al.*, 1998).

ρ_{Min}	ρ_1								
	0.1	0.2	0.3	0.4	0.5	0.6	0.7	0.8	0.9
$r = 2$									
0.0	616	152	70	36	22	15	10	7	5
0.1		592	143	61	33	20	12	8	5
0.2			544	129	53	28	16	10	6
0.3				477	109	44	22	12	7
0.4					394	87	33	16	8
0.5						301	63	22	9
0.6							206	40	12
0.7								118	19
0.8									46

4.15   Post-hoc sample size calculations

Sample size estimation and power calculation are essentially a priori, that is, before the data is collected. After we have carried out the study it is the observed data which will determine the size and direction of the treatment effect and the width of any confidence interval estimates for this treatment effect. The a priori power is immaterial to this. It is the size of the treatment effect and the width of the confidence intervals and their interpretation which are important. The width of the confidence interval depends on the precision or standard error of the estimated treatment effect, which is itself dependent on the variability of the outcome and the study sample size. The only parameter we need to consider from the initial power calculation is the size of the effect we considered to be clinically meaningful, δ, the minimum clinically important difference (MCID), and how our observed treatment effect and associated confidence intervals appear in relation to this MCID (Walters, 2009).

4.16   Conclusion: Usefulness of sample size calculations

A sample size calculation, with all its attendant assumptions, is better than no sample size calculation at all. The mere fact of a sample size calculation means that a number of fundamental issues have been thought about:

- What is the main outcome variable?

- What is a clinically important effect?

- How is it measured?

The investigator is also likely to have specified the method and frequency of data analysis. Thus, protocols that are explicit about sample size are easier to evaluate in terms of scientific quality and the likelihood of achieving objectives. If in doubt, do not be afraid to ask a medical statistician for help in study design and sample size estimation *before* the data are collected!

4.17   Further reading

There is an extensive literature about sample size estimation for a variety of study designs and types of outcome data. Machin and Campbell (2005) provide a good introduction to the design of studies for medical research. Machin *et al.* (2008) provides an extensive list of tables for the design of clinical trials. Computer-intensive simulation or bootstrap methods are useful alternatives that may be used to generate sample size estimates when formulae are unavailable; such methods are described by Walters and Campbell (2005).

Exercises

4.1 Suppose that we are planning a randomized controlled trial in patients with osteoarthritis of the knee to investigate the benefit of adding acupuncture to a course of advice and exercise delivered by physiotherapists for pain reduction.

One group will be given advice, exercise and acupuncture whilst the other control group will receive advice and exercise. The primary outcome will be the mean score on the WOMAC osteoarthritis index pain subscale at 6 months. The WOMAC pain domain is scored on a 0–20 scale, with a higher score indicating more pain.

We know from published data on the WOMAC pain dimension in total knee replacement patients (Mitchell *et al.*, 2005) that the baseline WOMAC pain score is 12.0 (SD 3.3). Suppose that the effect of the acupuncture will be considered important if it decreases the WOMAC pain subscale by at least 1.5 points compared with the control treatment at 6-month follow-up.

(a) How many patients would be needed for a two-sided significance of 5% and 80% power?

(b) How many patients would be needed for a two-sided significance of 5% and 90% power?

4.2 Brown *et al.* (2007) describe the results of an RCT, in 135 men, to evaluate the effectiveness of self-management as a first line intervention for men with lower urinary tract symptoms compared with standard care. The men were randomized either to attend a self-management programme in addition to standard care or to standard care alone.

One outcome measure was the International Prostate Symptom Score (IPSS), where higher scores represent a poorer outcome, at 3 months. At 3 months, the mean international prostate symptom score was 10.7 in the self-management group and 16.4 in the standard care group (difference = 5.7, 95% CI: 3.7 to 7.7). Suppose that we have developed a new modified self-care programme and wish to design a trial to see whether this new programme is an improvement on the original. Assume a difference (reduction) of 3 points on the IPSS, at follow-up, is worthwhile and considered to represent an improvement in symptoms that is meaningful to patients.

(a) Estimate the standard deviation (SD), for the IPSS at follow-up, from the quoted confidence interval.

(b) Use the estimated SD from part (a) to calculate how many patients would be needed, to detect a difference in IPSS of 3 points, at follow-up, with a two-sided significance of 5% and 90% power.

(c) If 20% of patients drop out by 3-month follow-up, how many patients will we need to recruit and randomize?

4.3 Suppose that we are planning a randomized controlled trial in patients undergoing hip replacement surgery following a fractured hip to compare a new artificial replacement hip joint with the usual standard hip joint. The primary outcome will be hip function as measured by the Harris Hip score 12 months after surgery. The Harris Hip scale score ranges from 0 to 100, with a higher score indicating better functioning. We know from published data on the Harris Hip score in hip fracture patients (Frihagen *et al.*, 2007) that the baseline Harris Hip score is 84.0 (SD 15.0).

The effect of the new joint on hip functioning will be considered important if it increases the Harris Hip score at 12 months after surgery by at least 7.5 points compared with the control treatment.

(a) How many patients would be needed for a two-sided significance of 5% and 90% power?

The investigators decide that they would like to treat twice as many hip fracture patients using the new hip than with the standard replacement hip joint. They decide that patients will be randomized in the ratio 2:1, that is, two patients are to be allocated the new hip joint for every one allocated the existing replacement hip joint.

(b) How many patients would be needed for 2:1 randomization with a two-sided significance of 5% and 90% power?

(c) If 20% of patients drop out by 12-month follow-up, how many patients will we need to recruit and randomize (assuming 2:1 randomization)?

4.4 Suppose that we are planning a randomized controlled trial in new mothers identified as at high risk of postnatal depression (PND) to see if a new psychological intervention will lead to an improved QoL compared with usual care offered by health visitors (HV). Health visitors trained in detecting depressive symptoms at 6–8 weeks after childbirth, using the Edinburgh Postnatal Depression Scale (EPDS) and clinical assessment, will offer 'at-risk women' a psychological intervention of one hour per week for 8 weeks.
The primary outcome will be the mean EPDS score at 6 months after childbirth. The EPDS is a single-domain, 10-item condition-specific QoL questionnaire assessing depressive symptoms on a 0–30 scale, with a higher score indicting more symptoms. From a previous study of 229 women, the EPDS score at 6 months after childbirth was 6.6 with a standard deviation of 5.6 (Morrell et al., 2000). Approximately 19.7% (45/229) scored 12 or more on the EPDS and were regard as at greater risk of PND.

(a) How many women would need to be individually randomized per group to have an 80% chance of detecting a difference of at least 2 points in mean 6-month EPDS scores between the intervention and control groups as statistically significant at the 5% (two-sided) level?

(b) Suppose that the primary outcome is binary: a 6-month EPDS score of 12 or more vs. less than 12. Let us assume that approximately 20% of new mothers in the control group will have a 6-month EPDS score of 12 or more and are at higher risk of PND. We anticipate that the new psychological intervention offered by health visitors will reduce (improve) this proportion to 10% having a score of 12 or more in the intervention group. How many women would be needed to detect this difference in proportions with 80% power and 5% (two-sided) significance?

(c) Express the absolute difference in proportions of 10% and 20% for 6-month EPDS scores of 12 or more in the intervention and control groups respectively (from (b)) as an odds ratio for the risk of a 6-month EPDS score of 12 more in the intervention group relative to the control group.

(d) Suppose that the continuous EPDS is recoded into a four-category ordinal variable. The four new EPDS categories are 0–5.99, 6–11.99, 12–17.99 and 18 or more. Assume proportions of 0.50, 0.30, 0.15 and 0.05 in the four EPDS categories in the control group and the same odds ratio as in (c). How many women would be needed to detect this odds ratio with 80% power and 5% (two-sided) significance?

Suppose we believe that since the health visitors deliver the intervention they may behave differently with women under their care individually randomized to the control group. Therefore we believe a cluster randomized design is more appropriate, that is, health visitors rather than individual women will be randomized to deliver the psychological intervention or usual care. Let us assume that health visitors will recruit about 10 women from their caseload during the trial period and the intra-cluster correlation for the EPDS outcome is 0.05.

(e) Re-estimate the sample size from (a) to take into account the clustered nature of the design. How many HV (and women) would need to be randomized per group to have an 80% chance of detecting a difference of at least 2 points in mean 6-month EPDS scores between the intervention and control groups as statistically significant at the 5% (two-sided) level?

(f) Re-estimate the sample size from (b), treating the EPDS as a binary outcome, to take into account the clustered design. How many HV (and women) would be needed to detect this difference in proportions (of 20% vs. 10%) with 80% power and 5% (two-sided) significance?

(g) Re-estimate the sample size from (d), treating the EPDS as an ordered categorical outcome, to take into account the clustered design. How many HV (and women) would be needed to detect this odds ratio with 80% power and 5% (two-sided) significance?

4.5 Suppose that we are planning a postal questionnaire survey of patients with lung cancer to estimate their overall QoL one year after diagnosis and treatment. We propose to use a variety of QoL measurements, including the EQ-5D, SF-36 and EORTC QLQ-C30. The primary outcome, for the purposes of sample size estimation, will be the score on the global QoL scale of the EORTC QLQ-C30. From a study of 305 lung cancer patients, the mean global QoL score before treatment was 56.7, with a standard deviation of 23.5 (Aaronson et al., 1993).

(a) Suppose that we wish to estimate the mean EORTC QLQ-C30 global QoL score in the sample with a precision of ±5 points with 95% confidence. How many survey responders would we require to have this degree of precision for our outcome, the estimated mean EORTC QLQ-C30 global QoL score?

(b) If we anticipate a response rate of 50% to the postal survey, how many questionnaires will we need to send out to achieve the number of responders from (a)?

4.6 Suppose that we are planning case–control study in patients who have recently suffered a heart attack or myocardial infarction (MI) to compare their QoL with an age- and sex-matched control group. The primary outcome will be the EQ-5D utility score. This will be measured approximately 6-weeks post MI for the cases. From a previous study of 222 patients recovering from an acute MI, the mean EQ-5D score was 0.683 (SD 0.233) 6 weeks post MI (Lacey and Walters, 2003). A mean difference of 0.05 points or more, on the EQ-5D, between the MI cases and controls would be regarded as clinically and practically important.

(a) Assume that the between-persond standard deviation of 0.233 is the same as the standard deviation of the difference ($s_{Difference}$) between the EQ-5D measurements on the MI case and the matched control. Calculate how many patients would be needed to detect a 0.05 point difference in mean EQ-5D scores, between the MI cases and controls, with a two-sided significance of 5% and 80% power.

(b) If we assume a correlation $\rho = 0.60$ between the EQ-5D values of the cases and their age- and sex-matched controls, estimate the standard deviation of the differences, $s_{Difference}$, between the cases and their paired controls.

(c) Use the estimated SD from (b) to calculate how many patients would be needed to detect a 0.05 point difference in mean EQ-5D scores, between the MI cases and controls, with a two-sided significance of 5% and 80% power.

4.7 Underwood et al. (2008) describe the results of an RCT, in 247 people aged 50 or more, with chronic knee pain, comparing the topical and oral application of a non-steroidal anti-inflammatory drug (NSAID). The aim of the RCT was to demonstrate the equivalence of the two forms of application, oral and topical. The primary outcome was the change in global WOMAC scores from baseline to 12 months. In the randomized trial the difference (topical minus oral) was 2.0 (95% CI: -2 to 6). Suppose that a new topical cream, based on the original NSAID, has been developed and we wish to design a trial to compare the equivalence of the new topical NSAID cream with the existing NSAID cream. The primary outcome will again be the change in global WOMAC scores from baseline to 12 months. Assume that the two treatments will be regarded as equivalent if the difference in mean change in global WOMAC scores, from baseline to 12 months, between the two treatment groups is less than 2 points.

(a) Estimate the standard deviation (SD), for the change in global WOMAC score, from baseline to 12 months, from the quoted confidence interval.

(b) Use the estimated SD from (a) to calculate how many patients would be needed to demonstrate the equivalence of the two treatments (assuming the two will be considered equivalent if the difference in global WOMAC scores, from baseline to 12 months, is less than 2 points), with a two-sided significance of 5% and 80% power.

(c) If 20% of patients drop out by 12-month follow-up, how many patients will we need to recruit and randomize?

5

Reliability and method comparison studies for quality of life measurements

Summary

A basic requirement of a QoL measurement is that it is repeatable. If the same measurement is made on a second occasion, and nothing has changed, then we would expect to obtain the same answer, within experimental error. In QoL research, measurements are often made which need to be validated. Many studies with QoL instruments start with a proposed method of measuring something, in a specific population, and the important question is whether the instrument measures what it purports to measure in this population. This chapter describes the statistical methods to assess the repeatability or reliability of QoL measures and how to assess the internal consistency of QoL items and scales. Graphical methods for assessing agreement between two QoL measurements are also discussed. This chapter emphasizes that we are not testing whether something is reliable but rather measuring how reliable it is.

5.1   Introduction

A basic requirement of a QoL measurement, on an individual subject, is that it is repeatable. If the same measurement is made on a second occasion, and nothing has changed, then we would expect it to give the same answer, within experimental error. Assessment of reliability consists of determining that the process used for measurement yields reproducible and consistent results. Any QoL measurement, whether on a numerical scale or by more subjective means, should yield reproducible or similar values if it is used repeatedly on the same subject whilst the subject's condition has not changed materially. In these circumstances, reliability concerns the level of agreement between two or more repeated measures. This is sometimes known as test–retest reliability.

Quality of Life Outcomes in Clinical Trials and Health-Care Evaluation   Stephen J. Walters
© 2009 John Wiley & Sons, Ltd

If the measuring instrument is a questionnaire, perhaps to measure patient quality of life, then during the development stage of the questionnaire itself reliability of the scales to be ultimately used is of particular concern. Thus for scales containing multiple items, all the items should have internal reliability and therefore be consistent in the sense that they should all measure the same thing. Just as with any quantitative measurement, the final questionnaire should also have test–retest reliability. It is important to note that tests of statistical significance are rarely appropriate for reliability studies (Campbell *et al.*, 2007).

5.2   Intra-class correlation coefficient

In the QoL context, if a patient is in a stable condition, a QoL instrument should yield repeatable and reproducible results if it is used repeatedly on that subject. This is usually assessed using a test–retest study, with subjects who are thought to have stable disease and who are not expected to experience changes due to treatment effects or toxicity. The subjects are asked to complete the same QoL questionnaire on several occasions. The level of agreement between the occasions is a measure of the reliability of the instrument. It is important to select subjects whose QoL or condition is stable, and to choose carefully a between-assessments time-gap that is neither too short nor too long. Too short a period might allow subjects to recall their earlier responses, and too long a period might allow a true change in the status of the subject (Campbell *et al.*, 2007).

With repeated QoL assessments on a number of subjects there are two sources of variability that must be taken into account when assessing repeatability. The first source is the *between-subjects variability* ($\sigma^2_{\text{Subjects}}$), since different subjects will have different QoL. The second source of variability, since we are now taking repeated measurements on the same individuals, is the random error (σ^2_{Error}) of the QoL measurement on the individual subject or the *within-subject variability* in the repeated QoL assessments. In these circumstances, repeatability can be assessed by the intra-class correlation coefficient (ICC). This measures the strength of agreement between repeated QoL measurements, by assessing the proportion of the between-subjects variance ($\sigma^2_{\text{Subjects}}$) to the total variance, comprising the sum of both the within-subject and between-subjects variation ($\sigma = \sigma^2_{\text{Subjects}} + \sigma^2_{\text{Error}}$). Thus the ICC, denoted here by ρ, is given by

$$\rho = \frac{\sigma^2_{\text{Subjects}}}{\sigma^2_{\text{Subjects}} + \sigma^2_{\text{Error}}}. \tag{5.1}$$

If we only have one observation per person we cannot estimate the within-person standard deviation, σ_{Error}. If we have more than one observation per person, we can estimate the standard deviation for each person and take the average variance, across all the subjects, as an estimate of σ^2_{Error}. We can estimate the between-persons variance $\sigma^2_{\text{Subjects}}$ from the variance of the means for each person.

If the ICC is large (close to 1), then the within-subject (or random error) variability is low and a high proportion of the variance in the observations is attributable to variation between the different subjects. The measurements are then described as having high reliability. Conversely, if the ICC is low (close to 0), then the random error variability dominates and the measurements have low reliability. If the error variability is regarded as 'noise' and the true value of raters' scores as the 'signal', then the ICC measures the signal-to-noise ratio.

The error variability in equation (5.1) can be further separated into two more components, one due to random error (σ^2_{Error}) and the other due to repeated assessments with the same subject ($\sigma^2_{Repeats}$):

$$\rho = \frac{\sigma^2_{Subjects}}{\sigma^2_{Subjects} + \sigma^2_{Repeats} + \sigma^2_{Error}}. \tag{5.2}$$

The ICC can be estimated from an analysis of variance (ANOVA) model. The ANOVA model is described in more detail in Chapter 7. Basically, the ANOVA model splits up the total variance into several separate components according to the source of the variability. Table 5.1 shows an ANOVA table in which n subjects repeat the same QoL assessment on r occasions.

Substituting the Mean Square (MS) estimates for the variances from Table 5.1 into equation (5.2) and simplifying and rearranging gives the more general form of the ICC for repeated assessments:

$$ICC = \frac{MS_{Subjects} - MS_{Error}}{MS_{Subjects} + (r-1)MS_{Error} + \frac{r}{n}(MS_{Repeats} + MS_{Error})}. \tag{5.3}$$

For $r = 2$ repeated assessments on the same individuals, the ICC can be obtained as follows. Let x_{i1} and x_{i2} be the QoL scores at time 1 and time 2 respectively for subject i. Let $t_i = x_{i1} + x_{i2}$ and $d_i = x_{i1} - x_{i2}$ be the sum and difference of a pair of values. Calculate the mean difference, $\bar{d}$, and the standard deviations of t_i and d_i, s_t and s_d respectively. Then

$$ICC = \frac{s_t^2 - s_d^2}{s_t^2 + s_d^2 + \frac{2}{n}(n\bar{d}^2 - s_d^2)}. \tag{5.4}$$

A worked example, of how to calculate the ICC is given at the end of this chapter in Section 5.7.1.

Table 5.1   ANOVA table to estimate the intra-class correlation.

Source of variation	Sums of squares (SS)	Degrees of freedom (df)	Mean square (MS)	Expected MS (variances)
Between subjects	$SS_{Subjects}$	$n-1$	$MS_{Subjects} = \dfrac{SS_{Subjects}}{n-1}$	$r\sigma^2_{Subjects} + \sigma^2_{Error}$
Repeats (within subjects)	$SS_{Repeats}$	$r-1$	$MS_{Repeats} = \dfrac{SS_{Repeats}}{r-1}$	$n\sigma^2_{Repeats} + \sigma^2_{Error}$
Error	SS_{Error}	$rn-r-n+1$	$MS_{Error} = \dfrac{SS_{Error}}{rn-r-n+1}$	σ^2_{Error}
Total	SS_{Total}	$rn-1$		

Example: Estimating test–retest reliability

Ruta *et al.* (1998) evaluated the two week test–retest reliability of the SF-36 for a sample of ($n = 31$) patients with rheumatoid arthritis who reported that their arthritis and overall health had remained the same during this time. The corresponding ICC values are shown in Table 3.4, and all are above 0.76. These findings suggest that the SF-36 has high test–retest reliability in stable patients.   □

5.2.1   Inappropriate method

Despite the ICC being the appropriate measure to use, sometimes the Pearson correlation coefficient (see Chapter 7) is mistakenly used in this context. Clearly, if duplicate measures are made on n subjects, then the Pearson correlation coefficient can be calculated. However, repeated measurements may have a correlation close to 1 and so be highly correlated yet may be systematically different. For example, if the subject records consistently higher values on the first occasion than on the second by (say) exactly 5 units on whatever QoL measuring instrument is being used, then there would be zero agreement between the two QoL assessments (see Figure 5.1). Despite this, the correlation coefficient would be 1, indicating perfect association. So as well as good association, good agreement is required, which implies near equality of the measures being taken (Campbell *et al.*, 2007).

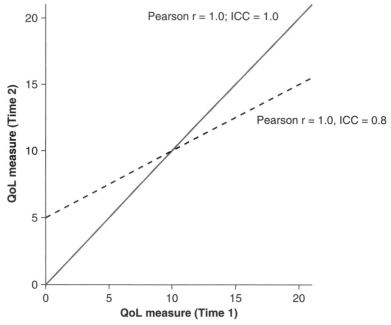

Figure 5.1   Typical graph of test–retest reliability scores, showing difference between Pearson correlation and intra-class correlation.

5.3   Agreement between individual items on a quality of life questionnaire

The ICC is mainly used to assess agreement or reliability between the dimension scores on a QoL instrument for two or more repeated assessments on the same subject. It can also be used to assess the agreement or reliability between individual items on the questionnaire for two or more repeated assessments on the same subject. However, as the items on most QoL questionnaires have categorical (binary or ordinal) responses rather than continuous responses, a more appropriate measure of reliability or agreement is the proportion of agreement or kappa.

5.3.1   Binary data: Proportion of agreement

Binary responses to QoL items include ratings such as yes/no, present/absent, or positive/negative. The simplest method of assessing agreement or repeatability is the proportion of agreement when the same instrument or item is assessed on two occasions. When subjects are assessed twice, the resulting responses and data can be displayed as in Table 5.2.

The number of subjects who respond in the same way on both assessments is $x_{11} + x_{22}$, and so the proportion of agreements is

$$P_{\text{Agree}} = \frac{x_{11} + x_{22}}{N_{\text{Repeat}}}. \tag{5.5}$$

5.3.2   Binary data: Kappa

If the response options to the QoL item are binary, then there are a very limited number of options (only two) for each item so that if subjects made their repeated response at random, rather than their true response to the item, these will agree some of the time. Jacob Cohen developed the kappa (κ) statistic in 1960 to allow for chance agreements of this kind. It is essentially the proportion of times that the two assessments agree minus the proportion of times they are likely to agree by chance, scaled so that if the assessments

Table 5.2   Notation for repeated binary data, with two assessments on the same N subjects.

Second assessment	First assessment Positive	Negative	Total
Positive	x_{11}	x_{12}	r_1
Negative	x_{21}	x_{22}	r_2
Total	c_1	c_2	N_{Repeat}

Table 5.3   Guideline values of κ to indicate the strength of agreement. Adapted by permission from Fayers, P.M., Machin, D., *Quality of Life: The Assessment, Analysis and Interpretation of Patient-reported Outcomes*. 2nd edition. John Wiley & Sons Ltd, Chichester. © 2007 John Wiley & Sons Ltd.

κ	Agreement
<0.20	Poor
0.20 to <0.40	Slight
0.40 to <0.60	Moderate
0.60 to <0.80	Good
0.80 to 1.00	Very High

agree all the time, then $\kappa = 1$. Thus if $\kappa = 1$, there is perfect agreement, and when $\kappa = 0$ the agreement is no better than chance. Negative values indicate an agreement that is even less than what would be expected by chance.

The expected proportion of chance agreements is

$$P_{\text{Chance}} = \frac{\dfrac{c_1 r_1}{N_{\text{Repeat}}} + \dfrac{c_2 r_2}{N_{\text{Repeat}}}}{N_{\text{Repeat}}} = \frac{c_1 r_1 + c_2 r_2}{N_{\text{Repeat}}^2}. \tag{5.6}$$

This leads to Cohen's kappa index of agreement

$$\kappa = \frac{P_{\text{Agree}} - P_{\text{Chance}}}{1 - P_{\text{Chance}}}. \tag{5.7}$$

Interpretation of κ is subjective, but Altman (1991) and Fayers and Machin (2007) suggest using the guideline values in Table 5.3. A worked example of how to calculate κ is given in Section 5.7.2.

5.3.3   Ordered categorical data: Weighted kappa

QoL items are frequently measured using ordered categorical responses. For example, items from some instruments are scored with $k = 4$ categories from 1 (not at all) to 4 (very much). In this case the results of two assessments may be summarized in a square $k \times k$ contingency table where k is the number of possible categorical responses to the question. So if we construct a $k \times k$ two-way table of frequencies similar to Table 5.2 we obtain

$$P_{\text{Agree}} = \frac{\sum_{i=1}^{k} x_{ii}}{N_{\text{Repeat}}} \quad \text{and} \quad P_{\text{Chance}} = \frac{\sum_{i=1}^{k} r_i c_i}{N_{\text{Repeat}}^2}. \tag{5.8}$$

Equation (5.7) is then used to calculate κ for a $k \times k$ contingency table.

Kappa was developed for categorical classifications, where disagreement is equally likely between categories. When the categories are ordered, disagreement between more extreme categories is less likely. One can extend the concept of κ and give less weight to the more extreme disagreements. For example, a difference between QoL item scores of 1 and 3 on the two occasions would be considered of greater importance than a difference between 1 and 2. Values that are off the diagonal in row i and column j of the $k \times k$ contingency table are given weights according to their distance from the diagonal. These weights correspond to the degree of disagreement. Two commonly use weights are *linear*,

$$w_{ij} = 1 - \frac{|i - j|}{k - 1}.$$ (5.9a)

where $|i - j|$ is the absolute difference between i and j, ignoring the sign of the difference, and *quadratic*,

$$w_{ij} = 1 - \left(\frac{i - j}{k - 1}\right)^2.$$ (5.9b)

Fayers and Machin (2007) suggest that quadratic weights are to be preferred, and this leads to

$$P^W_{Agree} = \frac{\sum_{i=1}^{k} \sum_{j=1}^{k} w_{ij} x_{ij}}{N_{Repeat}} \text{ and } P^W_{Chance} = \frac{\sum_{i=1}^{k} \sum_{j=1}^{k} w_{ij} r_i c_j}{N^2_{Repeat}}.$$ (5.10)

Equation (5.11) is then applied to give the weighted kappa,

$$\kappa_W = \frac{P^W_{Agree} - P^W_{Chance}}{1 - P^W_{Chance}}.$$ (5.11)

A worked example of how to calculate κ_W is given in Section 5.7.3.

Kappa and weighted kappa have a number of limitations (Campbell *et al.*, 2007):

(i) The maximum value of $\kappa = 1$ is only obtainable when the measurements on the first and second assessments agree completely.

(ii) For a given level of agreement, κ increases when the number of categories decreases, and so should only be used for comparisons when the number of categories is the same.

(iii) κ depends on the marginal distributions (the values of r_1, r_2, c_1 and c_2 in Table 5.2) so one can get the same values of κ but different apparent agreements if in one comparison one observer has a systematic bias, but in the other there is more random disagreement.

(iv) Some computer programs give a P-value associated with κ. These should be ignored since the null hypothesis they are testing has no meaning.

Despite these limitations, when analysing individual items in a QoL questionnaire, which only have a few ordered categories, κ or κ_W remains the most suitable measure for assessing agreement between the two items or between the two repeated assessments (Fayers and Machin, 2007). If quadratic weights are used then weighted κ is exactly identical to the ICC (Streiner and Norman, 2003).

Example: Estimating test–retest reliability

Ruta *et al.* (1998) evaluated the two-week test–retest reliability of the SF-36 for a sample of ($n = 31$) patients with rheumatoid arthritis who reported that their arthritis and overall health had remained the same during this time. Kappa was calculated for the three SF-36 scales (Social Functioning, Role Physical and Role Emotional). The corresponding kappa values are shown in Table 3.4. The values for kappa were low, less than 0.59, indicating poor test–retest reliability.   □

5.4   Internal consistency and Cronbach's alpha

Some QoL questionnaires, such as those used to assess concepts like anxiety and depression in patients, often comprise a series of questions. Each question is then scored, and the scores are combined in some way to give a single numerical value. Often this is done by merely summing the scores for each answer to give an overall scale score. The internal validity of each of the component questions of the scale is indicated if they are all positively correlated with each other; a lack of correlation of two such items would indicate that at least one of them was not measuring the concept in question. Alternatively, one might frame a question in two different ways, and if the answers are always similar, then the questions are *internally consistent*.

A measure of internal consistency is Cronbach's alpha, α_{Cronbach} (see Cronbach, 1951). It is essentially a form of correlation coefficient. A value of 0 would indicate that there was no correlation between the items that make up a scale, and a value of 1 would indicate perfect correlation.

If a QoL questionnaire or a specific dimension on the QoL instrument has k items, and this has been administered to a group of subjects, then the standard deviation (s_i) of the ith item and the standard deviation (s_T) of the sum score T of all the items are required. Then

$$\alpha_{\text{Cronbach}} = \frac{k}{k-1}\left(1 - \frac{\sum_{i=1}^{k} s_i^2}{s_T^2}\right). \tag{5.12}$$

For comparing groups, α_{Cronbach} values of 0.7 to 0.8 are regarded as satisfactory, although for clinical applications much higher values are necessary. However, a value of 1 would indicate that most of the questions could in fact be discarded, since all the information is contained in just one of them. Cronbach's α is essentially a measure of how correlated items are. Clearly one would like items that all refer to a single concept such as pain to be related to each other. However, if they are too closely related then some of the questions are redundant. When constructing a questionnaire, one might omit items which have a weak or very strong correlation with other items in the domain of interest. A worked example of how to calculate α_{Cronbach} is given in Section 5.7.4.

Example: Cronbach's α

Walters *et al.* (2001a) examined the internal consistency of the items and dimensions in the SF-36 in a sample of 7011 older adults aged 65–101. The external consistencies of the items and scales in the SF-36 were assessed with Cronbach's α statistic. The

Table 5.4 Internal consistency of the items and dimensions in the SF-36 from three general population surveys (data from Walters *et al.*, 2001a).

Dimension	No. of items	Cronbach's alpha		
		Sheffield (aged 16–74) (min $n = 1514$)	OHLS (aged 18–64) (min $n = 8883$)	Elderly 65+ (min $n = 7011$)
Physical Functioning	10	0.93	0.90	0.94
Physical Functioning II*	13			0.95
Role Physical	4	0.96	0.88	0.89
Bodily Pain	2	0.85	0.82	0.89
General Health	5	0.80	0.80	0.89
Vitality	4	0.96	0.85	0.85
Social Functioning	2	0.73	0.76	0.78
Role Emotional	3	0.96	0.80	0.88
Mental Health	5	0.95	0.83	0.81

*Only this study used an extra three items for the Physical Functioning dimension.

rightmost column of Table 5.4 shows the results. Cronbach's α exceeded 0.8 for all dimensions except Social Functioning (0.78), which is similar to results reported in studies of younger populations (Brazier *et al.*, 1992; Jenkinson *et al.*, 1993). The result for Social Functioning may partly reflect the small number of items (two) in that dimension.   □

5.5   Graphical methods for assessing reliability or agreement between two quality of life measures or assessments

A common method of analysis is first to calculate the correlation coefficient between the two assessments and then to calculate a significance test for the null hypothesis of no association. Calculating the correlation coefficient to assess reliability or agreement between two reapeated QoL assessments is inappropriate for the following reasons (Campbell *et al.*, 2007):

(1) The correlation coefficient is a measure of *association* between two continuous variables. What is required here is a measure of *agreement*. We will have perfect association if the observations lie on any straight line, but there is only perfect agreement if the points lie on the line of equality $y = x$.

(2) The correlation coefficient observed depends on the range of measurements used. So one can increase the correlation coefficient by choosing widely spaced observations. Since investigators usually compare two methods over the whole range of likely values (as they should), a good correlation is almost guaranteed.

(3) Because of (2), data which have an apparently high correlation can, for individual subjects, show very poor agreement between the two assessments.

(4) The test of significance is not relevant since it would be very surprising if two repeated QoL assessments on the same individual were not related.

We shall illustrate the graphical methods of assessing agreement or reliability between two repeated QoL assessments by using data comparing two QoL assessments 2 weeks apart. New mothers were asked to complete the Edinburgh Postnatal Depression Scale (EPDS) at 6 weeks and 8 weeks after childbirth as part of a cluster randomized trial (Morrell *et al.*, 2009). The EPDS is a 10-item instrument assessing postnatal depression (PND). It is scored on a 0–30 scale with higher scores (12 or more) indicating a greater risk of PND.

Figure 5.2 shows a scatter diagram of the data. If the 6- and 8-week EPDS scores agreed exactly then all the points would lie on the line of equality (a line with a 45° slope passing through the origin of the horizontal and vertical axes). However, we can see that although some of the data are near the line of equality, for the majority of mothers the two EPDS scores differ considerably.

Bland and Altman (1986) argue that the correlation coefficient is inappropriate and recommend an alternative approach. As an initial step one should plot the data as in Figure 5.2, but omit the calculation of the corresponding correlation coefficient and the associated test of significance. Bland and Altman (1986) recommend an alternative, more informative plot to the simple scatter plot of Figure 5.2, as shown in Figure 5.3. Here the differences in EPDS scores between the two repeated assessments (first assessment minus second assessment) are plotted against the average of the two EPDS scores.Now we can much more easily see the size of the differences between reviewer QoL scores and also their distribution around zero. We can also check visually that the differences

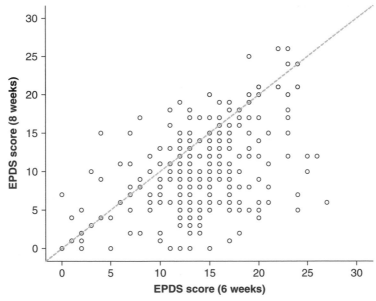

Figure 5.2   Scatter diagram of 8-week versus 6-week postnatal Edinburgh Postnatal Depression Scale score in 307 new mothers, with a line of equality superimposed (data from Morrell *et al.*, 2009).

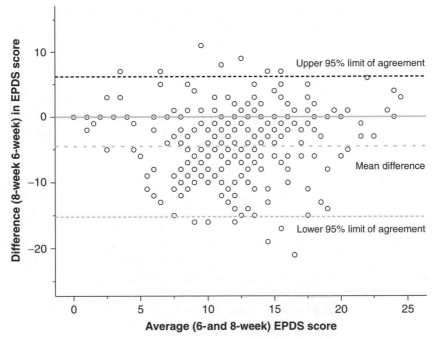

Figure 5.3 Difference between 6-week and 8-week postnatal EPDS scores versus average EPDS score from ($n = 307$) new mothers, plus the observed mean difference and 95% limits of agreement (data from Morrell *et al* 2009).

are not related to the size of the measurement (for this purpose the average of the two reviewers' scores acts as our best estimate of the true unknown value.)

We could use a one-sample t-test of the differences against zero (or, equivalently, a paired t-test on the original data; see Chapter 7) to see if the mean difference is significantly different from zero, but we are concerned with the degree of agreement between the two assessments, so that this problem is one of estimating the degree of agreement rather than performing a hypothesis test. So it is more important to quantify the spread or variability of the individual data points.

We want to know how well the two methods (or observers in our example) agree. Altman (1991) explains that there are two parts to the answer to this question:

1. The mean difference is an estimate of the average bias of one method relative to the other.

2. It is important to consider how well the methods are likely to agree for an individual, for which purpose we can use the standard deviation of the differences (SD_{diff}).

We could simply quote the mean difference and standard deviation of the differences, but Altman (1991) argues that it is much more useful to use the mean and standard deviation to construct a range of values which we expect to cover the agreement between the methods for most subjects. For a reasonably symmetric distribution, statistical theory tell us that we expect the range mean $\pm 2SD$ to include about 95% of the observations.

For a method comparison study we can therefore take the mean $\pm 2SD_{diff}$ as a 95% range of agreement for individuals. This range of values defines the *95% limits of agreement* (Altman, 1991).

For the EPDS data we get a range from

$$-4.48 - (2 \times 5.34) \text{ to } -4.48 \text{ to } (2 \times 5.34),$$

which is -15.2 to 6.2. In other words, we expect the 6- and 8-week EPDS scores of new mothers to differ on average by less than 4.5 points with limits of agreement of -15.2 to 6.2. These limits of agreement are shown in Figure 5.3 as dotted lines, along with the mean difference of -4.5.

In Figure 5.3, only 14 out of 307 or 4.6% of the observations are outside the 95% limits of agreement. However, there is considerable variability in the difference in 6- and 8-week EPDS scores of new mothers and the mean difference of 4.5 points is large (approximately 15% of the 30-point EPDS scale range). The limits of agreement are also wide, almost 21 points in either direction, which is over two-thirds the of the 30-point EPDS scale range. This suggests rather poor agreement between the 6- and 8-week EPDS assessments. The ICC estimate of 0.32 supports this conclusion.

It is important to note that the interpretation of the mean and standard deviation of the differences must depend on the clinical circumstances. As Altman (1991) states: 'It is not possible to use statistics to define acceptable agreement.'

5.6   Further reading

The formulae for the ICC described in this chapter are not the only ones. They are for only one form of it and there are several different versions of the ICC, depending on the various assumptions we make and what we want to look for. The interested reader is referred to Streiner and Norman (2003) for more details.

5.7   Technical details

5.7.1   Calculation of ICC

Suppose that we have developed a new QoL instrument to measure fatigue in cancer patients. The scale has three items with four ordered responses coded 0, 1, 2 and 3. The items are summed to generate a fatigue dimension with scores ranging for 0 (not fatigued) to 9 (very fatigued). Table 5.5 shows the fatigue scale scores in nine cancer patients who were assessed 2 weeks apart.

For two repeated assessments on the same individuals the ICC can be obtained by using equation (5.4). The mean difference, $\bar{d} = 0.22$, and the standard deviations of t_i and d_i, s_t and s_d, are 5.39 and 1.99 respectively. Then

$$ICC = \frac{5.39^2 - 1.99^2}{5.39^2 + 1.99^2 + \dfrac{2}{9}(9 \times 0.22^2 - 1.99^2)} = 0.78.$$

This is high and suggests the measurements of fatigue are repeatable.

Table 5.5 Fatigue for nine cancer patients measured on two occasions.

Subject (i)	Fatigue scale (0–9) 2-week retest 1st Occasion (x_{i1})	2nd Occasion (x_{i2})	Difference $(d_i = x_{i1} - x_{i2})$	Average	Sum $(t_i = x_{i1} + x_{i2})$
1	0.0	2.0	2.0	1.0	2.0
2	5.0	3.0	−2.0	4.0	8.0
3	0.0	3.0	3.0	1.5	3.0
4	3.0	5.0	2.0	4.0	8.0
5	9.0	9.0	0.0	9.0	18.0
6	7.0	4.0	−3.0	5.5	11.0
7	7.0	6.0	−1.0	6.5	13.0
8	3.0	3.0	0.0	3.0	6.0
9	7.0	8.0	1.0	7.5	15.0
Mean	4.56	4.78	0.22	4.67	9.33
SD	3.24	2.44	1.99	2.69	5.39
Variance	10.53	5.94	3.94	7.25	29.00

Table 5.6 Four by four contingency table for fatigue question on problems sleeping at night for nine cancer patients measured on two occasions.

		2nd Assessment: Problems sleeping at night 0–Not at all	1–A little bit	2–Quite a bit	3–Very much	Total
1st Assessment:	0–Not at all	2	0	0	0	2
Problems	1–A little bit	1	2	0	0	3
sleeping at night	2–Quite a bit	0	1	2	0	3
	3–Very much	0	0	0	1	1
Total		3	3	2	1	9

5.7.2 Calculation of kappa

Suppose that one of the three items in the new fatigue scale described above asks subjects about problems sleeping at night. The item has four ordered responses coded 0 (not at all), 1 (a little bit), 2 (quite a bit) and 3 (very much). Table 5.6 shows the responses to the sleep item for nine cancer patients assessed 2 weeks apart.

From equation (5.5), the estimated probability that the patient's responses on the first and second assessments agree is

$$P_{\text{Agree}} = \frac{\sum_{i=1}^{k} x_{ii}}{N_{\text{Repeat}}} = \frac{7}{9} = 0.778.$$

From equation (5.6), the proportion of responses expected to agree by chance alone is

$$P_{\text{Chance}} = \frac{\sum_{i=1}^{k} r_i c_i}{N_{\text{Repeat}}^2} = \frac{(2 \times 3) + (3 \times 3) + (3 \times 2) + (1 \times 1)}{9^2} = \frac{22}{81} = 0.272.$$

Cohen's κ is then given by equation (5.7):

$$\kappa = \frac{P_{\text{Agree}} - P_{\text{Chance}}}{1 - P_{\text{Chance}}} = \frac{0.778 - 0.272}{1 - 0.272} = 0.695.$$

Using Table 5.3, this suggests good agreement between the responses to this item after two repeated assessments.

5.7.3   Calculation of weighted kappa

The four responses to the sleep item in the contingency table (Table 5.6) are clearly ordered. Therefore the use of weighted kappa is more appropriate than the simple unweighted kappa. We have $k = 4$ categories so, using equation (5.9b), the quadratic weights w_{ij} for 0, 1, 2 and 3 categories of disagreement are 1.0000, 0.8889, 0.5556 and 0.0000, respectively.

From equation (5.11), the estimated probability that the patient's responses on the first and second assessments agree is

$$P_{\text{Agree}}^{W} = \frac{\sum_{i=1}^{k} \sum_{j=1}^{k} w_{ij} x_{ij}}{N_{\text{Repeat}}}$$

$$= \frac{(1.0000 \times 7) + (0.8889 \times 2) + (0.5556 \times 0) + (0.0000 \times 0)}{9}$$

$$= \frac{8.778}{9} = 0.975$$

The calculation of the responses expected to agree by chance alone is more difficult, but using Table 5.7 and equation (5.10) we can estimate

$$P_{\text{Chance}}^{W} = \frac{\sum_{i=1}^{k} \sum_{j=1}^{k} w_{ij} r_i c_j}{N_{\text{Repeat}}^{2}} = \frac{22.0000 + 31.1115 + 10.564 + 0.0000}{9^2}$$

$$= \frac{63.6667}{81} = 0.786.$$

Finally, equation (5.11) is applied to give

$$\kappa_W = \frac{P_{\text{Agree}}^{W} - P_{\text{Chance}}^{W}}{1 - P_{\text{Chance}}^{W}} = \frac{0.975 - 0.786}{1 - 0.786} = 0.885.$$

Again using Table 5.3, this suggests very high agreement between the responses to this item after two repeated assessments.

5.7.4   Calculation of Cronbach's alpha

Suppose that a new QoL questionnaire has a fatigue dimension section based on three items, which measure aspects of fatigue, each of which can have a score between 0 (not at all) and 3 (very much). The three items are summed to give the total score for a particular dimension of the questionnaire. Table 5.8 shows the responses to the three items and a total scale score for 10 cancer patients.

Table 5.7 Calculation of P_{Chance}^{W} for 4×4 contingency table.

Categories of disagreement	r_i	c_j	w_{ij}	$w_{ij}r_ic_j$	$\sum w_{ij}r_ic_j$
0	2	3	1.0000	6	
	3	3	1.0000	9	
	3	2	1.0000	6	
	1	1	1.0000	1	22.0000
1	3	3	0.8889	8.0001	
	3	3	0.8889	8.0001	
	2	1	0.8889	1.7778	
	2	3	0.8889	5.3334	
	3	2	0.8889	5.3334	
	3	1	0.8889	2.6667	31.1115
2	3	3	0.5556	5.0004	
	1	3	0.5556	1.6668	
	2	2	0.5556	2.2224	
	3	1	0.5556	1.6668	10.5564
3	2	1	0.0000	0.0000	
	1	3	0.0000	0.0000	
	3	1	0.0000	0.0000	0.0000

Table 5.8 Responses to three fatigue questions and total scale score for 10 subjects.

	Q1	Q2	Q3	Total
Subject	Feeling weak	Feeling tired	Problems sleeping at night	Fatigue scale (0–9)
1	1	1	0	2
2	1	1	1	3
3	1	2	0	3
4	1	1	1	3
5	1	1	1	3
6	2	2	0	4
7	2	2	1	5
8	2	2	2	6
9	3	3	2	8
10	3	3	3	9
Mean	1.70	1.80	1.10	4.60
SD	0.82	0.79	0.99	2.37

If a questionnaire has k items, and this has been administered to a group of subjects, then if s_i is the standard deviation of the ith item, T is the sum score of all the items, and s_T is the standard deviation of T, then Cronbach's alpha, α_{Cronbach}, is given by equation (5.12).

Thus for our data $k = 3$, $\sum s_i^2 = 0.82^2 + 0.79^2 + 0.99^2 = 2.28$, and $s_T^2 = 2.37^2 = 5.62$, so $\alpha_{\text{Cronbach}} = 1.5[1 - (2.28/5.62)] = 0.89$.

The reason why α_{Cronbach} is a measure of correlation is as follows (Campbell et al., 2007). If $X_1, \ldots, X_k$ are independent random variables and $T = X_1 + \ldots + X_k$ is their sum, then the variance of T, $\text{Var}(T) = \text{Var}(X_1) + \cdots + \text{Var}(X_k)$. Hence the numerator and denominator in the brackets in equation (5.12) for α_{Cronback} are the same and so $\alpha_{\text{Cronback}} = 0$. If $X_1, \ldots, X_k$ are perfectly correlated so that $X_1 = X_2 = \cdots = X_k$ then $T = kX_1$ and $\text{Var}(T) = k^2\text{Var}(X_1)$, whereas $\sum \text{Var}(X_i) = k\text{Var}(X_1)$. Thus the ratio in the brackets is now $1/k$ and so $\alpha_{\text{Cronback}} = 1$.

Exercises

5.1 Suppose that we have developed a new QoL instrument to measure family and social issues in cancer patients. The scale has four items with four ordered responses coded 0 (not at all), 1 (a little bit), 2 (quite a bit) and 3 (very much). The items are summed to generate a family and social issues scale with scores ranging for 0 (no issues) to 12 (many issues). Table 5.9 shows the family and social issues scale scores in nine cancer patients assessed 2 weeks apart.

(a) Draw a scatter plot of the difference between the first and second assessments in family and social issues scale scores (on the vertical axis) versus the average score (on the horizontal axis) for the nine cancer patients.

Table 5.9 Family and social issues scale scores for nine cancer patients measured on two occasions.

| Subject | Family and social issues scale (0–12) 2–week retest | | | | |
	1st Occasion	2nd Occasion	Difference	Average	Sum
1	0	1	−1	0.5	1
2	2	2	0	2	4
3	0	1	−1	0.5	1
4	1	1	0	1	2
5	2	3	−1	2.5	5
6	3	3	0	3	6
7	3	3	0	3	6
8	0	0	0	0	0
9	1	1	0	1	2
Mean	1.33	1.67	−0.33	1.50	3.00
SD	1.22	1.12	0.50	1.15	2.29
Variance	1.50	1.25	0.25	1.31	5.25

Table 5.10   Responses to four family and social issues questions and total scale score for nine cancer patients.

Subject	Q1 Feeling that people do not understand what you want	Q2 Worrying about the effect that your illness is having on your family	Q3 Lack of support from your family or others	Q4 Needing more help than your family or others could give	Total
1	0	0	0	0	0
2	1	1	0	0	2
3	0	0	0	0	0
4	0	1	0	0	1
5	0	2	0	0	2
6	1	1	0	1	3
7	0	3	0	0	3
8	0	0	0	0	0
9	0	1	0	0	1
Mean	0.25	1.00	0.00	0.13	1.38
SD	0.46	1.07	0.00	0.35	1.30
Variance	0.21	1.14	0.00	0.13	1.70

Table 5.11   Four by four contingency table for family and social issues question on worrying about the effect that your illness is having on your family for nine cancer patients measured on two occasions.

	2nd assessment: Worrying about the effect that your illness is having on your family				Total
	0–Not at all	1–A little bit	2–Quite a bit	3–Very much	
1st assessment: 0–Not at all	2	1	0	0	3
Worrying about 1–A little bit	0	3	1	0	4
the effect that 2–Quite a bit	0	0	0	1	1
your illness is 3–Very much	0	0	0	1	1
having on your					
family					
Total	2	4	1	2	9

(b) Calculate the 95% limits of agreement and show these, plus the observed mean difference on the scatter plot.

(c) From the graph does there appear to be a relationship between the two variables?

(d) Calculate and comment on the test–retest reliability ICC for the data in Table 5.9.

5.2 Suppose that we have developed a new QoL instrument to measure family and social issues in cancer patients. The scale has four items with four ordered responses coded 0 (not at all), 1 (a little bit), 2 (quite a bit) and 3 (very much). The items are summed to generate a family and social issues scale with scores ranging for 0 (no issues) to 12 (many issues). Table 5.10 shows the responses to the four items of the family and social issues scale and the total scale score in nine cancer patients.

(a) What do you notice about the responses to question 3?

(b) Calculate and comment on the value of $\alpha_{Cronbach}$.

5.3 Question 2 of the four items for the new family and social issues scale described in Exercises 5.1 and 5.2 asks cancer patients if they are worried about the effect that their illness is having on their family. This item has four ordered responses coded 0 (not at all), 1 (a little bit), 2 (quite a bit) and 3 (very much). Table 5.11 shows the responses to this item for nine cancer patients assessed 2 weeks apart.

(a) Calculate Cohen's kappa and interpret it.

(b) Calculate weighted kappa (using quadratic weights) and interpret it.

(c) Compare the weighted and unweighted kappa calculated for (a) and (b).

6

Summarizing, tabulating and graphically displaying quality of life outcomes

Summary

This chapter describes how to graphically display and summarize QoL data. Three summary measures of central tendency or location are described (mean, median and mode) as well as three measures of spread or variability (range, interquartile range and standard deviation). Graphical methods for displaying QoL data such as dot plots, histograms and box-and-whisker plots are discussed. The chapter also shows how to present QoL data and results in tables and graphs for comparing two groups.

6.1 Introduction

QoL measures are usually measured or scored on an ordered categorical (ordinal) scale. This means that responses to individual questions or items are usually classified into a small number of response categories which can be ordered (e.g. poor, moderate and good). In planning and analysis, the question responses are often analysed by assigning equally spaced numerical scores to the ordinal categories (e.g. $0 =$ poor, $1 =$ moderate, $2 =$ good). The scores across similar questions are then summed to generate a QoL measurement. These 'summated scores' gives the appearance that the QoL instruments are continuous measurements. However, the skewed, discrete and bounded distribution of QoL measures leads to several problems in determining sample size and analysing the data (Walters *et al.*, 2001b; see Box 6.1).

There are advantages in being able to treat QoL scales as continuous for statistical analysis (in terms of simplifying the analysis and making the results easier to interpret).

Quality of Life Outcomes in Clinical Trials and Health-Care Evaluation   Stephen J. Walters
© 2009 John Wiley & Sons, Ltd

Box 6.1 Problems with scaling of QoL outcomes

1. The apparent continuum hides the fact that only a few discrete values are possible.

2. The scale may not be linear.

3. There is often a floor or ceiling effect.

4. Methods based on the Normal distribution (such as linear regression) assume that the outcome variable has a constant variance.

5. Normal approximations may not apply.

6. Missing values likely.

7. It is difficult to quantify an effect size.

Most researchers (and authors) tend to do this. However, a key question when analysing QoL data is to decide whether or not the data are ordinal or continuous.

If you fundamentally believe there is an underlying latent continuous QoL scale and you are measuring discrete values of this scale with your instrument then treat the data as continuous. This scale is shown at the bottom of Figure 6.1. An example is measuring age to the nearest year or in age bands rather than exact age (in years, days, hours, . . .).

Alternatively, if you fundamentally believe there is *not* an underlying latent continuous QoL scale, and the scale is like the top graph in Figure 6.1, then treat the data as ordinal. An example is measuring stage of cancer (0, I, II, III, IV). We know there is an ordering, but we do not think there is an underlying cancer continuum. The cancer staging describes the extent or severity of an individual's cancer based on the extent of the original (primary) tumour and the extent of spread in the body. Higher cancer stage numbers indicate more extensive disease: greater tumour size, and/or spread of the cancer to nearby lymph nodes and/or organs adjacent to the primary tumour.

My own experience is that the majority of QoL scales are developed under the belief that there is an underlying latent continuous scale for the outcome. Therefore I tend to treat the scales as continuous and use statistical analysis methods appropriate for continuous outcomes. This chapter and most of the subsequent chapters in this book will assume that QoL scales are continuous measurements.

6.2 Graphs

As a first step in any analysis of QoL outcomes it is useful to plot the data and examine them visually. This will show any extreme observations (outliers) together with any interesting patterns. In addition to being a useful preliminary step to analysis, information can also be displayed pictorially when summarizing the data and reporting results. Graphs are useful as they can be read quickly, and help particularly when presenting information to an audience. However, when using graphs for presentation purposes care must be taken to ensure that they are not misleading (see Box 6.2; Freeman *et al.*, 2008).

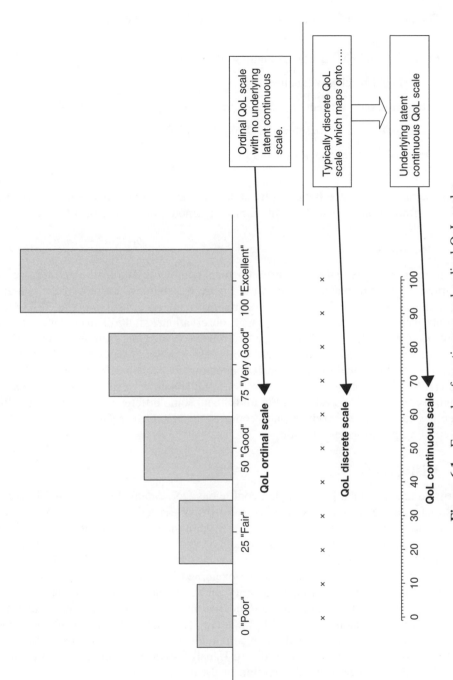

Figure 6.1 Example of continuous and ordinal QoL scales.

Box 6.2 Guidelines for good practice when constructing graphs

1. The amount of information should be maximized for the minimum amount of ink.

2. Figures should have a title explaining what is being displayed.

3. Axes should be clearly labelled.

4. Gridlines should be kept to a minimum.

5. Avoid 3-D charts as these can be difficult to read.

6. The number of observations should be included.

A fundamental principle for both graphs and tables is that they should maximize the amount of information presented for the minimum amount of ink used (Tufte, 1983).

6.2.1   Dot plots

There are several graphs that can be used for displaying QoL data. *Dot plots* are one of the simplest ways of displaying all the data. Figure 6.2 shows a dot plot of the general health, as measured by the SF-36v2, of a sample of male cancer survivors aged 25–45. These data were taken from a cross-sectional, observational study of male cancer cases and controls (Greenfield *et al.*, 2007). Each dot represents the QoL score for an individual and is plotted along a vertical axis, which in this case represents the General Health QoL scale of the SF-36v2, with a score of 100 equating to good health. Data for several groups can be plotted alongside each other for comparison; for example, data for cases and controls are plotted separately in Figure 6.2 and some differences in General Health between the cases (cancer survivors) and controls can clearly be seen, with more of the cases reporting poorer general health.

6.2.2   Histograms

The most common method for displaying continuous QoL data is the *histogram*. In order to construct a histogram the data range is divided into several non-overlapping equally sized categories, and the number of observations falling into each category counted. The categories are then displayed on the horizontal axis and the frequencies displayed on the vertical axis, as in Figure 6.3.

The way that data are distributed can be examined using a histogram. Occasionally they display the percentages in each category on the vertical axis rather than the frequencies and it is important that if this is done, the total number of observations that the percentages are based upon is included in the chart. The choice of number of categories is important: too few categories and much important information is lost, too many and any patterns are obscured by too much detail. Usually between 5 and 15 categories will be enough to gain an idea of the distribution of the data.

One useful feature of a histogram is that it makes it possible to see whether the distribution of the data is skewed or symmetric (and approximately Normally distributed). Figure 6.3 shows that the General Health QoL data in our male controls is left or

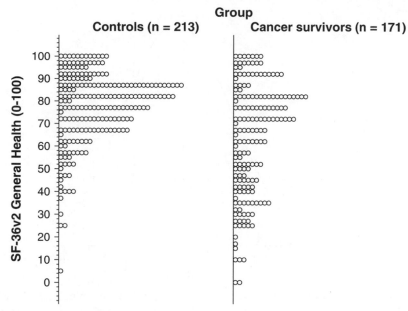

Figure 6.2   Dot plot showing SF-36 General Health by group (cancer survivor or control) for 384 men aged 25–45 (data from Greenfield *et al.*, 2007).

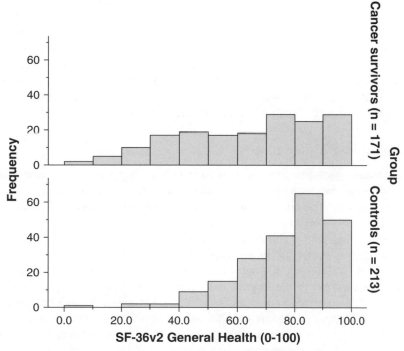

Figure 6.3   Histogram of SF-36 General Health by group (cancer survivor or control) for 384 men aged 25–45 (data from Greenfield *et al.*, 2007).

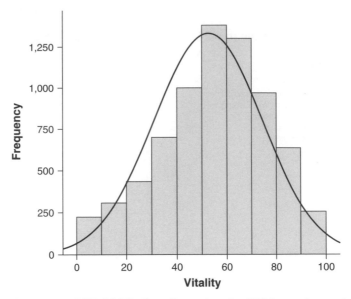

Figure 6.4 Histogram of SF-36 Vitality dimension for 7213 people aged 16–101 who responded to a general population survey of Sheffield, United Kingdom, residents (data from Walters *et al.*, 2001a).

negatively skewed, with the bulk of the data over to the right and a long tail to the left. The histogram of Normally distributed data will have a classic 'bell' shape, with a peak in the middle and symmetrical tails, such as that in Figure 6.4 for the Vitality dimension of the SF-36, taken from 7213 people aged 16–101 who responded to a general population survey of Sheffield, United Kingdom, residents, displayed here with a theoretical Normal distribution curve (Walters *et al.*, 2001a). The Normal distribution (sometimes called the Gaussian distribution) is one of the fundamental distributions of statistics, and its properties underpin many of the methods explored later.

6.2.3   Box-and-whisker plot

Another extremely useful method of plotting continuous data is the *box-and-whisker* or *box plot*. Box plots can be particularly useful for comparing the distribution of the data across several groups. The box contains the middle 50% of the data, with lowest 25% of the data lying below it and the highest 25% of the data lying above it. In fact the upper and lower edges represent a particular quantity called the interquartile range (described later). The median is shown by the horizontal line across the box (this is described later, but briefly it is the value such that half of the observations lie below it and half lie above it). The whiskers extend to the largest and smallest values, excluding the outlying and extreme values. The outlying values are those values between 1.5 and 3 box lengths from the upper or lower edges of the box, and are represented as the dots outside the whiskers. Extreme values are cases with values more than 3 box lengths from the upper or lower edge of the box, and are represented as the asterisks outside the whiskers.

Figure 6.5 shows box plots of the SF-36 General Health score by group (cancer survivor or control) for 384 men aged 25–45 (data from Greenfield *et al.*, 2007). The group

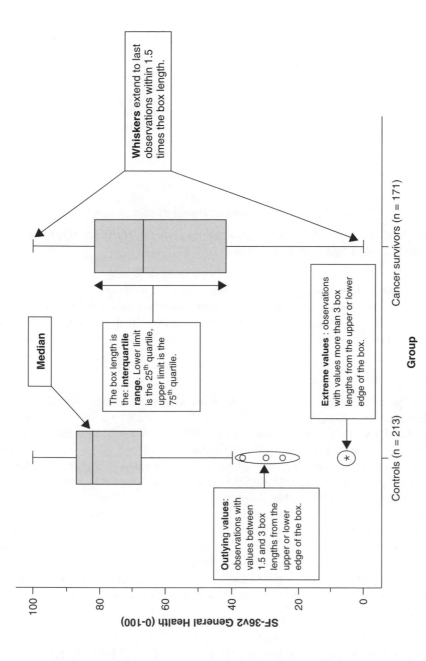

Figure 6.5 Box-and-whisker plot of SF-36 General Health by group (cancer survivor or control) for 384 men aged 25–45 (data from Greenfield *et al.*, 2007).

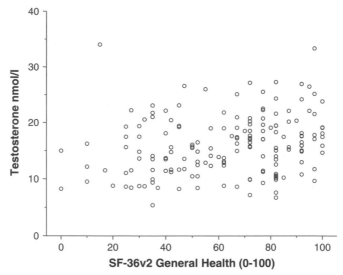

Figure 6.6 Scatter plot of testosterone versus SF-36 General Health for 170 male cancer survivors aged 25–45 (data from Greenfield *et al.*, 2007).

differences in QoL are immediately obvious from this plot, with the controls having the better general health, and this illustrates the main advantage of the box plot over histograms when looking at multiple groups. Differences in the distributions of data between groups are much easier to spot with box plots than with dot plots and histograms.

6.2.4   Scatter plots

The association between two continuous variables can be examined visually by constructing a *scatter plot*. The values of one variable are plotted on the horizontal axis (sometimes known as the X-axis) and the values of another are plotted on the vertical axis (Y-axis). If it is known (or suspected) that the value of one variable (independent) influences the value of the other variable (dependent), it is usual to plot the independent variable on the horizontal axis and the dependent variable on the vertical axis (the reason for this will be explained later in this chapter).

The cross-sectional, observational study of male cancer survivors aged 25–45 also measured their testosterone hormone levels. Figure 6.6 shows the scatter plot of testosterone against QoL, each dot representing the testosterone and QoL values for an individual. Testosterone is plotted on the vertical axis and QoL is plotted on the horizontal axis, although the variables could legitimately be plotted the other way around. It is clear from the scatter plot that general health and testosterone are not associated in this sample of male cancer survivors.

6.3   Describing and summarizing quality of life data

As it can be difficult to make sense of a large number of QoL observations, an initial approach would be to calculate summary measures, to describe the *location* (a measure of the 'middle value') and the *spread* (a measure of the dispersion of the values) of the collected QoL data. These are of great interest, particularly if a comparison between groups is to be made or the results of the study are to be generalized to a larger group, and so it is necessary to find reliable ways of determining their values (Campbell *et al.*, 2007).

6.3.1   Measures of location

There are three commonly used measures of location, the so-called three Ms: mean, median and mode.

6.3.1.1   Mean

The arithmetic *mean* or average of n observations $\bar{x}$ (pronounced 'x bar') is simply the sum of the observations divided by their number; thus

$$\bar{x} = \frac{\text{Sum of all sample values}}{\text{Size of sample}} = \frac{\sum_{i=1}^{n} x_i}{n}.$$

In the above equation, x_i represents the individual sample values and $\sum_{i=1}^{n} x_i$ their sum. The Greek letter 'Σ' (sigma) is the Greek capital 'S' and stands for 'sum' and simply means 'add up the n observations x_i from the first to the last (nth)'.

Example: Calculation of mean QoL

Consider the following 10 QoL scores on the General Health dimension of the SF-36 randomly selected from the young male cancer survivors, aged 25–45, from the Greenfield *et al.*, (2007) study.

$$25, 42, 52, 57, 62, 72, 82, 85, 95, 100$$

The sum of these 10 QoL observations is $25 + 42 + 52 + 57 + 62 + 72 + 82 + 85 + 95 + 100 = 672$. Thus the sample mean QoL, $\bar{x} = 672/10 = 67.2$. It is usual to quote 1 more decimal place for the mean than for the data recorded.   □

The major advantage of the mean is that it uses all the data values, and is, in a statistical sense, efficient. The main disadvantage of the mean is that it is vulnerable to what are known as *outliers*. Outliers are single observations which, if excluded from the calculations, have noticeable influence on the results. For example, if we had entered '1' instead of '100', for the General Health of the 10th subject, we would find the mean QoL changed from 67.2 to 57.3. It does not necessarily follow, however, that outliers should be excluded from the final data summary, or that they result from an erroneous measurement.

6.3.1.2   Median

The *median* is the middle observation, when the data are arranged in order of increasing value. It is the value that divides the data into two equal halves. If there are an even number of observations then the median is calculated as the average of the two middle observations. For example, if there are 11 observations the median is simply the 6th observation, but if there are 10 observations the median is found by summing the 5th and 6th observations and dividing by 2.

Example: Calculation of median QoL

Consider the 10 QoL scores on the General Health dimension of the SF-36 randomly selected from the young male cancer survivors, aged 25–45, from the Greenfield *et al.*, (2007) study, given in the previous example. This time the ten QoL observations in the sample, are ranked or ordered from the smallest to the largest.

Rank Order	QoL
1	25
2	42
3	52
4	57
5	62
6	72
7	82
8	85
9	95
10	100

⟸ Median (between rank 5 and 6)

Since the number of QoL observations, $n = 10$, is even, then there is no unique middle value that splits the data set into two halves. Therefore the median QoL is the average of the 5th and 6th ordered observations i.e. $(62 + 72)/2 = 67.0$. ☐

The median is not sensitive to the behaviour of outlying data, thus if the smallest value was even smaller, or the largest value even bigger, it would have no impact on the value of the median. So, for example, the median in the data would be unaffected by replacing '25' with '1'. However, it is not statistically efficient, as it does not make use of all the individual data values.

6.3.1.3   Mode

A third measure of location is termed the *mode*. This is the value that occurs most frequently, or, if the data are grouped, the grouping with the highest frequency. It is not used much in statistical analysis, since its value depends on the accuracy with which the data are measured; although it may be useful for categorical data to describe the most frequent category.

The mode can be an appropriate summary measure for QoL data, since many QoL outcomes are typically scored in discrete categories. For example, the Role Physical dimension of the first version of the SF-36 is scored on a 0–100 scale but it can actually only take five possible discrete values of 0, 25, 50, 75 or 100. However, the mode is rarely used in summarizing QoL outcomes as it not very amenable to statistical analysis.

Example: Modal General Health for male cancer survivors and controls

The dot plots of the General Health data in Figure 6.2 show that the mode is 87 for the 213 male controls and 82 for the 171 male cancer survivors. ☐

Generally the most useful measure of the central value of a set of data is the mean. It is calculated as the sum of all observations divided by the total number of observations. Each observation makes a contribution to the mean value and thus it is sensitive to the behaviour of outlying data: as the largest value increases this causes the mean value to increase, and conversely, as the value of the smallest observation becomes smaller the value of the mean decreases.

Both the mean and median can be useful, but they can give very different impressions when the distribution of the data is skewed, because of the relative contributions (or lack of, in the case of the median) of the extreme values. Skewed data are data that are not symmetrical. This is best illustrated by examining the shape of the histogram for General Health for the control subjects (Figure 6.3). There are few observations at lower levels of QoL, whilst the majority of observations are clustered at the higher levels of QoL. This is described as being negatively skewed, as there is a long left-hand tail at lower values. Data which have a long right-hand tail of higher values, but where the majority of observations are clustered at lower values are called positively skewed. There are no firm rules about which to use, but when the distribution is not skew it is usual to use the mean. However, if data are skew then it is better to use the median, as this is not influenced by the extreme values and may not be as misleading as the mean.

Means and medians convey different impressions of the location of data, and one cannot give a prescription as to which is preferable; often both give useful information. If the distribution is symmetric, then in general the mean is the better summary statistic, and if it is skewed then the median is less influenced by the tails. If the data are skewed, then the median will reflect the QoL of a 'typical' individual better.

6.3.2   Measures of spread

In addition to finding measures to describe the location of a data set, it is also necessary to be able to describe its spread. Just as with the measures of location, there are both simple and more complex possibilities.

6.3.2.1   Range

The simplest is the *range* of the data, from the smallest to the largest observation. The advantage of the range is that it is easily calculated, but its drawback is that it is vulnerable to outliers, extremely large and extremely small observations. Most QoL instruments have a bounded range of scores, that is, a maximum and minimum value, dependent on how subjects respond to the individual items in the questionnaire. For example, the dimensions of the SF-36 have a possible range of 0–100.

Example: Range of SF-36 General Health scores for male cancer survivors and controls

The dot plots of the General Health data in Figure 6.2 show that the range is 5–100 for the 213 male controls and 0–100 for the 171 male cancer survivors.

The theoretical minimum and maximum values for the SF-36 General Health dimension are 0 and 100, respectively. Hence none of the controls had a General Health score of 0.   □

6.3.2.2 Interquartile range

A more useful measure is to take the median value as discussed above and further divide the two halves of the data into halves again. These values are called the quartiles and the difference between the upper quartile (or 75th percentile) and lower quartile (or 25th percentile) is the *interquartile range* (IQR). The lower quartile is the observation below which the bottom 25% of the data lie, and the upper quartile is the observation above which the top 25% of the data lie. The middle 50% of the data lie between these limits. Unlike the range, it is not sensitive to the extreme values.

Example: Calculation of range, quartiles and interquartile range

Suppose we had 10 General Health QoL scores arranged in increasing order from the Greenfield *et al.*, (2007) study.

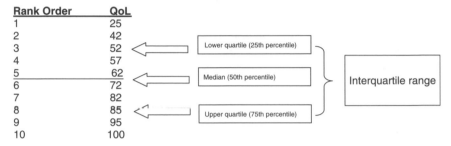

The range of QoL scores in these data is from 25 to 100 (simply the smallest and largest General Health scores).

The median is the average of the 5th and 6th observations $(62 + 72)/2 = 67$. The first half of the data has five observations so the lower quartile is the 3rd ranked observation, namely 52, and similarly the upper quartile would be the 8th ranked observation, namely 85. So the interquartile range is $85 - 52 = 33$.

The range (minimum and maximum values), median, quartiles and interquartile range can be shown on a box-and-whisker plot. Figure 6.5 shows the IQR for the General Health dimension of the SF-36 for the male cancer survivors is $82 - 42 = 40$. Strictly speaking the range and IQR are single numbers, but frequently the two values, minimum and maximum, or the 25% and 75% percentiles respectively, are reported as this can be more informative.   □

6.3.2.3 Standard deviation and variance

However, the most common measure of the spread of the data is the *standard deviation*. It provides a summary of the differences of each observation from the mean value. The standard deviation has units on the same scale as the original measurement, which is the case of QoL measures is unitless! The standard deviation (SD or s) is calculated as follows:

$$\text{SD} = s = \sqrt{\frac{\sum_{i=1}^{n} (x_i - \bar{x})^2}{n - 1}}.$$

The expression $\sum_{i=1}^{n} (x_i - \bar{x})^2$ may look complicated, but it is easier to understand when thought of in stages. From each x-value subtract the mean $\bar{x}$, square this difference, then add each of the n squared differences. This sum is then divided by $(n-1)$. This expression is known as the *variance*. The variance is expressed in square units, so we take the square root to return to the original units, which give the standard deviation, s. Examining this expression, it can be seen that if all the x-values were the same, then they would equal $\bar{x}$ and so s would be zero. If the x-values were widely scattered about $\bar{x}$, then s would be large. In this way s reflects the variability in the data. The standard deviation is vulnerable to outliers, so if the 100 was replaced by 1 we would get a very different result.

Example: Calculation of the standard deviation

Consider the following 10 QoL scores on the General Health dimension of the SF-36: 25, 42, 52, 57, 62, 72, 82, 85, 95, 100. The calculations to work out the standard deviation are given in Table 6.1.

We first find the mean QoL to be 67.2, then subtract this from each of the ten individual QoL observations in the sample to get the 'differences from the mean'. Note that the sum of this column is zero. This will always be the case: the positive deviations from the mean cancel the negative ones. A convenient method of removing the negative signs is by squaring the deviations, as given in the next column, which is then summed to get 5185.6. Note that around one third of this sum (34%) is contributed by one observation, the value

Table 6.1 Calculating the standard deviation of a set of QoL scores.

Subject	i	QoL x_i	Mean QoL $\bar{x}$	Differences from mean $x_i - x$	Square of differences from mean $(x_i - \bar{x})^2$
	1	25	67.2	−42.20	1780.84
	2	42	67.2	−25.20	635.04
	3	52	67.2	−15.20	231.04
	4	57	67.2	−10.20	104.04
	5	62	67.2	−5.20	27.04
	6	72	67.2	4.80	23.04
	7	82	67.2	14.80	219.04
	8	85	67.2	17.80	316.84
	9	95	67.2	27.80	772.84
	10	100	67.2	32.80	1075.84
Totals (sum)		672		0.00	5185.60
Mean		67.2		**Variance**	576.2 ⟵ Variance = 5185.6/9
n		10		**Standard deviation**	24.0
n − 1		9			⇧ SD = square root of the variance

25 from subject 1, which is the observation furthest from the mean. This illustrates that much of the value of a standard deviation is derived from the outlying observations. We now need to find the average squared deviation. Common sense would suggest dividing by n, but it turns out that this actually gives an estimate of the population variance which is too small. This is because we use the estimated mean $\bar{x}$ in the calculation in place of the true population mean. In fact we seldom know the population mean so there is little choice but for us to use its estimated value, $\bar{x}$, in the calculation. The consequence is that it is then better to divide by what are known as the *degrees of freedom*, which in this case is $n - 1$, to obtain the standard deviation.   □

As with the measures of location, when deciding which measure of spread to present it is necessary to know whether the data are skewed or not and this will also have a bearing on how the data will be analysed subsequently, as will be seen later on in this chapter. When the distribution is not skewed it is usual to use the standard deviation. However, if data are skewed then it is better to use the range or interquartile range.

6.4   Presenting quality of life data and results in tables and graphs

Some basic graphs for displaying QoL data were described in Section 6.2. As stated, plotting data can be a useful first stage to any analysis as this will show extreme observations together with any interesting patterns. Graphs are useful as they can be read quickly, and are particularly helpful when presenting information to an audience such as at a seminar or conference. Although there are no hard and fast rules about when to use a graph and when to use a table, when presenting the results in a report or a paper it is often best to use tables so that the reader can scrutinize the numbers directly. Tables can be useful for displaying information about many variables at once, whilst graphs can be useful for showing multiple observations on groups or individuals (such as a dot plot or a histogram). As with graphs, there are a few basic rules of good practice when presenting data in tables (see Box 6.3; Freeman *et al.*, 2008).

6.4.1   Tables for summarizing QoL outcomes

Data on continuous variables, such as QoL, can be summarized using a measure of central tendency or location along with a measure of spread or variability (Campbell *et al.*, 2007). If the QoL measurements have a symmetric distribution then the mean and standard deviation are the preferred summary statistics. Alternatively, if the QoL measurements have a skewed distribution then the median and a percentile range, such as the IQR, are the preferred summary statistics.

The Greenfield *et al.*, (2007) cross-sectional study of young male cancer survivors also recorded the type of cancer the patient was diagnosed with. Table 6.2 reports mean self-reported QoL, as measured by the SF-36 General Health dimension, by cancer types. In Table 6.2 the rows (cancer type) have been placed in descending numerical order of mean General Heath, with the best QoL, for leukaemia patients, presented first. The table has a title explaining what is being displayed and the columns and rows are clearly labelled. As with Table 6.2, the sample size for each cancer type group is reported in the

---

Box 6.3 Summary of good practice when presenting data in tables

1. The amount of information should be maximized for the minimum amount of ink.

2. Numerical precision should be consistent throughout a paper or presentation, as far as possible.

3. Avoid spurious accuracy. Bear in mind the precision of the original data. Numbers should be rounded to two effective digits.

4. The number of observations on which the data being presented are based should always be displayed.

5. Quantitative data should be summarized using either the mean and standard deviation (for symmetrically distributed data) or the median and IQR or range (for skewed data). The number of observations on which these summary measures are based should be included for each result in the table.

6. Categorical data should be summarized as frequencies and percentages. As with quantitative data, the number of observations should be included.

7. Tables should have a title explaining what is being displayed and columns and rows should be clearly labelled.

8. Gridlines in tables should be kept to a minimum.

9. Rows and columns should be ordered by size (if there is no natural ordering).

---

final column of the table as this improves the table's readability. It is good practice to put the variable of most interest, in this table the mean, in the first data column as it can be immediately read with its associated group label. The footnote to the table also explains how the SF-36 is scaled. The units and scale of QoL may be unfamiliar to many readers (unlike other outcomes such as birthweight) and the footnote helps in the understanding and interpretation of the mean SF-36 dimension scores. Most QoL measures generate a scale or scores that have no natural units and have varying scale ranges: for some a high score implies good QoL and for others a high score implies poor QoL. With outcomes with unfamiliar scales or units of measurement it is recommended to add a footnote to tables, explaining the scale of measurement to help interpretation of the data presented.

Alternatively, if an initial graphical examination (e.g. histograms or dot plots) of the data in Table 6.2 showed that the distribution of QoL outcome was skewed in all four cancer types then the median and quartiles could replace the mean and standard deviation as the most appropriate summary measures for the data. It is common that some groups will have fairly symmetric QoL data and others will have skewed QoL data. In these circumstances a practical or pragmatic decision will have to be made to use either the mean (and standard deviation) or the median (and quartiles) as the summary measures for the groups and not a mixture of both. My own preference, in these circumstances,

Table 6.2 Self-reported QoL, SF-36 General Health, by cancer type for $n = 171$ men aged 20–45 (data from Greenfield et al., 2007).

		SF-36v2 General Health*		
		Mean	(SD)	n
Cancer type				
	Leukaemia	73.7	(21.1)	11
	Germ cell (testicular)	69.2	(23.4)	66
	Other	61.9	(26.1)	24
	Lymphoma	55.5	(24.2)	70
Total		62.9	(24.7)	171

*The SF-36 General Health outcome is measured on a 0 (poor QoL) to 100 (good) scale.

Table 6.3 Self-reported QoL, SF-36 General Health, by cancer type and testosterone level for $n = 171$ male cancer survivors aged 20–45 (data from Greenfield et al., 2007).

	Testosterone level					
	Normal ($> = 10$ nmol/l) SF-36v2 General Health*			Low (<10 nmol/l) SF-36v2 General Health*		
	Mean	(SD)	n	Mean	(SD)	n
Cancer type						
Lymphoma	57.7	(23.2)	60	42.7	(27.9)	10
Germ cell (testicular)	72.0	(21.7)	57	51.1	(27.4)	9
Other	64.9	(26.3)	21	41.3	(12.9)	3
Leukaemia	71.9	(23.1)	9	82.0	(.0)	2
Total	65.1	(23.8)	147	49.0	(26.5)	24

*The SF-36 General Health outcome is measured on a 0 (poor QoL) to 100 (good) scale.

is to report the mean (and standard deviation), as this is what most authors do in the literature (Fairclough, 2002; Fayers and Machin, 2007).

In many studies, comparisons are made between different groups. For example, two groups of patients may be given different treatments and the outcomes compared between these treatment groups. Table 6.3 shows an example of a more complex table with three variables: QoL (the outcome variable in this case); and two categorical variables or factors, testosterone level (normal or low) and cancer type. The QoL outcome, SF-36 General Health, is cross-classified by testosterone level and cancer type. In this example cancer type is ordered by the combined sample size for each cancer type.

6.4.2   Tables for multiple outcome measures

Many QoL measures have several or multiple dimensions. For example, the SF-36 contains 36 questions measuring health across eight dimensions, as described in Section 1.3: Physical Functioning; Role Physical; Social Functioning; Vitality; Bodily Pain; Mental Health; Role Emotional; and General Health. These eight dimensions are usually regarded as a continuous outcome and are scored on a 0–100 scale, where 100 indicates good health.

Table 6.4 Mean (SD) scores and samples sizes, for the eight dimensions of the SF-36 by age, $n = 5841$ (data from Walters *et al.*, 2001a)) *.

		Age (years)					Group Total
		65–69	70–74	75–79	80–84	85+	
Social Functioning	*Mean*	78.2	75.1	69.6	61.0	48.9	70.9
	SD	(28.4)	(29.8)	(31.1)	(33.1)	(32.8)	(31.5)
	n	1641	1720	1274	746	460	5841
Mental Health	*Mean*	72.2	71.7	70.4	67.8	65.9	70.6
	SD	(20.3)	(19.8)	(19.5)	(20.2)	(21.1)	(20.1)
	n	1641	1720	1274	746	460	5841
Bodily Pain	*Mean*	66.4	63.2	61.5	55.3	53.4	62.0
	SD	(27.7)	(27.8)	(28.5)	(28.6)	(29.4)	(28.5)
	n	1641	1720	1274	746	460	5841
Role Emotional	*Mean*	65.8	60.0	52.8	45.5	42.8	56.9
	SD	(42.4)	(43.8)	(44.7)	(44.3)	(45.8)	(44.5)
	n	1641	1720	1274	746	460	5841
Physical Functioning	*Mean*	65.4	59.5	52.6	42.0	27.6	54.9
	SD	(28.9)	(29.7)	(29.7)	(30.0)	(26.4)	(31.2)
	n	1641	1720	1274	746	460	5841
General Health	*Mean*	57.8	56.6	54.7	49.5	46.5	54.8
	SD	(24.1)	(23.6)	(22.9)	(23.2)	(21.4)	(23.6)
	n	1641	1720	1274	746	460	5841
Vitality	*Mean*	56.6	53.8	50.6	44.7	39.0	51.5
	SD	(23.1)	(22.5)	(21.9)	(22.7)	(21.7)	(23.1)
	n	1641	1720	1274	746	460	5841
Role Physical	*Mean*	55.6	46.8	41.2	30.2	25.2	44.2
	SD	(42.7)	(43.0)	(41.8)	(38.4)	(35.8)	(42.6)
	n	1641	1720	1274	746	460	5841

*The dimensions of the SF-36 are scored on a 0 (worst possible health) to 100 (best possible health) scale.

Table 6.4 shows SF-36 data from a postal survey of all patients aged 65 or over registered with 12 general practices. The survey aimed to assess the practicality and validity of using the SF-36 in a community-dwelling population over 65 years old, and obtain population scores in this age group (Walters *et al.*, 2001a). The table displays summary statistics (mean, standard deviation and sample size) for the eight SF-36 dimensions.

The columns contain the ordered age categories and the rows contain the eight SF-36 dimensions. The column variable, age, has a natural ordering so the columns are clearly ordered by the age categories. The row variables (the eight SF-36 dimensions) have no natural ordering; in this example they are ordered by the dimension with the highest overall mean score (Social Functioning).

The table has a title explaining what is being displayed and the columns and rows are clearly labelled. Enclosing the standard deviations in brackets helps distinguish the variability in the QoL data from the mean dimension score. The sample size for each age group is reported beneath the standard deviation. As the SF-36 dimensions are scored on a 0–100 scale, the means and SDs for the various dimensions are reported to one decimal place in the table to avoid the spurious numerical precision discussed earlier.

In many studies comparisons are made between different groups. We will now look at ways of tabulating and graphical displaying QoL outcome data when comparing two groups.

6.4.3   Tables and graphs for comparing two groups

Walters *et al.*, (2001a) report the results of a general population survey of 9700 residents of Sheffield, UK. The aim of this cross-sectional survey was to estimate the self-reported QoL, as measured by the SF-36, of Sheffield residents. In this study a comparison was also made between the QoL of men and women. The mean SF-36 dimension scores of people aged 16–101, by gender, are shown in Table 6.5. Data for the two genders are arranged in the columns; the rows correspond to the eight SF-36 dimensions, and are ordered by mean difference. The mean dimension scores (and their variability) are described separately for each group. A 95% confidence interval for the difference in mean scores, between the genders, is also reported. *P*-values are given in the last column of the table. A footnote to the table is included describing how the SF-36 is scaled and scored, what hypothesis test has been performed and how the mean difference should be interpreted. Since the SF-36 is scored on a 0–100 scale these data are reported to a precision of one decimal place. Note that as the number of observations varies considerably across the eight dimensions a second table could also be produced for those individuals who had data on all dimensions. Further details of how to calculate the mean difference and it associated confidence interval and *P*-value are given in the next chapter.

Table 6.5   Mean SF-36 dimension scores of people aged 16–101, by gender, from a general population survey (data from Walters *et al.*, 2001a).

							Gender Group			
SF-36		Male			Female		Mean			
Dimension[1]	*n*	Mean	(SD)	*n*	Mean	(SD)	Diff[2]	95% CI	*P*-value[3]
Physical Functioning	3767	64.9	(31.3)	4862	55.0	(32.8)	9.9	(8.5 to 11.3)	<0.0001
Role Physical	3936	53.2	(43.5)	5093	45.0	(43.6)	8.2	(6.4 to 10.0)	<0.0002
Role Emotional	3888	63.8	(43.2)	5003	55.7	(44.6)	8.0	(6.2 to 9.9)	<0.0003
Mental Health	3998	74.5	(18.9)	5227	67.1	(20.2)	7.4	(6.5 to 8.2)	<0.0004
Bodily Pain	4074	68.0	(28.0)	5432	61.0	(29.1)	7.0	(5.8 to 8.1)	<0.0005
Social Functioning	4046	75.8	(30.1)	5326	69.3	(31.9)	6.4	(5.2 to 7.7)	<0.0006
Vitality	4012	55.7	(21.7)	5247	49.3	(21.7)	6.4	(5.5 to 7.3)	<0.0007
General Health	3803	58.6	(24.2)	4860	56.1	(23.9)	2.5	(1.5 to 3.6)	<0.0008

CI: Confidence interval
[1] The SF-36 dimensions are scored on a 0 (poor) to 100 (good health) scale.
[2] A positive mean difference indicates that the men have the better QoL than the women.
[3] *P*-value from two independent samples *t*-test.

The SF-36 is also an example of a profile QoL measure since it generates eight separate scores for each dimension of health. The scores on the eight dimensions are not independent – they are linked to the same subject. One way of graphically displaying such data is by a *radar plot* or *spider's web plot*.

Figure 6.7 shows a radar plot for the overall mean SF-36 dimension scores from the survey, by gender, for the data in presented in Table 6.5. The plot has eight spokes corresponding to the eight QoL dimensions of the SF-36, with the centre point of the plot indicating a score of zero. The spokes are linked by lines, which clearly show that the outcomes are related and are not independent. The radar plot in Figure 6.7 clearly shows that the male responders to the survey reported better QoL than the females for all eight dimensions of the SF-36.

Figure 6.7 conceals the fact that the sample size for each dimension varies considerably. We could also report the number of subjects for each outcome. A better strategy is to report the mean scores on the spokes for subjects who have data on all the outcomes. Figure 6.8 shows the radar plot with the mean scores for all 7213 subjects who provided data on all eight dimensions of the SF-36. Figure 6.7 is very similar to Figure 6.8. In this example, it is unlikely that excluding subjects from the analysis will affect the mean dimension scores to any appreciable extent.

The radar plots of Figures 6.7 and 6.8 clearly display the mean SF-36 dimension scores by gender. However, for a randomized controlled trial or any other two-group comparison, what is required is the contrast or difference in outcomes between the groups and the associated uncertainty or confidence interval around this estimated difference or treatment effect.

The mean difference and its associated confidence interval can be shown graphically as in Figure 6.9. Figure 6.9 shows the estimated difference (mean difference in SF-36 scores between the male and female groups) and the corresponding confidence interval, for the eight dimensions of the SF-36 (Walters *et al.*, 2001a). A similar plot to this is

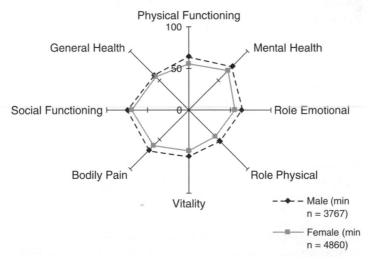

Figure 6.7   Radar plot with mean scores of people aged 16–101, for the eight dimensions of the SF-36, by gender, $n = 9506$, from a general population survey of Sheffield, UK, residents (data from Walters *et al.*, 2001a).

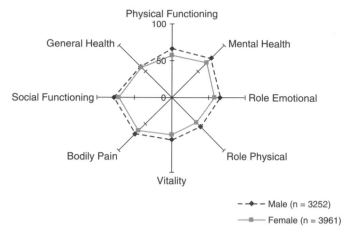

Figure 6.8 Radar plot with mean scores of people aged 16–101, for the eight dimensions of the SF-36, by gender, $n = 7213$, from a general population survey of Sheffield, UK, residents (data from Walters *et al.*, 2001a).

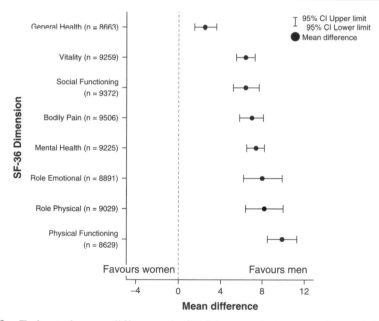

Figure 6.9 Estimated mean difference in SF-36 scores between males and females and the corresponding confidence interval, $n = 9506$, from a general population survey of Sheffield, UK, residents (data from Walters *et al.*, 2001a).

known as a *forest* plot, which is commonly used for displaying the results of systematic reviews and meta-analyses. These are discussed in Freeman *et al.*, (2008).

Figure 6.9 is visually very impressive, and the difference in QoL between males and females across all eight dimensions is readily apparent. It can be useful in conference presentations. However, much of the data present in Table 6.5 is not shown. For example,

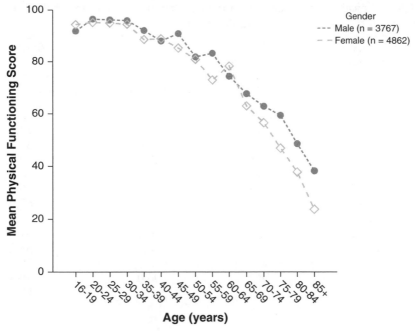

The PF Dimension is scored on a 0 to 100 (good health) scale

Figure 6.10   Profile of mean SF-36 Physical Functioning scores by age and gender (data from Walters *et al.*, 2001a).

the sample size per group and mean SF-36 scores (and their variability) for each group are omitted. These are important results, and this information should be reported. Hence, for presentation in a scientific report or paper, Table 6.5 is preferred.

6.4.4   Profile graphs

The SF-36 data presented in Table 6.5 can be further cross-classified by age or age group. In Table 6.5 the SF-36 dimension scores are combined or aggregated over the whole age range and not reported in separate age groups (as in Table 6.4). The age group and gender data in Tables 6.4 and 6.5 for each SF-36 dimension can be plotted as a series of line graphs (Figure 6.10), with a separate line for each gender group. Figure 6.10 clearly shows how physical functioning declines with age and varies between the genders across all age groups. Since the data are cross-sectional and not longitudinal, it is important that the points are not joined using solid lines, since we are not measuring the same people in each age group. If the study had been longitudinal and the plot had been only for those individuals who had data at each time point/age group it would be legitimate to join the mean physical function scores together with solid lines.

Exercises

6.1 Table 6.6 shows a selection of the clinical and QoL data for a random sample of 15 young male cancer survivors from the Greenfield *et al.*, (2007) study.

Table 6.6   Clinical and QoL data for a random sample of 15 young male cancer survivors from the Greenfield *et al.* (2007) study.

	Testosterone (nmol/l)	Total Body fat mass (kg)	SF-36v2 Physical Functioning (0–100)	SF-36v2 Norm-based (US 1998 popn) scoring: Physical Component Summary
1	9.96	38.8	85.0	52.4
2	11.66	32.9	80.0	38.4
3	13.01	29.0	100.0	59.6
4	14.96	40.7	30.0	34.6
5	16.27	42.8	65.0	45.6
6	17.11	16.5	100.0	62.9
7	17.49	13.0	100.0	60.0
8	19.12	31.9	100.0	61.6
9	19.40	34.3	50.0	33.2
10	19.50	30.4	85.0	50.1
11	20.26	14.5	100.0	58.8
12	21.58	11.1	100.0	59.9
13	21.65	28.4	100.0	53.8
14	21.79	47.9	75.0	46.3
15	27.17	17.6	100.0	58.9

The clinical data include the testosterone levels and total body fat mass and the QoL data consist of the SF-36v2 Physical Functioning dimension and SF-36v2 Physical Component Summary (PCS) score.

(a) Draw a dot plot and a histogram for the SF-36v2 Physical Functioning dimension. Is this distribution symmetric or skewed?

(b) Calculate the mean, median and mode for the SF-36v2 Physical Functioning dimension score. Which of these measures is best at describing the location or central tendency of this data?

(c) Calculate the range, interquartile range and standard deviation for the SF-36v2 Physical Functioning score. Which of these summary measures is better to describe the variability of these data?

6.2 Table 6.6 shows the total body fat mass (in kg) and SF-36v2 PCS score of 15 young male cancer survivors.

(a) Draw a scatter plot of total body fat mass versus SF-36v2 Physical Functioning dimension score.

(b) From the graph does there appear to be a relationship between the two variables?

Table 6.7 Median scores and quartiles, for the eight dimensions of the SF-36 by gender ($n = 7213$).

SF-36 dimension *	Gender					
	Female ($n = 3961$)			Male ($n = 3252$)		
	Median	25th Percentile	75th Percentile	Median	25th Percentile	75th Percentile
Role Emotional	66.7	.0	100.0	100.0	33.3	100.0
Social Functioning	77.8	44.4	100.0	88.9	66.7	100.0
Mental Health	68.0	56.0	84.0	80.0	64.0	92.0
Physical Functioning	65.0	30.0	85.0	75.0	40.0	90.0
Bodily Pain	66.7	44.4	88.9	77.8	44.4	100.0
General Health	60.0	40.0	77.0	62.0	40.0	77.0
Vitality	50.0	35.0	65.0	60.0	45.0	70.0
Role Physical	50.0	.0	100.0	75.0	.0	100.0

*The SF-36 dimensions are scored on a 0 (poor) to 100 (good health) scale.

6.3 Table 6.6 also shows the SF-36v2 Physical Functioning score and SF-36v2 PCS score of 15 young male cancer survivors.

(a) Draw a scatter plot of SF-36v2 Physical Functioning score versus SF-36v2 PCS score.

(b) From the graph does there appear to be a relationship between the two variables?

6.4 Table 6.7 reports the median scores and 25th and 75th percentiles (quartiles) for the eight dimensions of the SF-36 by gender from a general population survey of 7213 Sheffield residents (Walters *et al.*, 2001a).

(a) Use the median summary data presented in Table 6.7 to construct a radar plot of the eight SF-36 dimensions, with a separate line for each gender.

(b) From the graph, does there appear to be a difference in median QoL scores between the two genders?

7

Cross-sectional analysis of quality of life outcomes

Summary

This chapter describes the statistical methods used to compare QoL outcomes between two groups in an observational study or cross-sectional survey where QoL is assessed at a single common time point. It considers the comparison of QoL outcomes for two independent groups, such as men and women, in a cross-sectional survey and the comparison of QoL outcomes for matched pairs of subjects. The chapter ends with a discussion of the use of multiple linear regression to compare QoL outcomes between groups and adjust for potential confounding variables such as age and gender.

7.1 Introduction

It is rarely possible to obtain information on an entire population, and usually data are collected on a sample of individuals from the population of interest. The main aim of statistical analysis is to use the information from the sample to draw conclusions (make inferences) about the population of interest. For example, the study of young male cancer survivors aged 25–45 (Greenfield *et al.*, 2007) was conducted as it was not possible to study all young male cancer survivors. Instead a sample of cancer survivors from a hospital outpatient clinic was recruited along with a control sample of men aged 25–45 years with no history of malignant disease or testosterone therapy. The controls were recruited by advertisement in the community and from general practitioner surgeries by selecting men who fitted the age criteria. This was in order to compare the QoL of young male cancer survivors with a control group of healthy young men of similar age. The two main approaches to statistical analysis, hypothesis testing and estimation, are outlined in the following sections.

Quality of Life Outcomes in Clinical Trials and Health-Care Evaluation   Stephen J. Walters
© 2009 John Wiley & Sons, Ltd

7.2 Hypothesis testing (using *P*-values)

Before examining the different techniques available for analysing data, it is first essential to understand the process of hypothesis testing and its key principles, such as what a *P*-value is and what is meant by the phrase 'statistical significance'. Box 7.1 describes the four main steps in the process of hypothesis testing.

At the outset it is important to have a clear research question and know what the outcome variable to be compared is. Once the research question has been stated, the null and alternative hypotheses can be formulated. The null hypothesis (H_0) assumes that there is no difference in the outcome of interest between the study groups, in the population. The study or alternative hypothesis (H_A) states that there is a difference between the study groups, in the population. In general, the direction of the difference (e.g. that treatment A is better than treatment B) is not specified.

For the survey of QoL of young male cancer survivors and their controls, the research question of interest is: do young male cancer survivors, aged 25–45, have a different QoL (as measured by the SF-36 General Health dimension) than young men of a similar age with no history of cancer? The null hypothesis is:

> H_0: There is no difference in QoL between the cancer survivors and control group.

The alternative hypothesis is:

> H_A: There is a difference in QoL between the cancer survivors and control group.

Having set the null and alternative hypotheses, the next stage is to carry out a significance test. This is done by first calculating a test statistic using the study data. This test statistic is then used to obtain a *P*-value. For the comparison above, Table 7.1 shows that patients in the cancer survivor group had, on average, a 14.4 point lower SF-36 General

---

Box 7.1 Hypothesis testing – the main steps

1. State your *null hypothesis* (H_0), the statement you are looking for evidence to disprove.
   State your *alternative hypothesis* (H_A).

2. Choose a *significance level* (α) for the test.

3. Conduct the study, collect the data, observe the outcome and compute the probability of observing your results, or results more extreme, if the null hypothesis is true (*P*-value).

4. Use your *P*-value to make a decision about whether to reject, or not reject, your null hypothesis. That is, if the *P*-value is less than or equal to α, conclude that the data are not consistent with the null hypothesis; if the *P*-value is greater than α, do not reject the null hypothesis, and view it as 'not yet disproved'.

Table 7.1   Computer output from the two independent samples *t*-test.

Group Statistics					
	Group	*n*	Mean	SD	SE
SF-36v2 General Health	Cancer survivors	171	62.9	24.7	1.9
	Controls	213	77.3	16.5	62.9

> The standard deviations for the two groups are different, but the ratio of the two SDs is less than 2.

Independent samples *t*-test

			t-test for Equality of Means					
	t	*df*	*P*-value	Mean difference	SE difference	95% Confidence Interval of the difference	
						Lower	Upper
SF-36v2 General Health (0-100)	−6.815	382	<0.001	−14.4	2.1	−18.6	−10.3

> The *P*-value is <0.001. Thus the results are unlikely when the null hypothesis (that there is no difference between the groups) is true. The result is said to be statistically significant because the *P*-value is less than the significance level (α) set at 5% or 0.05 and there is sufficient evidence to reject the null hypothesis and accept the alternative hypothesis, that there is a difference in mean General Health between the Cancer Survivors and Control groups.

Health dimension score than the control group mean and the *P*-value associated with this difference was less than 0.001.

The final and most crucial stage of hypothesis testing is to make a decision based upon the *P*-value. In order to do this it is necessary to understand first what a *P*-value is and what it is not, and then understand how to use it to make a decision about whether to reject or not reject the null hypothesis.

So what does a *P*-value mean? A *P*-value is the probability of obtaining the study results (or results more extreme) if the null hypothesis is true. Common misinterpretations of the *P*-value are that it is either the probability of the data having arisen by chance or the probability that the observed effect is not a real one. The distinction between these incorrect definitions and the true definition is the absence of the phrase 'if the null hypothesis is true'. The omission of 'if the null hypothesis is true' leads to the incorrect belief that it is possible to evaluate the probability of the observed effect being a real one. The observed effect in the sample is genuine, but what is true in the population is not known. All that can be known with a *P*-value is, if there truly is no difference in the population, how likely is the result obtained (from the study data).

It is important to remember that a *P*-value is a probability and its value can vary between 0 and 1. A 'small' *P*-value, say close to zero, indicates that the results obtained are unlikely when the null hypothesis is true and the null hypothesis is rejected. Alternatively, if the *P*-value is 'large', then the results obtained are likely when the null hypothesis is true and the null hypothesis is not rejected. But how small is small? Conventionally the cut-off value or significance level for declaring that a particular result is statistically significant is set at 0.05 (or 5%). Thus if the P-value is less than this value the null hypothesis (of no difference) is rejected and the result is said to be statistically significant at the 5% or 0.05 level (Box 7.2). For the example above, of the difference in SF-36 General Health scores between cancer survivors and controls, the P-value is less than 0.001. As this is less than the cut-off value of 0.05 there is said to be a statistically significant difference in General Health, as measured by the SF-36, between the two groups at the 5% level.

Though the decision to reject or not reject the null hypothesis may seem clear-cut, it is possible that a mistake may be made, as can be seen from the shaded cells of Box 7.3. Whatever is decided, this decision may correctly reflect what is true in the population: the null hypothesis is rejected when it is in fact false, or the null hypothesis is not rejected, when in fact it is true. Alternatively, it may not reflect what is true in the population: the

---

Box 7.2 Statistical significance

	P-value ≤ 0.05	P-value > 0.05
Result is	Statistically significant	Not Statistically significant
Decide	That there is sufficient evidence to reject the null hypothesis and accept the alternative	That there is insufficient evidence to reject the null hypothesis

We cannot say the null hypothesis is true, only that there is not enough evidence to reject it.

Box 7.3 Possible errors arising when performing a hypothesis test

		The null hypothesis is actually:	
		False	True
Decide to:	Reject the null hypothesis	Correct	Type1 error (α) (false positive error)
	Not reject the null hypothesis	Type 2 error (β) (false negative error)	Correct

null hypothesis is rejected when it is in fact true (false positive or Type I error, α); or the null hypothesis is not rejected when it is in fact false (false negative, Type II error, β). Minimizing the probability or chance of Type I or Type II error is one of the key issues when designing and study and is the basis of the sample size equations described in Chapter 4.

The probability that a study will be able to detect a difference, of a given size, if one truly exists is called the *power* of the study and is the probability of rejecting the null hypothesis when it is actually false. It is usually expressed in percentages, so for a study which has 80% power, there is a likelihood of 80% of being able to detect a difference, of a given size, if there genuinely is a difference in the population. This is the basis for most of the sample size calculations outlined in Chapter 4.

7.3   Estimation (using confidence intervals)

Statistical significance does not necessarily mean the result obtained is clinically significant or of any practical importance. A P-value will only indicate how likely the results obtained are when the null hypothesis is true. It can only be used to decide whether the results are statistically significant or not; it does not give any information about the likely size of the effect. Much more information, such as whether the result is likely to be of clinical importance, can be gained by calculating a confidence interval. A confidence interval may be calculated for any estimated quantity (from the sample data), such as the mean, median, proportion, or even a difference, for example the mean difference in QoL between two groups. It is a measure of the precision (accuracy) with which the quantity of interest is estimated (in this case the mean difference in SF-36 General Health dimension scores between the cancer survivors and control groups).

Technically, the 95% confidence interval is the range of values within which the true population quantity would fall 95% of the time if the study were to be repeated many times. Crudely speaking, the confidence interval gives a range of plausible values for the quantity estimated; although not strictly correct, it is usually interpreted as the range of values within which there is 95% certainty that the true value in the population lies. For the cancer survivors example above, the quantity estimated was the mean difference in SF-36 General Heath dimension scores between the cancer survivors and control groups; this was 14.4 points (see Table 7.1). The 95% confidence interval for this difference was 10.3 to 18.6 points. Thus, whilst the best available estimate of the mean difference was 14.4, it could be as low as 10.3 or as high as 18.6, with 95% certainty. The P-value associated with this difference was less than 0.001, and in the previous section it was concluded that this difference was statistically significant at the 5% level. Whilst the P-value will give an indication of whether the result obtained is statistically significant, it gives no other information; the confidence interval is more informative as it gives a range of plausible values for the estimated quantity. Provided this range does not include the value for no difference (in this case 0), it can be concluded that there is a difference between the groups being compared. In this example, the cancer survivors had significantly worse general health than the control group subjects.

Box 7.4 What type of statistical test? Five key questions to ask

1. What are the aims and objectives of the study?

2. What is the hypothesis to be tested?

3. What type of data are the outcome data?

4. How are the outcome data distributed?

5. What is the summary measure for the outcome data?

Box 7.5 Three common problems in statistical inference

1. Comparison of independent groups, e.g. groups of patients given different treatments.

2. Comparison of the response for paired observations, e.g. in a cross-over trial, or for matched pairs of subjects.

3. Investigation of the relationship between two variables measured on the same sample of subjects.

7.4   Choosing the statistical method

The type of statistical analysis chosen depends on the answers to five key questions (Box 7.4). It depends fundamentally on what the main purpose of the study is, and, in particular, on the main question to be answered. The data type for the outcome variable will also govern how it is to be analysed, as an analysis appropriate to continuous data would be completely inappropriate for binary data. In addition to what type of data the outcome variable is, its distribution is important, as is the summary measure to be used. Highly skewed data require a different analysis compared to data which are Normally distributed.

The choice of method of analysis for a problem depends on the comparison to be made and the data to be used. The rest of this chapter outlines the methods appropriate for the three most common problems in statistical inference as outlined in Box 7.5. However, before beginning any analysis it is important to examine the data, using the techniques described earlier in Chapter 6. Adequate description of the data should precede and complement the formal statistical analysis. For most studies and for randomized controlled trials in particular, it is good practice to produce a table or tables that describe the initial or baseline characteristics of the sample.

7.5   Comparison of two independent groups

Before comparing two independent groups it is important to decide what type of data the outcome is and how it is distributed, as this will determine the most appropriate analysis. This section describes, for different types of data, the statistical methods available for comparing two independent groups, as outlined in Figure 7.1.

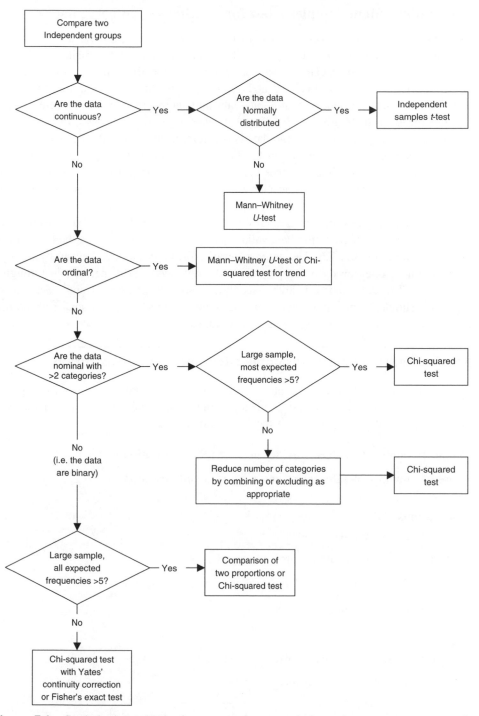

Figure 7.1 Statistical methods for comparing two independent groups or samples. Reproduced with permission from Campbell, M.J., Machin, D., Walters, S.J., *Medical Statistics: A Text Book for the Health Sciences*. 4th edition. John Wiley & Sons Ltd, Chichester. © 2007 John Wiley & Sons Ltd.

7.5.1   Independent samples t-test for continuous outcome data

The independent samples t-test is used to test for a difference in the mean value of a continuous variable between two groups. For example, one of the main questions of interest in the young male cancer survivors study was whether there was a difference in QoL between the cancer survivors and control groups. If we assume that the SF-36 General Health scale produces continuous data and there are two independent groups, assuming the data are Normally distributed in each of the two groups, then the most appropriate summary measure for the data is the sample mean and the best comparative summary measure is the difference in the mean SF-36 General Health scores between the two groups. In these circumstances Figure 7.1 would suggest using the independent samples t-test to compare the SF-36 General Health dimension scores between the two groups.

When conducting any statistical analysis it is important to check that the assumptions which underpin the chosen method are valid. The assumptions underlying the two-sample t-test are outlined in Box 7.6. The assumption of Normality can be checked by plotting two histograms, one for each sample; these do not need to be perfect, just roughly symmetrical. The two standard deviations should also be calculated and as a rule of thumb, one should be no more than twice the other. At this stage, we shall assume that the outcome is Normally distributed in both groups.

Box 7.6   Independent two-sample t-test for comparing means

Suppose that we wish to test the null hypothesis, H_0, that the means from two populations, estimated from two independent samples, are equal, against the alternative hypothesis, H_A, that the population means are not equal.

Sample 1: number of subjects n_1, mean $\bar{x}_1$, standard deviation s_1.

Sample 2: number of subjects n_2, mean $\bar{x}_2$, standard deviation s_2.

Assumptions
1. The groups are independent.
2. The variables of interest are continuous.
3. The data in both groups have similar standard deviations.
4. The data is Normally distributed in both groups.

Steps
1. First calculate the mean difference between groups $\bar{x}_1 - \bar{x}_2$.
2. Calculate the pooled standard deviation

$$\text{pooled SD} = \sqrt{\frac{(n_1 - 1)s_1^2 + (n_2 - 1)s_2^2}{n_1 + n_2 - 2}}.$$

3. Then calculate the standard error of the difference between two means $SE(\bar{x}_1 - \bar{x}_2) = $ pooled $SD \times \sqrt{\frac{1}{n_1} + \frac{1}{n_2}}$.

4. Calculate the test statistic

$$t = \frac{\bar{x}_1 - \bar{x}_2}{SE(\bar{x}_1 - \bar{x}_2)}.$$

5. Compare the test statistic with the t distribution with $n_1 + n_2 - 2$ degrees of freedom. This gives us the probability of the observing the test statistic t or a more extreme value under the null hypothesis.

6. The $100(1 - \alpha)\%$ confidence interval for the mean difference in the population is:

$$(\bar{x}_1 - \bar{x}_2) - [t_{df,\alpha} \times SE(\bar{x}_1 - \bar{x}_2)] \text{ to } (\bar{x}_1 - \bar{x}_2) + [t_{df,\alpha} \times SE(\bar{x}_1 - \bar{x}_2)],$$

where $t_{df,\alpha}$ is taken from the t distribution with $df = n_1 + n_2 - 2$.

In this example a suitable null hypothesis is that there is no difference in mean SF-36 General Health dimension scores between the cancer survivors and control groups, that is, $\mu_{\text{Cancer\_survivors}} - \mu_{\text{Control}} = 0$ (note that this refers to the difference in the population). The alternative hypothesis is that there is a difference in mean SF-36 General Health dimension scores between the cancer survivors and control groups, i.e. $\mu_{\text{Cancer\_survivors}} - \mu_{\text{Control}} \neq 0$.

The summary statistics for the SF-36 General Health dimension for the cancer survivors and control groups are shown in the top half of the computer output in Table 7.1. We have a mean difference between the groups, $\bar{x}_1 - \bar{x}_2 = 62.9 - 77.3 = -14.4$ and the standard error of this mean difference is $SE(\bar{x}_1 - \bar{x}_2) = 2.1$. In this example the degrees of freedom are $df = n_1 + n_2 - 2$ or $171 + 213 - 2 = 382$. The test or t statistic is $t = -14.4/2.1 = -6.815$. This value is then compared to values of the t distribution with $df - 383$. From Table B.2 in Appendix B, the closest tabulated value is with $df = 30$ but with such large df we can use the final row of the table which has infinite degrees of freedom, suggesting a P-value less than 0.001. This is clearly less than 0.05. The computer output in Table 7.1 shows that the P-value is < 0.001.

The $100(1 - \alpha)\%$ confidence interval for the mean difference in the population is

$$(\bar{x}_1 - \bar{x}_2) - [t_{df,\alpha} \times SE(\bar{x}_1 - \bar{x}_2)] \text{ to } (\bar{x}_1 - \bar{x}_2) + [t_{df,\alpha} \times SE(\bar{x}_1 - \bar{x}_2)],$$

where $t_{df,\alpha}$ is taken from the t distribution with $df = n_1 + n_2 - 2$. For a 95% CI $t_{383,0.05} = 1.960$. Thus the 95% CI for the mean difference is from $-14.4 - (1.960 \times 2.1)$ to $14.4 + (1.960 \times 2.1)$ or from -18.6 to -10.3.

Table 7.1 shows the computer output for comparing general health between the two groups using the two independent samples t-test. It can be seen that there is a significant difference between the groups; the 95% CI for the difference suggests that that patients in the cancer survivor group have between -18.6 and -10.3 poorer or worse general health, as measured by the SF-36, than subjects in the control group and the best estimate is a mean difference of -14.4 points.

When conducting any statistical analysis it is important to check that the assumptions which underpin the chosen method are valid. For the two independent samples t-test, the assumption that the outcome is Normally distributed in each group can be checked by plotting two histograms, one for each sample. Figure 6.2 in the previous chapter shows two histograms for the SF-36 General Health dimension outcome. The outcome in both groups is clearly not Normally distributed and both distributions appear negatively skewed. Hence in these circumstances it looks like the two-independent samples t-test is not the most appropriate test. The flow diagram of Figure 7.1 suggests that the Mann–Whitney U-test may be a more suitable alternative.

Example: Two independent samples t-test

Akehurst *et al.* (2002) used the two independent samples t-test to compare QoL, as measured by the SF-36, between a group of primary care patients with irritable bowel syndrome (IBS) and a control group of non-IBS patients of similar age, gender and social status. Table 7.2 gives the mean SF-36 dimension score for each group, the mean difference and its associated confidence interval and P-value. The differences on all eight dimensions were statistically significant, with IBS patients reporting lower or worse QoL than the control group. The SF-36 data presented in Table 7.2 could also be presented as a radar plot or forest plot as described in Chapter 6.   □

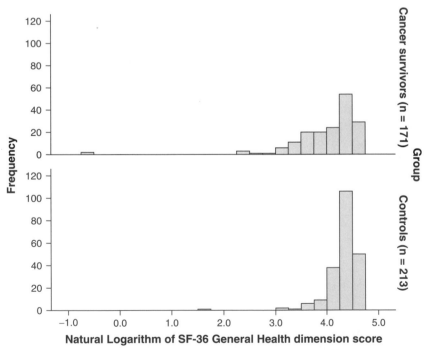

Figure 7.2 Histogram of the natural logarithm of SF-36 General Health by group for 384 men aged 25–45 (data from Greenfield *et al.*, 2007).

Table 7.2 Comparison of IBS sample and control group SF-36 scores at baseline (data from Akehurst *et al.*, 2002).

SF-36 dimension[1]	IBS sample			Control group			Mean difference[2]	95% CI	P-value[3]
	n	Mean	SD	n	Mean	SD			
Physical Functioning	151	74.9	27.1	208	83.3	23.1	−8.1	(−13.5 to −3.1)	0.002
Social Functioning	158	69.9	26.5	210	83.2	23.8	−13.3	(−18.5 to −8.2)	0.001
Role Physical	154	52.3	43.4	209	78.1	37.1	−25.8	(−34.2 to −17.5)	0.001
Role Emotional	154	60.8	41.8	210	76.4	37.1	−15.5	(−23.7 to −7.4)	0.001
Bodily Pain	158	52.1	24.1	211	73.4	25.2	−21.3	(−26.4 to −16.2)	0.001
Mental Health	155	60.7	19.7	209	72.1	19.2	−11.4	(−15.4 to −7.4)	0.001
Vitality	158	42.7	22.1	209	57.4	20.6	−14.7	(−19.1 to −10.3)	0.001
General Health	156	51.9	23.3	207	71.6	21.2	−19.6	(−24.3 to −15.0)	0.001

SD = standard deviation; CI = confidence interval
[1] The SF-36 is scored on a 0 (poor health) to 100 (good health) scale.
[2] A negative mean difference indicates the IBS group had a worse QoL than the control group.
[3] P-value from independent samples *t*-test

7.5.2 Mann–Whitney U-test

There are several possible approaches when at least one of the requirements for the t-test is not met. The data may be transformed (e.g. the logarithm transformation can be useful particularly when the variances are not equal) or a non-parametric method can be used. Non-parametric or distribution-free methods do not involve making assumptions about the manner in which the data are distributed (e.g. that the data are Normally distributed). An important point to note is that it is the test that is parametric or non-parametric, not the data.

As many QoL variables have skewed distributions, they may require a mathematical transformation to make the data appropriate for analysis. In such circumstances the natural logarithmic (log) transformation is often applicable. The SF-36, in common with many other QoL outcomes, is scored on a 0 to 100 scale. Unfortunately, the natural logarithm of 0 does not exist. Therefore other transformations (such as the square root or reciprocal) may be more suitable. Alternatively, a practical solution is to add a small constant, say 0.5, to all the raw QoL data and then take the natural logarithm of this data. After analysis it is desirable to convert the results back into the original scale for reporting. If a transformation is used it is important to check that the desired effect (such as an approximately Normal distribution) is achieved.

Figure 7.2 shows the results of adding 0.5 to the individual SF-36 General Health data and taking the natural logarithm of this new value. Figure 7.2 clearly shows that sometimes taking natural logarithms does not make QoL data more symmetric or Normally distributed. In my experience of analysing QoL data this is fairly common, and transforming QoL data, which have a skewed distribution, rarely makes them more symmetric. So if you are really worried about the assumptions of the parametric tests, such as the t-test, then my practical advice is use a non-parametric test on the raw untransformed QoL data.

When the assumptions underlying the t-test are not met, then the non-parametric equivalent, the Mann–Whitney U-test, may be used. There are two derivations of the test, one due to Wilcoxon and the other to Mann and Whitney. It is better to call the method the Mann–Whitney U-test in order to avoid confusion with the paired test due to Wilcoxon.

The Mann–Whitney test (see Box 7.7) requires all the observations to be ranked as if they were from a single sample. We can now use two alternative test statistics, U and W. The statistic W (due to Wilcoxon) is simply the sum of the ranks in the smaller group and is easier to calculate by hand. The statistic U (due to Mann and Whitney) is more complicated. U is the number of all possible pairs of observations comprising one from each sample for which the value in the first group precedes a value in the second group.

Whilst the independent samples t-test is specifically a test of the null hypothesis that the groups have the same mean value, the Mann–Whitney U-test is a more general test of the null hypothesis that the distribution of the outcome variable in the two groups is the same; it is possible for the outcome data in the two groups to have similar measures of central tendency or location, such as mean and medians, but different distributions.

Examining the output from the Mann–Whitney U-test in Table 7.3, there is sufficient evidence to reject the null hypothesis and accept the alternative hypothesis that there is a difference in General Health between the cancer survivors and control groups.

Box 7.7 Mann–Whitney U-test

Suppose we wish to test the null hypothesis that two samples or groups have the same distribution in the population (i.e. they come from the same population), against the alternative hypothesis that the two groups have different distributions in the population. The data are at least ordinal and from two independent groups of size n_1 and n_2, respectively.

Assumptions

1. The groups are independent.

2. The variables of interest are at least ordinal (i.e. can be ranked).

Steps

1. Combine the two groups and rank the entire data set of $N(= n_1 + n_2)$ values in increasing order (smallest observation to the largest) from 1 to N. If some of the observations are numerically equal, they are given tied ranks equal to the mean of the ranks which would otherwise have been used.

2. Sum the ranks for one of the groups. Let W be the sum of the ranks for the n_1 observations in this group.

3. If there are no ties or only a few ties, calculate the test statistic

$$z = \frac{W - \dfrac{n_1(n_1 + n_2 + 1)}{2}}{\sqrt{\dfrac{n_1 n_2 (n_1 + n_2 + 1)}{12}}}.$$

4. Under the null hypothesis that the two samples come from the same population, the test statistic, z, is approximately Normally distributed with mean 0 and standard deviation 1, and can be referred to Table B.1 to calculate a P-value.

Many textbooks give special tables for the Mann–Whitney U-test, when sample sizes are small, that is, when n_1 and n_2 are less than 20. However, the above expression is usually sufficient. The formula is not very accurate if there any many ties in the data. The reader is referred to Armitage et $al.$ (2002) in such situations.

However, this example illustrates that the t-test is very robust to violations of the assumptions of Normality and equal variances, particularly for moderate to large sample sizes, as the P-values and conclusions from both the t-test and Mann–Whitney test are the same, despite the non-Normal distribution of the data.

Example: Mann–Whitney test

Brazier et $al.$ (1999) used the Mann–Whitney test to compare WOMAC pain, stiffness and physical function scores between 65 patients with mild/moderate and 45 patients with

Table 7.3   Computer output from the Mann–Whitney U-test.

Ranks

	Group	n	Mean Rank	Sum of Ranks
SF-36v2 General Health	Controls	213	221.58	47196.50
	Cancer survivors	171	156.28	26723.50
	Total	384		

Test Statistics

	SF-36v2 General Health
Mann-Whitney U	12017.5
Wilcoxon W	26723.5
Z	−5.744
P-value	<0.001

P value: probability of observing the statistic, W or U, under the null hypothesis. As the value of 0.001 is less than the significance level (α) set at 0.05 or 5% this means that the result obtained is unlikely when the null hypothesis is true. Thus there is sufficient evidence to reject the null hypothesis and accept the alternative hypothesis that there is a difference in General Health between the Cancer Survivors and Control groups.

severe knee osteoarthritis in a rheumatology clinic. The P-values for all three tests were less than 0.001. In the paper the authors reported that 'Mean score differences between patients with a clinical assessment of mild/moderate vs. severe disease were highly significant for all three dimensions of the WOMAC questionnaire'. Strictly speaking, as mentioned previously in Box 7.7, the Mann–Whitney test is a test of the null hypothesis that the two samples or groups have the same distribution in the population (i.e. they come from the same population), against the alternative hypothesis that the two groups have different distributions in the population. Otherwise the authors' interpretation of the data is correct.   □

7.6   Comparing more than two groups

The methods outlined above can be extended to more than two groups. For the independent samples t-test, the analogous method for more than two groups is called the analysis of variance (ANOVA) and the assumptions underlying it are similar. The non-parametric equivalent for the method of ANOVA when there are more than two groups is called the Kruskal–Wallis test.

For example, consider the data presented in Table 6.2 on 171 young male cancer survivors. These data were taken from a cross-sectional, observational study of male cancer cases and controls (Greenfield et al., 2007). Table 6.2 describes the mean General Health, as measured by the SF-36, of four different types of cancer survivors: germ cell (testicular), lymphoma, leukaemia and other. Suppose that we wish to compare the mean QoL across the four different cancer groups. We could perform a series of six hypothesis tests, using the t-test or MW test described previously, to compare the means in each pair of groups. However, this may result in a high Type I error rate, because of the large number of comparisons, and this may mean that we draw incorrect conclusions from the test. Therefore, it may be preferable to carry out a single global test to determine whether the means differ in any of the groups.

7.6.1   One-way analysis of variance

One-way ANOVA separates the total variability in the data into several components. One component is the variability in the data that can be attributed to differences between the individuals from the different groups. This is known as the *between-groups variation*. A second component is the random variation between the individuals within each group. This is known as the *within-group variation*, although it is sometimes referred to as the *unexplained* or *residual* variation. The components are measured using variances (see Chapter 6), hence the name 'analysis of variance'. Under the null hypothesis that the group means are the same, the between-groups variance will be similar to the within-group variance. If, however, there are differences between the groups, then the between-groups variance will be larger than the within-group variance. The ANOVA test statistic or F test is based on the ratio of these two variances.

The calculations involved in ANOVA are complex (see Box 7.8) and are best left to a computer. Most computer packages will output the values directly in an ANOVA table, which will usually include the F-ratio and a P-value.

Box 7.8 One-way analysis of variance

Suppose that there are g $(g \geq 2)$ independent groups of observations on a variable y and let y_{ij} denote the jth observation in the ith group. The sample size, means and standard deviations in each group are n_i, $\bar{y}_i$ and s_i respectively $(i = 1, 2, \ldots, g)$. The total sample size is $N = n_1 + n_2 + \cdots + n_g = \sum_{i=1}^{g} n_i$. We wish to test the null hypothesis that the all group means in the population are equal. against the alternative hypothesis that at least one group mean in the population differs from the others.

Assumptions

   1. The groups are independent.

   2. The variable of interest is continuous.

   3. The data in the groups have similar variances or standard deviations.

   4. The data are Normally distributed in each group.

Steps

   1. Calculate:

$\bar{y}_i$ = mean of observations in the ith group;

$S_i = \sum_{i=1}^{n_i} (y_i - \bar{y}_i)^2$ = sum of squares of observations in the ith group;

$T = \sum_{i=1}^{g} n_i \bar{y}_i$ = sum of all observations;

$S = \sum_{i=1}^{g} S_i$ = sum of squares of all observations.

2. Calculate the overall or total variability of the data about its overall mean, $\bar{y}$, called the *total sum of squares*:

$$SS_{Total} = \sum_{i,j} (y_{ij} - \bar{y})^2 = S - \frac{T^2}{N}.$$

3. Calculate the within-group variability, called the *within-group sum of squares*:

$$SS_{Within} = S - \sum_{i=1}^{g} n_i \bar{y}_i^2.$$

4. Calculate the between-groups variability or the *between-groups sum of squares*:

$$SS_{Between} = \sum_{i=1}^{g} n_i \bar{y}_i^2 - T^2/N.$$

5. Calculate the mean squares ($MS_{Between}$ and MS_{Within}) by dividing the sums of squares by the degrees of freedom.

6. Calculate the variance ratio or F-test statistic by dividing $MS_{Between}$ by MS_{Within}.

7. Compare the test statistic with the F distribution with $(g-1, N-1)$ degrees of freedom in the numerator and denominator, respectively (see Table B.3). This gives us the probability of the observing the test statistic F or more extreme values under the null hypothesis.

One-way ANOVA table to compare g group means

Source of variation	Sums of squares (SS)	Degrees of freedom (df)	Mean square (MS) or Variances	Variance ratio F
Between groups	$SS_{Between} = \sum_{i=1}^{g} n_i \bar{y}_i^2 - \frac{T^2}{N}$	$g - 1$	$MS_{Between} = \frac{SS_{Between}}{g-1}$	$F = \frac{MS_{Between}}{MS_{Within}}$
Within groups	$SS_{Within} = S - \sum_{i=1}^{g} n_i \bar{y}_i^2$	$N - g$	$MS_{Within} = \frac{SS_{Within}}{N-g}$	
Total	$SS_{Total} = S - \frac{T^2}{N}$	$N - 1$		

Table 7.4 shows the computer output for comparing General Health between the four cancer groups using a one-way ANOVA. The F statistic, 4.453, shows that the between-groups variation is about four times the within-group variation. When compared to the F distribution on 3 and 167 degrees of freedom, this results in a P-value of 0.005. This is statistically significant so we can reject the null hypothesis and accept the alternative hypothesis that at least one cancer group has different mean General Health score from the other three groups.

If we obtain a significant result at this initial stage, we may consider performing a series of specific pairwise *post-hoc* comparisons. We can use one of a number of special tests devised for this purpose or we can use the two independent samples t-test (described previously) adjusted for multiple hypothesis testing (see Chapter 11). We can also calculate a confidence interval for each individual group mean. Note that we use a pooled estimate of the variance of the values from all the groups when calculating confidence intervals and performing t-tests. Most software packages refer to this estimate of the variance as the residual variance or the residual mean square. It is found in the ANOVA table. The square root of the within-group mean square is the residual standard deviation. The example in Table 7.4 shows a residual variance of 576.9 or residual standard deviation of $\sqrt{576.9} = 24.0$.

Although independent sample t-test and ANOVA appear to be different, they will give the same results when there are only two groups. Like the t-test, ANOVA is relatively robust to moderate departures from Normality. It is not as robust to unequal variances.

Table 7.4 Computer output from the one-way ANOVA.

Descriptive statistics

SF-36v2 General Health (0–100)

	n	Mean	SD
Germ cell (testicular)	66	69.2	23.4
Lymphoma	70	55.5	24.2
Leukaemia	11	73.7	21.1
Other	24	61.9	26.1
Total	171	62.9	24.7

The F-test statistic is compared to the F distribution on (3, 167) degrees of freedom.

ANOVA

SF-36v2 General Health (0–100)

	Sum of Squares	df	Mean Square	F	P-value.
Between groups	7708.007	3	2569.336	4.453	.005
Within groups	96346.625	167	576.926		
Total	104054.632	170			

P-value: probability of observing the F statistic under the null hypothesis that all four group means in the population are equal. As the value of 0.005 is less than the significance level (α) set at 0.05 or 5%, this means that the result obtained is unlikely when the null hypothesis is true. Thus there is sufficient evidence to reject the null hypothesis and accept the alternative hypothesis that at least one cancer group has different mean General Health score from the other three groups.

Therefore before carrying out the analysis we should check for Normality and whether the variances are similar by graphical methods (histograms, dot plots, box-and-whisker plots) described in Chapter 6 or by simply eyeballing the standard deviations. The descriptive statistics computer output of Table 7.4 suggests that standard deviations are broadly similar across the four cancer groups. If the assumptions are not satisfied, we can either transform the data or use the non-parametric equivalent of one-way ANOVA, the Kruskal–Wallis test.

Example: One-way ANOVA

Walters *et al.* (1999) used a one-way ANOVA to compare the mean change in QoL, as measured by the SF-36, between three groups of patients with venous leg ulcers. The three groups were based on the perceived health change over 3 months, classified as same, better or worse. Table 7.5 shows that the means on six out of the eight of the SF-36 dimensions were statistically significantly different between the three groups.   □

7.6.2   The Kruskal–Wallis test

This is a non-parametric extension of the Mann–Whitney U-test. Under the null hypothesis of no differences in the distributions between the groups, the sums of the ranks in each of the groups should be comparable after allowing for any differences in sample size. The steps for performing a Kruskal–Wallis test are described in Box 7.9.

Table 7.6 shows the computer output for the Kruskal–Wallis test. The test statistic is 12.88 (with allowance for tied ranks), which is very similar to the value of 12.84 using the formulae in Box 7.9 with no allowance for ties, suggesting the effect of tying in the ranks is negligible. The conclusions from the analysis are very similar to those from the analysis of variance example in Table 7.4: the differences are statistically significant. Thus there is sufficient evidence to reject the null hypothesis and accept the alternative hypothesis that each cancer type group does not have the same distribution of SF-36 General Health scores.

Example: Kruskal–Wallis test

Brazier *et al.* (1999) used a Kruskal–Wallis test to compare the change in WOMAC pain, stiffness and physical function scores, over a 6-month period, between three groups of patients with osteoarthritis of the knee. The three groups were based on the perceived health change over 6 months, classified as same, better or worse. The P-values from the Kruskal–Wallis test for the WOMAC pain, stiffness and physical function scores were 0.05, 0.04 and 0.02, respectively. This suggests that the three groups do not have the same distribution of WOMAC scores.   □

7.7   Two groups of paired observations

When there is more than one group of observations it is vital to distinguish the case where the data are paired from that where the groups are independent. Paired data may arise

Table 7.5 Mean score differences[1] on the SF-36 between initial assessment and 3-month follow-up in relation to self-perceived health change (data from Walters et al., 1999).

SF-36:	Perceived health change by 3-month follow-up									
	Worse			Same			Better			
	n	Mean difference	SD	n	Mean difference	SD	n	Mean difference	SD	P-value[2]
Physical Functioning	21	−3.3	31.7	129	−0.6	22.6	50	−0.1	22.4	0.25
Role Physical	21	−22.6	33.5	128	−12.1	43.4	49	−5.1	43.9	0.28
Bodily Pain	20	−16.1	22.9	128	−0.9	28.6	51	13.7	27.2	0.0001
General Health	19	−18.3	21.9	127	−9.0	17.8	51	−2.4	16.2	0.004
Vitality	19	−23.7	21.2	128	−7.7	19.4	49	2.9	20.1	0.0001
Social Functioning	20	−25.0	33.4	128	−5.8	28.4	50	−2.9	23.1	0.009
Role Emotional	21	−22.2	71.0	127	−11.5	46.3	48	4.2	44.9	0.07
Mental Heath	20	−13.0	31.4	128	−2.1	17.5	50	6.7	18.8	0.0005

[1] A mean difference greater than 0 indicates a health improvement.
[2] P-value from one-way ANOVA to compare mean score differences by self-perceived health change group.

Box 7.9 Kruskal–Wallis test

Suppose that we wish to test the null hypothesis that g ($g \geq 2$) samples or groups come from the same population (i.e. each group has the same distribution of values in the population), against the alternative hypothesis that each group does not have the same distribution of values in the population. The data are at least ordinal and from g independent groups of size $n_1, n_2, \ldots, n_g$, respectively. The total sample size is $N = \sum_{i=1}^{g} n_i$, where n_i is the number of observations in group i.

Assumptions

1. The groups are independent.

2. The variables of interest are at least ordinal (can be ranked).

Steps

1. Combine the data in all g groups and rank the entire data set, of N values, in increasing order (smallest observation to largest) from 1 to N. If some of the observations are numerically equal, they are given tied ranks equal to the mean of the ranks which would otherwise have been used.

2. Separately sum the ranks for each of the g groups. Let R_i be the sum of the ranks for the n_i observations in group i.

3. If there are no ties or only a few ties, calculate the test statistic

$$H = \frac{12}{N(N+1)} \sum_{i=1}^{g} \left\{ \frac{R_i^2}{n_i} - 3(N+1) \right\}.$$

4. Under the null hypothesis that the g samples come from the same population, the test statistic, H follows a chi-squared distribution with $g - 1$ degrees of freedom and can be referred to Table B.4 to calculate a P-value.

The formula is not very accurate if there any many ties in the data. The reader is referred to Armitage *et al.* (2002) in such situations.

---

when the same individuals are studied more than once, usually in different circumstances, or when individuals are paired, as in a case–control study.

For example, Parry *et al.* (2007) describe the results of a case–control cross-sectional survey to compare the health status or QoL of a group of Gypsies and Travellers (GT) in England with a control group. The GT responders were individually matched by age and sex to a comparison sample of non-Gypsies/Travellers from rural communities, deprived inner-city white residents and ethnic minority populations. QoL of life was measured by the EQ-5D utility measure. In this example the individuals in the two groups are clearly not sampled independently of each other and the data are regarded as being matched or paired. Therefore the methods of analysis for independent groups, described earlier in this chapter, are not appropriate. Methods of analysis for matched or paired samples, like this example, are summarized in Figure 7.3.

Table 7.6   Computer output from the Kruskal–Wallis test.

Ranks

	Cancer type	*n*	Mean Rank	Sum of ranks
SF-36v2 General Health (0–100)	Germ cell (testicular)	66	98.53	6503
	Lymphoma	70	71.11	4978
	Leukaemia	11	108.45	1193
	Other	24	84.67	2032
	Total	171		

Kruskal-Wallis Test Statistic

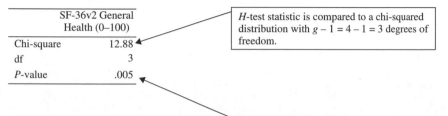

	SF-36v2 General Health (0–100)
Chi-square	12.88
df	3
P-value	.005

H-test statistic is compared to a chi-squared distribution with $g - 1 = 4 - 1 = 3$ degrees of freedom.

P-value: probability of observing the statistic under the null hypothesis that each group has the same distribution of values in the population. As the value of 0.005 is less than the significance level (α) set at 0.05 or 5%, this means that the result obtained is unlikely when the null hypothesis is true. Thus there is sufficient evidence to reject the null hypothesis and accept the alternative hypothesis that each cancer type group does not have the same distribution of SF-36 General Health scores.

7.7.1   Paired *t*-test

The EQ-5D QoL outcome is regarded as a continuous variable and the data are matched or paired as measurements are made on a Gypsy/Traveller age and sex matched to another non-Gypsy/Traveller individual. Therefore, interest is in the mean of the paired differences in EQ-5D scores between the matched subjects and not the difference between the two means for each group. If we assume that the paired differences are Normally distributed, then the most appropriate summary measure for the data is the sample mean, for each group, and the best comparative summary measure is the mean of the paired difference in QoL between the GT and their age-sex matched control. In these circumstances Figure 7.3 would suggest using the paired *t*-test to compare the EQ-5D scores between the GT group and the control group. Box 7.10 outlines the assumptions and steps for carrying out a paired *t*-test on the data.

Table 7.7 shows there were 260 Gypsies/Travellers who were matched by age and sex to 260 control subjects. Examining the computer output for the comparison of EQ-5D scores for these 260 matched subjects shows that the result is statistically significant (Table 7.7), with a *P*-value of 0.001. It appears that Gypsies/Travellers are reporting significantly lower mean EQ-5D scores, 0.75 vs. 0.87, than their corresponding age- and sex-matched controls. The 95% confidence interval of the difference suggests that we are 95% confident that the matched control subjects have EQ-5D scores between 0.07 and 0.16 points better or higher than Gypsies/Travellers and the best estimate is a mean difference of 0.12 points.

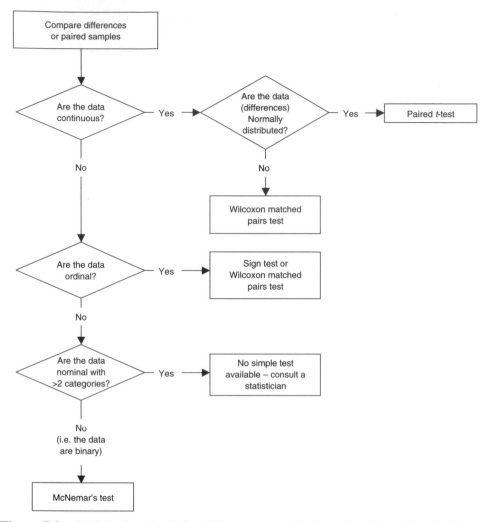

Figure 7.3   Statistical methods for differences or paired samples. Reproduced with permission from Campbell, M.J., Machin, D., Walters, S.J., *Medical Statistics: A Text Book
for the Health Sciences*. 4th edition. John Wiley & Sons Ltd, Chichester. © 2007 John
Wiley & Sons Ltd.

The assumptions underlying the use of the paired *t*-test are outlined in Box 7.10.
Figure 7.4 shows a histogram of the difference in EQ-5D scores between the Gyp-
sies/Travellers and their age- and sex-matched controls. The distribution of these paired
differences appears to be slightly skewed and non-Normally distributed. If the differences
do not follow a Normal distribution then one of the assumptions underlying the paired
t-test is not satisfied. We can either transform the data or use a non-parametric test.
Figure 7.3 shows that the non-parametric alternative to the paired *t*-test is the Wilcoxon
signed rank sum test.

Box 7.10 Paired t-test

We have two groups of paired observations, $x_{11}, x_{12}, \ldots, x_{1n}$ in group 1 and $x_{21}, x_{22}, \ldots, x_{2n}$ in group 2, such that x_{1i} is paired with x_{2i} and the difference between them is $d_i = x_{1i} - x_{2i}$. The null hypothesis is that the mean difference in the population equals zero, and the alternative hypothesis is that the mean difference in the population does not equal zero.

Assumptions

1. The d_i are plausibly Normally distributed. It is not essential for the original observations to be Normally distributed.

2. The d_i are independent of each other.

Steps

1. Calculate the differences $d_i = x_{1i} - x_{2i}$, $i = 1, \ldots, n$.

2. Calculate the mean $\bar{d}$ and standard deviation, s_d, of the differences d_i.

3. Calculate the standard error of the mean difference,

$$\mathrm{SE}(\bar{d}) = \frac{s_d}{\sqrt{n}}.$$

4. Calculate the test statistic

$$t = \frac{\bar{d}}{\mathrm{SE}(\bar{d})}.$$

5. Under the null hypothesis, the test statistic, t, is distributed as Student's t, with degrees of freedom $df = n - 1$.

6. The $100(1 - \alpha)\%$ confidence interval for the mean difference in the population is:

$$\bar{d} - [t_{df,\alpha} \times \mathrm{SE}(\bar{d})] \text{ to } \bar{d} + [t_{df,\alpha} \times \mathrm{SE}(\bar{d})],$$

where $t_{df,\alpha}$ is taken from the t distribution with $df = n - 1$ degrees of freedom.

Example: Paired t-test

Akehurst et al. (2002) used a paired t-test to compare the change in QoL over a 3-month period, as measured by the IBS-QoL, in a group of 120 primary care patients with irritable bowel syndrome. The IBS-QoL is scored on a 0 (very affected) to 100 (not affected) scale. The baseline overall IBS-QoL score was 71.6 (SD 18.5) and the 3-month follow-up score was 71.5 (SD 19.8), a difference of -0.1 (95% CI: -1.9 to 1.7, $P = 0.89$). The authors' stated that 'There was no statistically significant change between the baseline and follow-up questionnaires'. □

Table 7.7 Computer output from paired *t*-test.

Paired Samples Statistics

	Mean	*n*	SD	SE
Control: EQ-5D score	.87	260	.23	.01
Gypsy Traveller: EQ-5D score	.75	260	.36	.02

Paired Samples *t*-test

	Paired Differences					*t*	df	*P*-value
	Mean	SD	SE	95% Confidence Interval of the Difference				
				Lower	Upper			
Control: EQ-5D - Gypsy Traveller: EQ-5D score	.12	.38	.02	.07	.16	4.928	259	<0.001

The EQ-5D is scored on a −0.6 to 1.00 (good health) scale

The *P*-value is the probability of observing the *t* statistic under the null hypothesis that the paired mean difference in the population is zero. As the value of 0.001 is less than the significance level (α) set at 0.05 or 5%, this means that the result obtained is unlikely when the null hypothesis is true. Thus there is sufficient evidence to reject the null hypothesis and accept the alternative hypothesis that the mean difference is non-zero and that Gypsies and Travellers have a different mean EQ-5D score to the control group subjects.

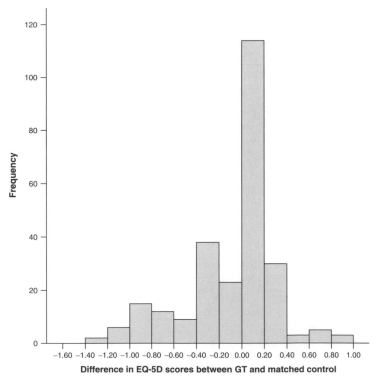

Figure 7.4 Histogram of difference in EQ-5D scores between GT and age- and sex-matched controls (*n* = 260) (data from Parry *et al.*, 2007).

Box 7.11 Wilcoxon (matched pairs) signed rank test

We have two groups of paired observations, $x_{11}, x_{12}, \ldots, x_{1n}$ in group 1 and $x_{21}, x_{22}, \ldots, x_{2n}$ in group 2, such that x_{1i} is paired with x_{2i} and the difference between them is $d_i = x_{1i} - x_{2i}$. The null hypothesis is that the *median* difference in the population equals zero, and the alternative hypothesis is that the median difference in the population does not equal zero.

Assumptions

1. The d_i come from a population with a symmetric distribution.

2. The d_i are independent of each other.

Steps

1. Calculate the differences $d_i = x_{1i} - x_{2i}$, $i = 1, \ldots, n$.

2. Ignoring the signs of the differences, rank them in order of increasing magnitude form 1 to n', with zero values being ignored (so n' is the number of non-zero differences, which may be less than the original sample size n). If some of the observations are numerically equal, they are given tied ranks equal to the mean of the ranks which would otherwise have been used.

3. Calculate, T^+, the sum of the ranks of the positive values.

4. Calculate the test statistic
$$z = \frac{T^+ - \dfrac{n'(n' + 1)}{4}}{\sqrt{\dfrac{n'(n' + 1)(2n' + 1)}{24}}}.$$

5. Under the null hypothesis, z has an approximately Normal distribution, with mean $n'(n' + 1)/4$ and variance $n'(n' + 1)(2n' + 1)/24$.

7.7.2 Wilcoxon test

Box 7.11 outlines the steps for carrying out a paired Wilcoxon signed rank sum test. Table 7.8 shows the computer output for the Wilcoxon (matched pairs) signed rank test carried out on our GT data. The Z test statistic is -4.609 and the P-value is less than 0.001. The conclusions from the analysis are very similar to those from the paired t-test in Table 7.7: the differences are statistically significant. Thus there is sufficient evidence to reject the null hypothesis and accept the alternative hypothesis that there is a difference in EQ-5D scores between the GT and the controls.

7.8 The relationship between two continuous variables

Many statistical analyses are undertaken to examine the relationship between two continuous variables within a group of subjects (Table 7.9). Two of the main purposes of such analyses are:

Table 7.8 Computer output from Wilcoxon test.

		n	Mean rank	Sum of ranks
	Ranks			
GT: EQ-5D Overall Utility	Negative ranks	105(a)	94.26	9897.00
(Tariff) - Control: EQ-5D	Positive ranks	62(b)	66.63	4131.00
Overall Utility (Tariff)	Ties	93(c)		
	Total	260		

a GT: EQ-5D score < Control: EQ-5D score
b GT: EQ-5D score > Control: EQ-5D score
c GT: EQ-5D score = Control: EQ-5D score

Test Statistics

	GT: EQ-5D - Control:EQ-5D
Z	−4.609
P-value	<0.001

The P-value is the probability of observing the Z statistic under the null hypothesis that the paired mean difference in the population is zero. As the value of 0.001 is less than the significance level (α) set at 0.05 or 5%, this means that the result obtained is unlikely when the null hypothesis is true. Thus there is sufficient evidence to reject the null hypothesis and accept the alternative hypothesis that the mean difference is non-zero and that Gypsies and Travellers have a different mean EQ-5D score than the control group subjects.

1. To assess whether the two variables are associated. There is no distinction between the two variables and no causation is implied, simply association.

2. To enable the value of one variable to be predicted from any known value of the other variable. One variable is regarded as a response to the other predictor variable, and the value of the predictor variable is used to predict what the response would be.

For the first of these, the statistical method for assessing the association between two continuous variables is known as *correlation*, whilst the technique for the second, prediction of one continuous variable from another is known as *regression*. Correlation and regression are often presented together, and it is easy to get the impression that they are inseparable. In fact, they have distinct purposes and it is relatively rare that one is genuinely interested in performing both analyses on the same set of data. However, when preparing to analyse data using either technique it is always important to construct a scatter plot of the values of the two variables against each other. By drawing a scatter plot it is possible to see whether or not there is any visual evidence of a straight-line or linear association between the two variables.

Table 7.9 Statistical methods for relationships between two variables measured on the same sample of subjects.

	Continuous, Normal	Continuous, non-Normal	Ordinal	Nominal	Binary
Continuous, Normal	Regression Correlation (Pearson's r)	Regression Rank correlation (Spearman's r_s)	Rank correlation (Spearman's r_s)	One-way ANOVA	Independent samples t-test
Continuous, non-Normal		Regression Rank correlation (Spearman's r_s)	Rank correlation (Spearman's r_s)	Kruskal–Wallis test	Mann–Whitney U-test
Ordinal			Rank correlation (Spearman's r_s)	Kruskal–Wallis test	Mann–Whitney U-test
Nominal				Chi-squared test	Chi-squared test for trend
Binary					Chi-squared test Fisher's exact test

7.9 Correlation

The cross-sectional survey of the QoL of male cancer survivors was also interested in looking at the relationship between QoL and levels of the male hormone testosterone. Figure 7.5 shows a scatter plot of SF-36 Physical Component Summary (PCS) score against testosterone for 170 male cancer survivors aged 25–45. There is some sugges-tion of a positive linear relationship between QoL at testosterone, with higher values of testosterone being associated with higher PCS scores. However, this relationship is not obviously apparent from the scatter plot.

In order to examine whether there is an association between the two variables, QoL and testosterone, the correlation coefficient can be calculated. At this point, no assump-tions are made about whether the relationship is causal, that is, whether one variable is influencing the value of the other variable. The standard method (often ascribed to Pearson) leads to a statistic called r (see Box 7.12). In essence r is a measure of the scatter of the points around an underlying linear trend: the greater the spread of points, the lower the correlation. Pearson's correlation coefficient r must be between -1 and $+1$, with -1 representing a perfect negative correlation, $+1$ representing perfect positive correlation and 0 representing no linear trend.

The assumptions underlying the validity of the hypothesis test associated with the correlation coefficient are outlined in Box 7.12. The easiest way to check the validity of the hypothesis test is by examining a scatter plot of the data. This plot should be produced as a matter of routine when correlation coefficients are calculated, as it will give a good indication of whether the relationship between the two variables is roughly linear and thus whether it is appropriate to calculate a correlation coefficient. If the data do not have a Normal distribution, or a non-linear relationship between the variables

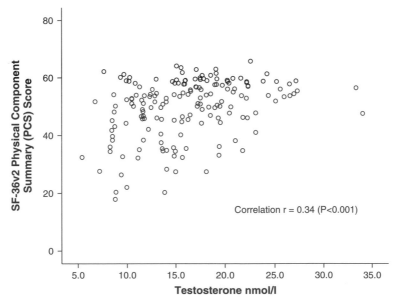

Figure 7.5 Scatter plot of SF-36 Physical Component Summary score versus testos-terone for 170 male cancer survivors aged 25–45 (data from Greenfield *et al.*, 2007).

Box 7.12 Pearson's correlation coefficient

The correlation coefficient can be calculated for any data set with two continuous variables.

Assumptions

1. For a valid hypothesis test the two variables are observed on a random sample of individuals, and the data for at least one of the variables should have a Normal distribution in the population.

2. For the calculation of a valid confidence interval for the correlation coefficient both variables should have a Normal distribution.

3. There is a linear relationship between the variables.

Steps

For a set of n pairs of observations (x_1, y_1), (x_2, y_2), ..., (x_n, y_n), with means $\bar{x}$ and $\bar{y}$ respectively, the Pearson correlation coefficient, r, is given by

$$r = \frac{\sum_{i=1}^{n} (y_i - \bar{y})(x_i - \bar{x})}{\sqrt{\sum_{i=1}^{n} (y_i - \bar{y})^2 \sum_{i=1}^{n} (x_i - \bar{x})^2}}.$$

The null hypothesis is that population correlation, ρ (the Greek letter rho) equals zero, against the alternative hypothesis that the population correlation does not equal zero. To test whether r is significantly different from zero, calculate

$$t = \frac{r}{\sqrt{(1 - r^2)/(n - 2)}}.$$

This is compared with the t distribution of Table B.2 with $df = n - 2$.

---

is suspected, then a non-parametric correlation coefficient, Spearman's rho (ρ_s), can be calculated (see Box 7.13).

From Figure 7.5 it can be seen that the Pearson correlation coefficient between SF-36 PCS score and testosterone is 0.34 and that this is statistically significant ($P < 0.001$). However, it is important to note that if the sample size is large, as in this example, then the null hypothesis (that the population correlation ρ is zero) may be rejected even if the sample estimate, r, is quite close to zero. Alternatively, even if r is large, H_0 may not be rejected if the sample size is small. For this reason, it is particularly important to look at the absolute value of the correlation coefficient r; Table 7.10 provides a guide to interpreting the value of the observed correlation in the sample. In this example the correlation of 0.34 suggests only a weak relationship between QoL and testosterone.

Another helpful way to interpret the correlation coefficient is to calculate r^2, the proportion of the total variance of one variable explained by its linear relationship with the other variable. Note that r^2 is the proportion of the variance of one variable 'explained' by the other. For example, $r = 0.34$ and $P < 0.001$ for a sample size of 170, but the relationship between QoL and testosterone is only explaining 12% ($= 0.34^2 \times 100$) of the variability of one variable.

Box 7.13 Spearman's rank correlation coefficient

Suppose we have a set of n pairs of observations $(x_1, y_1), (x_2, y_2), \ldots, (x_n, y_n)$.

Assumptions

At least one of the variables, x or y, is measured on an ordinal scale.

Neither x nor y is Normally distributed.

We require a measure of association between the two variables when their relationship is non-linear.

Steps

To estimate the population value of Spearman's rank correlation coefficient ρ_s, by its sample value, r_s:

1. Rank the x observations in order of increasing magnitude from 1 to n. If some of the observations are numerically equal, they are given tied ranks equal to the mean of the ranks which would otherwise have been used.

2. Rank the y observations in order of increasing magnitude from 1 to n. If some of the observations are numerically equal, they are given tied ranks equal to the mean of the ranks which would otherwise have been used.

3. Spearman's rank correlation, r_s, is calculated from Pearson's correlation coefficient on the *ranks* of the data.

4. An alternative, and easier to calculate, formula is

$$r_{\text{Spearman}} = 1 - \frac{6 \sum d_i^2}{n^3 - n},$$

where d_i is the difference in ranks for the ith individual.

Table 7.10   Interpretation of the values of the sample estimate of the correlation coefficient.

$|r| \geq 0.8$	very strong relationship
$0.6 \leq |r| < 0.8$	strong relationship
$0.4 \leq |r| < 0.6$	moderate relationship
$0.2 \leq |r| < 0.4$	weak relationship
$|r| < 0.2$	very weak relationship

$|r|$ denotes the modulus or absolute value of r (i.e. ignoring the sign in front of the correlation coefficient).

For the 170 male cancer survivors Spearman's rank correlation coefficient, r_s, between the SF-36 PCS score and testosterone, was calculated (as shown in Box 7.13) to be 0.33. This is very similar to Pearson's correlation coefficient estimate, r, of 0.34.

When presenting correlation, it is good practice to show a scatter diagram of the data wherever possible (Freeman *et al.*, 2008). The value of the correlation coefficient should be reported to a precision of two decimal places, together with a *P*-value if a hypothesis test is carried out. The number of observations that the correlation coefficient is based on should also be reported. If it is necessary to display the correlation between all pairs of a set of three or more variables, this should be done by means of correlation matrix or the preferred graphical equivalent (see the following example).

Example: Pearson correlation coefficient

Greenfield (*et al* 2007) calculated the Pearson correlation coefficients between testosterone and QoL, as measured by the SF-36, for a sample of young male cancer survivors aged 25–45. Table 7.11 shows correlations between testosterone and four dimensions of the SF-36. The largest observed correlation between QoL and testosterone was 0.34 (for the PCS score). The largest correlation, of 0.89, was between the Physical Functioning dimension score and the PCS score. Figure 7.6 makes it clear that there is a strong correlation between PCS and Physical Functioning, and far weaker relationships between the other variables. □

Example: Spearman correlation coefficient

Brazier *et al.* (1996) calculated Spearman correlation coefficients between SF-36 scores at baseline and 6 months later, for a sample of 79 women aged 75 and over. Table 7.12 shows the correlations between the eight dimensions of the SF-36 at baseline and 6 months later. The largest observed correlation, 0.70, was between the baseline and 6-month

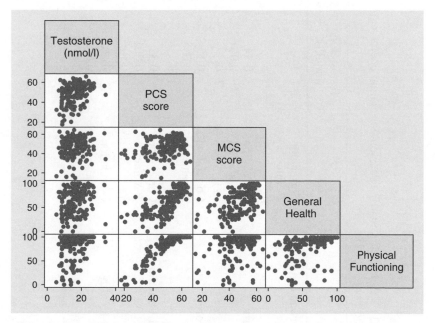

Figure 7.6 Scatter diagram matrix showing each of the two-way relationship between QoL and testosterone for 175 young male cancer survivors (data from Greenfield *et al* 2007).

Table 7.11 Correlation matrix (Pearson correlation coefficients) for QoL and Testosterone for 175 male cancer survivors (data from Greenfield et al., 2007).

		Testosterone (nmol/l)	PCS score	MCS score	Physical Functioning	General Health
Testosterone (nmol/l)	Correlation	1				
	P-value					
	n	175				
PCS score	Correlation	0.34	1			
	P-value	0.001				
	n	170	171			
MCS score	Correlation	0.15	0.36	1		
	P-value	0.058	0.001			
	n	170	171	171		
Physical Functioning	Correlation	0.32	0.89	0.39	1	
	P-value	0.001	0.001	0.001		
	n	170	171	171	171	
General Health	Correlation	0.26	0.70	0.52	0.50	1
	P-value	0.001	0.001	0.001	0.001	
	n	170	171	171	171	171

Table 7.12   Spearman's rank correlation coefficients, r_s, between SF-36 dimension scores at initial assessment and 6-month follow-up for a sample of 79 women aged 75 or more (data from Brazier *et al.*, 1996).

SF-36	r_s	n
Physical Functioning	0.62***	77
Social Functioning	0.28*	79
Role Physical	0.49***	68
Role Emotional	0.38**	67
Bodily Pain	0.66***	79
Mental Health	0.63***	74
Vitality	0.70***	71
General Health	0.58***	66

*$P < 0.05$ **$P < 0.01$ ***$P < 0.001$

SF-36 Vitality dimension scores. The smallest correlation, 0.28, was between the Social Functioning dimension scores. □

7.10   Regression

It is often of interest to quantify the relationship between two continuous variables, and, given the value of one variable for an individual, to predict the value of the other variable. This is not possible from the correlation coefficient as it simply indicates the strength of the association as a single number; in order to describe the relationship between the values of the two variables, a technique called regression is used. Let us make the big assumption that the level of testosterone is influencing the value of the QoL, rather than the other way around. Then, using regression, the level of testosterone could be used to predict QoL or the PCS score. The level of testosterone is regarded as the *x* variable. It is also sometimes called the independent, predictor or explanatory variable, and it should be plotted on the horizontal axis of the scatter plot. The SF-36 PCS score is regarded as the *y* variable. It is also known as the dependent or response variable, and is plotted on the vertical axis of the scatter plot (Figure 7.5). Five important assumptions underlie regression analysis as outlined in Box 7.14.

Box 7.14 Linear regression

The equation which estimates the simple linear regression line is

$$y = a + bx, \tag{7.1}$$

where *a* and *b* are called the regression coefficients; *a* is the *intercept* (the value of the dependent *y* variable, when the independent *x* variable is equal to zero) and *b* is the *slope* or *gradient* (the average change in the dependent *y* variable for a unit change in the *x* variable).

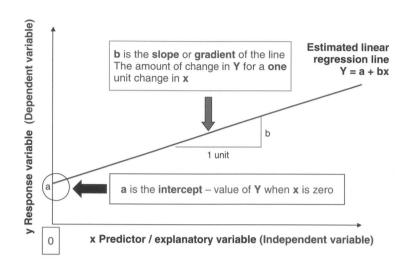

Assumptions

1. The values of the response variable y should have a Normal distribution for each value of the explanatory variable x.

2. The variance (or standard deviation) of y should be the same at each value of x, that is, there should be no evidence that as the value of y changes, the spread of the x-values changes.

3. The relationship between the two variables should be linear.

4. The observations in the sample are independent.

5. The variable x can be measured without error.

We perform a regression analysis using a sample of observations and obtain a and b, the sample estimates of the true population parameters α and β. The population regression model is $y = \alpha + \beta x$. The coefficients a and b are determined by the *method of least squares* (often called *ordinary least squares*, OLS) in such a way that the fit of the line $y = a + bx$ to the points in the scatter diagram is best. We determine the *line of best fit* by considering the *residuals*. The residuals are the vertical distance from each data point on the scatter diagram to the regression line: residual = observed y – fitted y. The line of best fit is chosen so that the sum of the squared residuals is a minimum. For simple linear regression the coefficients a and b can be calculated using the steps below.

Steps

Given a set of n pairs of observations (x_1, y_1), (x_2, y_2), ..., (x_n, y_n), with means $\bar{x}$ and $\bar{y}$ respectively (with $i = 1$ to n). The estimated slope, b, is given by

$$b = \frac{\sum_{i=1}^{n} (x_i - \bar{x})(y_i - \bar{y})}{\sum_{i=1}^{n} (x_i - \bar{x})^2}.$$

The intercept a, can be estimated by

$$a = \bar{y} - b\bar{x}.$$

If the first three assumptions hold, then the residuals should have a Normal distribution with a mean of zero. So we can check this by way of a histogram or dot plot of the residuals. We can also plot the residuals against the x-values. If the assumptions hold, then the points should be evenly scattered at all x-values. More details on how to check the assumptions are given in Section 7.14.

Regression slopes can be used to predict the response of a new patient with a particular value of the predictor/explanatory/independent variable. However, it is important that the regression model is not used to predict outside of the range of observations. In addition, it should not be assumed that just because an equation has been produced it means that x causes y. The results of regressing SF-36 PCS score on testosterone level are shown in Figure 7.7 and Table 7.13.

Looking at the table for the coefficients it can be seen that the slope coefficient for testosterone is 0.65 (P-value $= 0.001$), indicating that testosterone has a significant effect on PCS score. The value of r^2 is often quoted in published articles and indicates the proportion (sometimes expressed as a percentage) of the total variability of the outcome variable that is explained by the regression model fitted. In this case 11% of the total variability in PCS score is explained by testosterone level. This indicates that nearly 90% of the variability in PCS is unexplained.

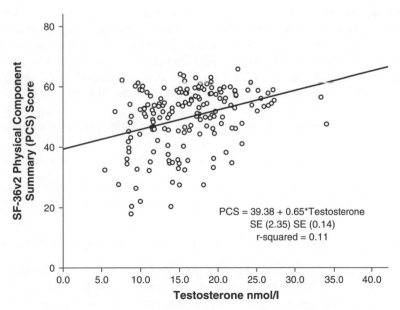

Figure 7.7 Linear regression relationship between SF-36 PCS score and testosterone for 170 male cancer survivors aged 25–45 (data from Greenfield et al., 2007).

Table 7.13 Estimated regression coefficients from the linear regression model to predict PCS from testosterone in 170 male cancer survivors (data from Greenfield *et al.*, 2007).

| | Regression Coefficients | | | | |
	b	SE(b)	t	P-value	95% CI for b
Intercept	39.38	(2.35)	16.74	.001	34.73 to 44.02
Testosterone (nmol/l)	0.65	(0.114)	4.64	.001	0.37 to 0.92

Y or Dependent Variable: PCS score
$r^2 = 0.11$
Residual SD = 9.56

The probability of observing this slope coefficient or more extreme under the null hypothesis (that $\beta = 0$) is 0.001.	We are 95% confident that the true population parameter for the slope or relationship between PCS score and testosterone lies somewhere between 0.37 and 0.92 and our best estimate is 0.65.

7.11 Multiple regression

Regression, as described above, involves the investigation of the effect of a single explanatory variable on the outcome of interest. However, there is usually more than one possible explanatory variable influencing the values of the outcome variable, and the method of regression can be extended to investigate the influence of more than one variable. In this case it is referred to as *multiple regression*, and several explanatory variables can be investigated simultaneously for their influence on the outcome of interest. For example, in the study of male cancer survivors, apart from testosterone level, age and previous treatment with chemotherapy may have a role to play influencing QoL, and these may be fitted into the model to examine what their influence on QoL is, over and above that exerted by testosterone alone.

There are three main reasons for carrying out a multiple regression analysis:

(i) to identify any explanatory variables that may be associated with the y variable;

(ii) to investigate the extent to which one or more explanatory variables are linearly related to the y variable after adjusting for other variables that may be related to it;

(iii) to predict the value of the y variable from the explanatory x variables.

The assumptions for multiple linear regression are the same as for simple linear regression (see Box 7.14). We just replace the single x variable with each of the x_i variables. The assumptions can be checked in the same way (see Section 7.14).

Suppose that we are interested in the effect of several explanatory variables, $x_1, x_2, \ldots, x_p$, on the response variable y. The estimated multiple regression equation, with p explanatory variables, would be

$$y = a + b_1x_1 + b_2x_2 + \ldots + b_px_p. \tag{7.2}$$

Here x_p is the pth explanatory variable or covariate; y is the estimated/predicted/expected mean or fitted value of y given a particular set of values of $x_1, x_2, \ldots, x_p$; a is the estimated intercept; a constant term; and is the value of Y when all the x_i ($i = 1, \ldots, p$) are zero. The b_i are the estimated regression coefficients. That is, b_1 represents the amount by which y increases on average if we increase x_1 by one unit, but keep all the other x_i constant (or adjust or control for them).

For the cancer survivor data the estimated multiple regression equation is

$$\text{PCS} = a + b_1\text{Testosterone} + b_2\text{Age} + b_3\text{Chemotherapy}. \tag{7.3}$$

Table 7.14 shows the estimated regression coefficients, b_1, b_2 and b_3, for testosterone, age and chemotherapy use respectively, and their associated confidence intervals and P-values. It appears that only testosterone level is significantly associated with PCS score.

As can be seen from Table 7.14, we can also carry out a multiple linear regression analysis using categorical explanatory variables. If we have a binary variable, say X_{Chemo} (previous chemotherapy treatment for cancer, coded as $0 = $ no and $1 = $ yes), and we increase X_{Chemo} by one unit, we are effectively changing from no previous chemotherapy treatment to being treated with chemotherapy. Thus the regression coefficient, b_{Chemo}, represents the difference in the estimated mean QoL between chemotherapy-treated cancer patients and non-chemotherapy-treated cancer patients after adjustment for the other x_i. So looking at the data in Table 7.14, the regression coefficient for the binary chemotherapy treatment variable suggests a difference or reduction of -6.94 in mean SF-36 PCS scores in patients treated with chemotherapy-treated compared with non-chemotherapy-treated cancer patients, after adjusting for age and testosterone level. However, the P-value of 0.112 is not statistically significant and the 95% confidence interval for the regression

Table 7.14 Estimated regression coefficients from the multiple linear regression model to predict PCS from testosterone in 170 male cancer survivors (data from Greenfield *et al.*, 2007).

	Regression Coefficients		t	P-value	95% CI for b	
	b	SE(b)			Lower Bound	Upper Bound
Intercept	50.25	7.14	7.040	0.001	36.16	64.34
Testosterone (nmol/l)	0.64	0.14	4.563	0.001	0.36	0.92
Age (years)	−0.11	0.13	−0.850	0.396	−0.36	0.14
Chemotherapy treatment for cancer (0 = No, 1 = Yes)	−6.94	4.34	−1.597	0.112	−15.51	1.64

Y or Dependent Variable: PCS score
$r^2 = 0.13$
Residual SD $= 9.53$

coefficient includes zero, suggesting the population value for the parameter is zero. If all the explanatory variables are categorical then an alternative, but equivalent, technique to multiple regression, is the *analysis of variance* (Campbell, 2006).

If we have a nominal categorical explanatory variable (e.g. type of cancer; see Table 7.4) with more than two categories of response, we have to create a number of dummy or indicator variables (coded as 0 or 1). In general, for a nominal variable with k categories, we create $k - 1$ binary dummy variables. We chose one category to be the reference category. Each dummy variable then allows us to compare one of the other $k - 1$ categories of the variable with the reference category.

For example, Table 7.4 used a one-way ANOVA to compare mean General Health scores between the four different cancer groups (germ cell, lymphoma, leukaemia and other). Suppose that we choose the lymphoma group (which has the largest sample size and lowest General Health score) to be the reference category. We have $k = 4$ types of cancer and need to create $k-1 = 3$ binary dummy variables. We generate one binary dummy variable to represent germ cell cancer patients. This takes the value 1 if the individual has germ cell cancer and 0 otherwise. We then generate two further binary dummy variables to identify leukaemia and other cancer patients. Those cancer patients with lymphoma can also be identified because these patients will have a code of 0 for each of the three binary dummy variables.

In the multiple regression model of Table 7.15, the regression coefficients for the three binary dummy variables represent the amount by which the General Health score (the y variable) differs on average among those with the relevant cancer type compared to patients with lymphoma. For example, leukaemia patients on average have a 18.2

Table 7.15   Estimated regression coefficients from the multiple linear regression model to predict SF-36 General Health from on cancer type in 171 male cancer survivors (data from Greenfield *et al.*, 2007).

	Regression Coefficients		t	P-value	95% CI for b	
	b	SE(b)			Lower Bound	Upper Bound
Intercept	55.53	2.87	19.34	.000	49.86	61.20
Germ cell vs. Lymphoma (0 = Lymphoma; 1 = Germ cell)	13.64	4.12	3.31	.001	5.50	21.77
Leukaemia vs. Lymphoma (0 = Lymphoma; 1 = Leukaemia)	18.20	7.79	2.34	.021	2.82	33.58
Other vs. Lymphoma (0 = Lymphoma; 1 = Other)	6.39	5.68	1.12	.262	−4.83	17.61

Y or Dependent Variable: General Health
$r^2 = 0.074$
Residual SD = 24.0

point higher General Health score than lymphoma cancer patients. The intercept of 55.53 in Table 7.15 provides an estimate of the mean GH score for male lymphoma cancer patients (when all the other dummy explanatory variables take the value of zero).

The term *covariate* is often simply used as an alternative name for explanatory variable, but perhaps more specifically to refer to variables that are not of primary interest in an investigation, but are measured because it is believed that they are likely to affect the response variable, and consequently need to be included in the analysis and model building. The term *factor* is also used in a variety of ways in statistics, but most commonly to refer to a categorical variable with a small number of levels, under investigation in an experiment as a possible source of variation. Essentially a factor is simply a categorical explanatory variable (e.g. gender or treatment group).

An extension of analysis of variance that allows for the possible effects of covariates on the response variable, in addition to the effect of the factor or treatment variables, is called *analysis of covariance* (ANCOVA). The covariates are assumed to be unaffected by treatments and, in general, their relationship to the response is assumed to be linear (e.g. age or baseline/pre-treatment outcome value). Inclusion of covariates decreases the error mean square and hence increases the sensitivity of the statistical tests used in assessing treatment differences. Such data can also be analysed using multiple linear regression techniques by creating one or more dummy binary variables to distinguish between the groups.

Example: Adjustment for confounders

Lacey and Walters (2003) used multiple regression to compare the QoL of men and women a year after discharge from hospital following a heart attack. Table 7.16 shows the QoL, as measured by the SF-36, at 1 year after discharge from hospital following a heart attack, by gender, adjusted for age and 6-week (baseline) QoL. Men reported significantly better health than women on three dimensions of the SF-36 after adjustment: Physical Functioning, Role Physical and Social Functioning.   □

7.12   Regression or correlation?

Regression is more informative than correlation. Correlation simply quantifies the degree of linear association (or not) between two variables. However, it is often more useful to describe the relationship between the two variables, or even predict a value of one variable for a given value of the other, and this is done using regression. If it is sensible to assume that one variable may be causing a response in the other then regression analysis should be used.

7.13   Parametric versus non-parametric methods

This chapter has described a variety of parametric and non-parametric tests for analysing QoL data. Since QoL outcomes tend to generate data with discrete, skewed and bounded distributions, there is a strong argument for using non-parametric methods to analyse QoL outcomes. This argument has much appeal. However, the overwhelming argument against the routine use of non-parametric tests is that they are not flexible enough (Campbell *et al.*,

Table 7.16 QoL at 1 year post discharge from hospital by gender, adjusted for age and baseline score, for heart attack patients (data from Lacey and Walters, 2003).

SF-36 dimension[1]	Males			Females			Difference (unadjusted) male to female			Difference (adjusted for age and six week baseline)		
	n	Mean	SD	n	Mean	SD	Mean diff[2]	CI	P-value[3]	Mean diff[2]	CI	P-value
Physical Functioning	163	66.5	26.2	52	49.9	27.1	16.7	8.4 to 25.0	0.000	11.0	4.2 to 17.8	0.002
Role Physical	155	50.6	44.2	48	37.0	45.3	13.6	−0.9 to 28.1	0.065	16.9	2.2 to 31.5	0.024
Bodily Pain	165	72.0	24.9	54	65.4	27.2	6.5	−1.4 to 14.4	0.106	5.3	−1.5 to 12.0	0.128
General Health	162	55.8	22.6	51	52.5	24.2	3.3	−4.0 to 10.6	0.370	0.7	−4.9 to 6.3	0.807
Vitality	164	52.0	22.0	53	41.8	24.9	10.2	3.1 to 17.3	0.005	4.4	−1.7 to 10.5	0.158
Role Emotional	166	64.6	24.8	55	58.2	26.3	6.4	−1.3 to 14.1	0.103	7.9	0.9 to 14.8	0.027
SF36-RE	155	66.2	41.4	47	53.9	47.4	12.3	−1.7 to 26.4	0.086	13.0	−0.8 to 26.8	0.065
Mental Health	165	72.6	19.7	53	67.2	22.5	5.4	−0.9 to 11.8	0.095	3.2	−2.1 to 8.5	0.239

SD = standard deviation; CI = confidence interval
[1] The SF-36 is scored on a 0 (poor health) to 100 (good health) scale.
[2] A positive mean difference indicates that the males had a better QoL than the females.
[3] P-value from independent samples t-test

2007). Non-parametric tests do not easily allow for analyses such as multiple regression or the estimation of confidence intervals for treatment effects and differences. Estimating confidence intervals for a treatment effect is very important, and is now regarded as good statistical practice (Altman *et al.*, 2000).

My own research experience suggests little difference between parametric and non-parametric methods when calculating standard errors, P-values and confidence intervals (Walters, 2003, 2004; Walters and Campbell, 2004, 2005). Therefore I tend to use standard statistical analysis methods (such as the t-test and multiple linear regression) to analyse QoL outcomes.

Heeren and D'Agostino (1987) have demonstrated the robustness of the two independent samples t-test when applied to three-, four- and five-point ordinal scaled data using assigned scores, in sample sizes as small as 20 subjects per group. Sullivan and D'Agostino (2003) have expanded this work to account for a covariate when the outcome is ordinal in nature. They again assign numeric scores to the distinct response categories and compare means between treatment groups, adjusting for a covariate reflecting a baseline assessment measured on the same scale. Their simulation study shows that in the presence of three-, four- and five-point ordinal data and small sample sizes (as low as 20 per group) both ANCOVA and the two independent sample t-test on difference scores are robust and produce actual significance levels close to the nominal significance levels.

Statistical theory says that if the distribution of x is Normal, so will be the distribution of the sample mean, $\bar{x}$. Much more importantly, even if the distribution of x is not Normal, that of the sample mean will become closer to the Normal distribution with mean μ and variance as n gets larger. This is a consequence of the Central Limit Theorem (CLT). The Normal distribution is strictly only the limiting form of the sampling distribution as n increases to infinity, but it provides a remarkable good approximation to the sampling distribution even when n is small and the distribution of x is far from Normal (Armitage *et al.*, 2002).

If the sample size is 'sufficiently large' the CLT guarantees that the sample means will be approximately Normally distributed (Hogg and Tanis, 1988). Thus, if the investigator is planning a large study and the sample mean is an appropriate summary measure of the outcome, then pragmatically there is no need to worry about the distribution of the outcome. Generally, if n is greater than 25, these approximations to Normality for sample means will be good. The work of Heeren and D'Agostino (1987) and Sullivan and D'Agostino (2003) supports the robustness of the two independent samples t-test and ANCOVA when applied to three-, four- and five-point ordinal scaled data using assigned scores, in sample sizes as small as 20 subjects per group.

7.14 Technical details: Checking the assumptions for a linear regression analysis

We defined the model or population linear regression line for the ith subject with a continuous QoL outcome, y_i, as

$$y_i = \alpha + \beta x_i + \varepsilon_i,$$

where x_j is an continuous or binary explanatory variable; ε_i is a Normally distributed random error term with mean 0 and variance σ_ε^2, and the correlation between the residuals, for any two individual subjects, i and k, is $\mathrm{Corr}(\varepsilon_i, \varepsilon_k) = 0$; α is the expected mean outcome when the explanatory variable x_i is zero; and β is the effect on the outcome for a one-unit increase in the explanatory variable x_i. For each observed value of x, the observed residual (e_i) is the observed y minus the corresponding fitted or predicted y, that is, $e_i = y_{\mathrm{obs}} - y_{\mathrm{fit}}$. Each residual may be positive or negative. The residuals should be Normally distributed with a mean or expected value of zero, and a variance of σ_{ε}^2. We can use the residuals to check the following assumptions underlying the linear regression model.

1. *The relationship between the two variables should be linear.* Either plot y against x (the data should approximate a straight line) or plot the residuals against x (this should produce a random scatter of points rather than any systematic pattern).
   Figure 7.7 shows a scatter plot of the relationship between PCS score and testosterone. The relationship between the two variables appears to be linear. Figure 7.8 shows a scatter plot of the relationship between the residuals from the linear regression of PCS on testosterone, and testosterone. The relationship between the two variables appears to be random and does not follow any systematic pattern.

2. *The values of the response variable y should have a Normal distribution for each value of the explanatory variable x.* This assumption means that the residuals are Normally distributed and should have a mean of zero. We can check this assumption by drawing a histogram, dot plot or box-and-whisker plot of the residuals and look at the results.
   Figure 7.9 shows a histogram of the residuals from the linear regression of PCS on testosterone for 170 male cancer survivors aged 25–45. The distribution of the residuals is approximately Normal.

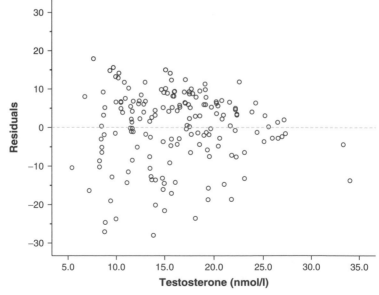

Figure 7.8 Scatter plot of residuals versus testosterone from the linear regression of PCS on testosterone for 170 male cancer survivors aged 25–45.

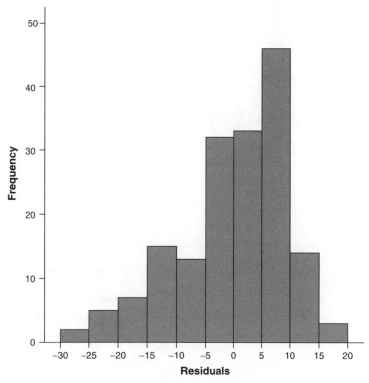

Figure 7.9 Histogram of the residuals from the linear regression of PCS on testosterone for 170 male cancer survivors aged 25–45.

3. *The variance (or standard deviation) of y should be the same at each value of x, that is, there should be no evidence that as the value of y changes, the spread of the x values changes.* This assumption means that the residuals have the same variability or constant variance for all the fitted values of y. We can check this assumption by a scatter plot of the residuals against the fitted or predicted Y values from the model. We should observe a random scatter of data points.
Figure 7.10 shows a scatter plot of the relationship between the residuals from the linear regression of PCS on testosterone and the fitted or predicted PCS values. The relationship between the two variables appears to be random and does not follow any systematic pattern. There is no tendency for the residuals to increase or decrease systematically with the fitted values. Therefore the constant variance assumption appears to be satisfied.

4. *The observations in the sample are independent.* The observations in the sample are independent if there is no more than one pair of observations on each subject.

5. *The variable x can be measured without error.* This is an almost impossible assumption to check and satisfy! The x variable is rarely measured without any error. We have to assume this error is small. Provided this is the case, then this is likely to have little effect on the model and the conclusions from the model.

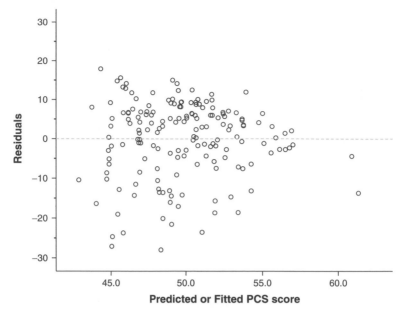

Figure 7.10   Scatter plot of residuals versus fitted or predicted PCS values from the linear regression of PCS on testosterone for 170 male cancer survivors aged 25–45.

Exercises

7.1 Table 7.17 shows the SF-36 Physical Functioning dimension scores for a random sample of 20 young male cancer survivors with normal and low levels of testosterone from the Greenfield *et al.* (2007) study. One of the aims of this study was to compare QoL between men with normal and low levels of testosterone.

(a) Write out a suitable null and alternative hypothesis for this problem and data set.

(b) Do these data suggest that men in the normal levels of testosterone group have a different level of physical functioning compared to men in the low testosterone group? Stating any assumptions you make, perform an appropriate hypothesis test to compare mean SF-36 Physical Functioning dimension scores between the groups of mean with normal and low levels of testosterone. Comment on the results of this hypothesis test.

(c) Calculate a 95% confidence interval for the difference in mean SF-36 Physical Functioning dimension scores between the groups of men with normal and low levels of testosterone. Discuss whether the confidence interval suggests that men in the normal testosterone group might have better physical functioning than men in the low testosterone group.

7.2 Table 7.18 shows the SF-36 Role Physical dimension scores for a random sample of 20 young male cancer survivors with normal and low levels of testosterone

Table 7.17   SF-36 Physical Functioning dimension scores in two groups of young male cancers survivors with normal and low levels of testosterone.

	Normal testosterone ($n = 10$)	Low testosterone ($n = 10$)
	100.0	80.0
	100.0	30.0
	95.0	0.0
	95.0	10.0
	50.0	45.0
	95.0	5.0
	95.0	100.0
	65.0	90.0
	100.0	75.0
	95.0	60.0
Mean	89.0	49.5
SD	17.1	36.9

Table 7.18   SF-36 Role Physical dimension scores in two groups of young male cancers survivors with normal and low levels of testosterone.

	Normal testosterone ($n = 10$) SF-36v2 Role Physical	Low testosterone ($n = 10$) SF-36v2 Role Physical
	100.0	75.0
	100.0	81.3
	100.0	25.0
	93.8	31.3
	50.0	56.3
	100.0	6.3
	93.8	100.0
	50.0	62.5
	100.0	50.0
	93.8	25.0
Mean	88.1	51.3
SD	20.3	29.4

from the Greenfield *et al.* (2007) study. One of the aims of this study was to compare QoL between men with normal and low levels of testosterone.

(a) Draw separate dot plots and/or histograms for the SF-36 Role Physical dimension for the normal and low testosterone groups, respectively. Do these graphs suggest that the distribution of the SF-36 Role Physical dimension is symmetric or skewed in the two groups?

(b) Do these data suggest that the young male cancer survivors with normal levels of testosterone have different SF-36 Role Physical dimension scores than men with low testosterone? Stating any assumptions you make, perform an appropriate hypothesis test to compare the SF-36 Role Physical dimension scores between the men with normal and low testosterone. Comment on the results of this hypothesis test.

(c) Calculate a 95% confidence interval for the difference in mean SF-36 Role Physical dimension scores between the groups of men with normal and low levels of testosterone. Discuss whether the confidence interval suggests that men in the normal testosterone group might have better Role Physical scores than men in the low testosterone group.

7.3 Table 7.19 shows the HAD Anxiety and Depression dimension scores for a random sample of 10 Gypsies/Travellers and their age- and sex-matched controls from the Parry *et al.* (2007) study. One of the aims of this study was to compare anxiety and depression levels between Gypsies/Travellers and their age- and sex-matched controls.

(a) Do these data suggest that the mean HAD anxiety scores between the Gypsy Travellers group and the age- and sex-matched control group is different? Stating any assumptions you make, perform an appropriate hypothesis test to compare mean HAD anxiety dimension scores between the Gypsies/Travellers and their age- and sex-matched controls in this sample of 10 pairs. Comment on the results of this hypothesis test.

(b) Calculate a 95% confidence interval for the difference in mean HAD Anxiety dimension scores between the Gypsies/Travellers group and the age- and sex-matched control group. Discuss whether the confidence interval suggests that Gypsies/Travellers might have higher levels of anxiety than their age- and sex-matched control counterparts.

Table 7.19   HAD Anxiety and Depression scores for 10 Gypsies/Travellers and their corresponding age- and sex-matched controls (data from Parry *et al.*, 2007).

Pair	GT: HAD Anxiety score	Control: HAD Anxiety score	Difference in HAD Anxiety scores between GT and matched control	GT: HAD Depression score	Control: HAD Depression	Difference in HAD Depression scores between GT and matched control
1	13	0	13.0	7	0	7.0
2	19	2	17.0	4	4	.0
3	21	5	16.0	15	2	13.0
4	10	4	6.0	5	3	2.0
5	4	2	2.0	2	3	−1.0
6	1	1	.0	8	2	6.0
7	19	4	15.0	11	1	10.0
8	4	2	2.0	3	0	3.0
9	11	5	6.0	12	2	10.0
10	20	1	19.0	10	2	8.0

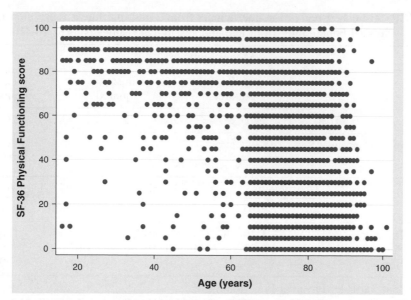

Figure 7.11 Scatter plot of SF-36 Physical Functioning dimension score versus age for 7213 subjects aged 18–101.

(c) Do these data suggest that the Gypsies/Travellers have different HAD depression dimension scores than an age- and sex-matched control group? Perform a Wilcoxon matched pairs hypothesis test to compare the HAD depression dimension scores between Gypsies/Travellers and their age- and sex-matched controls. Comment on the results of this hypothesis test.

7.4 Figure 7.11 shows a scatter plot of the SF-36 Physical Functioning score versus age for 7213 subjects aged 18–101.

(a) From the graph does there appear to be a relationship between the two variables?

(b) The Pearson correlation between age and Physical Functioning was −0.49, $P < 0.001$. What does this correlation say about the direction and strength of the relationship between age and SF-36 Physical Functioning score? What does $P < 0.001$ mean?

7.5 A survey was conducted on 7213 members of the general public using the SF-36 to measure their quality of life. Sex was coded 0 = female, 1 = male. The computer output from a multiple linear regression of age and sex on SF-36 Physical Functioning dimension score is shown in Table 7.20.

(a) Deduce the values of A and B.

(b) Are either age or sex significant predictors of Physical Functioning?

(c) What is the expected Physical Functioning score for a woman aged 45?

(d) What is the expected Physical Functioning score for a man aged 39?

Table 7.20 Estimated regression coefficients from a multiple linear regression model to predict Physical Functioning from age and sex in 7213 subjects aged 16–101.

		Model Summary		
Model	R	R squared	Adjusted R squared	Std. error of the estimate
1	0.507(a)	0.257	0.257	27.6051

a Predictors: (Constant), Sex, Age (years)

		Coefficients					
Model		Coefficients		t	P-value	95% CI for b	
		b	SE(b)			Lower bound	Upper bound
1	Intercept	123.90	1.46	84.732	0.001	121.03	126.77
	Age (years)	−0.98	0.02	A	0.001	−1.02	−0.94
	Sex	7.88	.65	12.061	0.001	B	9.17

a Dependent Variable: Physical Functioning

Table 7.21 Descriptive statistics for SF-36 Physical Functioning dimension by cancer type and ANOVA table for 171 young male cancer survivors (data from Greenfield et al., 2007).

Descriptive statistics for SF-36v2 Physical Functioning

Cancer type	n	Mean	Std. Deviation	Minimum	Maximum
Germ cell (testicular)	66	81.7	29.3	0	100.0
Lymphoma	70	81.7	23.6	0	100.0
Leukaemia	11	91.8	17.6	40.0	100.0
Other	24	79.0	29.0	5.0	100.0
Total	171	82.0	26.3	0	100.0

ANOVA Table

	Sum of Squares	df	Mean Square	F	Sig.
Between groups	1295.166	3	431.722	0.619	0.604
Within groups	116473.547	167	697.446		
Total	117768.713	170			

(e) Is the model a good fit to the data?

7.6 Table 7.21 shows some descriptive statistics for the SF-36 Physical Functioning dimension by cancer type and ANOVA table for 171 young male cancer survivors (Greenfield et al., 2007). Do these data suggest that the mean SF-36 Physical Functioning scores differ between the different types of cancer? Comment on the results of the analysis in the table.

8

Randomized controlled trials

Summary

Quality of life measures are becoming more frequently used in clinical trials and health services research, both as primary and secondary endpoints. This chapter emphasizes the importance of randomized controlled trials (RCTs) in evaluating alternative treatments or interventions. It shows how to analyse and present the QoL outcome data from RCTs. Different types of randomized trial, such as factorial, cluster and cross-over trials, are described and we distinguish between those to establish superiority and those that seek equivalence. A checklist of points to consider when presenting and reporting the results of an RCT is also included.

8.1 Introduction

A *clinical trial* is defined as a prospective study to examine the relative efficacy of treatments or interventions in human subjects. In many applications one of the treatments is a standard therapy (control) and the other a new therapy or intervention (test). Even with well-established and effective treatments it is well recognized that individual patients may react differently once these are administered. Thus aspirin will cure some people with headache speedily whilst others will continue with their headache. The human body is a very complex organism, whose functioning is far from completely understood, and so it is not surprising that it is often difficult to predict the exact reaction that a diseased individual will have to a particular therapy. Even though medical science might suggest that a new treatment is efficacious, it is only when it is tried in practice that any realistic assessment of its efficacy can be made and the presence of any adverse side-effects identified. Thus it is necessary to do comparative trials to evaluate the new treatment against the current standard (Campbell *et al.*, 2007). Quality of life measures are becoming more frequently used in clinical trials and health services research, both as primary and secondary endpoints.

Quality of Life Outcomes in Clinical Trials and Health-Care Evaluation   Stephen J. Walters
© 2009 John Wiley & Sons, Ltd

8.2   Randomized controlled trials

The key idea of a clinical trial is to compare groups of patients who differ only with respect to their treatment. If the groups differ in some other way then the comparison of treatments may be biased. The two treatments should be investigated concurrently, allocation of treatments to patients should be by a random process, and neither the patient nor the clinician should know which treatment was received. The *randomized double-blind controlled trial* is usually taken as the 'gold standard' against which to judge the quality of the design of a trial. Randomization is a method of allocating treatments to patients in a trial. It ensures that each patient has an equal chance of being allocated to the available treatments. It also ensures that the treatment to be given cannot be predicted.

8.3   Protocols

One essential aspect of planning a randomized controlled trial is to write a study *protocol*. This is a formal document specifying how the study is to be conducted. A protocol is necessary when applying for a grant to carry out the study. Most of the information will also be required by the local ethics committee. A protocol will aid carrying out the study and make writing up the results easier. The drawing up of a protocol is strongly recommended for any research project, not just an RCT.

There are three fundamental aspects of study design which must be precisely defined at an early stage:

1. Which patients are eligible?

2. Which treatments are to be evaluated?

3. How is each patient's response to be assessed?

For any study to fulfil the protocol specification there must be adequate financial support and sufficient skilled staff. Pocock (1983) lists the main features of a study protocol as shown in Box 8.1.

It is important that RCTs are reported adequately, since they have considerable potential to affect patient care. Concern over the variability in the quality of the reporting of RCTs in the medical literature led to the development of the Consolidation of Standards for Reporting Trials (CONSORT) statement. The CONSORT statement is a research tool designed to improve the quality of reports of clinical trials (Moher *et al.*, 2001). It consists of a flow diagram and a checklist of items which should be reported in the paper (see Table 8.1). The checklist identifies 22 items that should be incorporated in the title, abstract, introduction, methods, results and conclusions of every randomized clinical trial. More details can be found at http://www.consort-statement.org.

8.4   Pragmatic and explanatory trials

One can draw a useful distinction between trials that aim to determine the exact mechanism of action of a treatment (*explanatory* trials) and trials that aim to determine the efficacy of a treatment as used in day-to-day clinical practice (*pragmatic* trials). Explanatory studies seek to evaluate the comparative efficacy of a treatment or service and to help

---

Box 8.1 Main features of a study protocol.

1. Background and general aims

2. Specific objectives

3. Patient selection criteria

4. Treatment schedules

5. Methods of patient evaluation

6. Trial design

7. Registration and randomization of patients

8. Patient consent

9. Required size of study

10. Monitoring of trial progress

11. Forms and data handling

12. Protocol deviations

13. Plans for statistical analysis

14. Administrative responsibilities

Reproduced with permission from Pocock, SJ. *Clinical Trials: A Practical Approach*.
John Wiley & Sons Ltd, Chichester. © 1983 John Wiley & Sons Ltd.

---

explain why the treatment or service is effective or not. Explanatory trials try to answer the question whether the treatment or service works in principle. Pragmatic studies seek to evaluate the comparative effectiveness of a treatment or service, and aid decisions about which services or treatments should be provided. Pragmatic trials try to answer the question whether the treatment works in real life.

8.5 Intention-to-treat and per-protocol analyses

In many trials some patients will not have followed the protocol, either on purpose or by accident. This may include patients who actually receive the wrong treatment (i.e. not the one they were randomly allocated to) and patients who do not take their treatment. Also it is sometimes discovered after the trial has started that a patient was not after all eligible for entry into the trial. The only safe way to deal with all of these situations is to keep all randomized patients in the trial and to 'analyse as you randomise' (Altman, 1991). The analysis is based on the groups as randomized, and is known as an *intention-to-treat* analysis. Any other policy towards protocol violations will involve subjective decisions and will create an opportunity for bias. It is sometimes helpful to carry out an additional analysis of only those patients who adhered to the protocol, a *per-protocol* analysis. The analysis of the groups as randomized must be considered the main analysis for the trial (Altman, 1991).

Table 8.1   CONSORT checklist of items to include when reporting a randomized trial.

	Item no.	Descriptor
Title and abstract **Introduction**	*1*	How patients were allocated to interventions.
Background	2	Scientific background and explanation of rationale.
Methods *Participants*	*3*	Eligibility criteria for participants and the settings and locations where the data were collected.
Interventions	4	Precise details of the interventions intended for each group and how and when they were actually administered.
Objectives	5	Specific objectives and hypotheses.
Outcomes	6	Clearly defined primary and secondary outcome measures and, when applicable, any methods used to enhance the quality of measurements (e.g. multiple observations, training of assessors).
Sample size	7	How sample size was determined and, when applicable, explanation of any interim analyses and stopping rules.
Randomization		
Sequence generation	8	Method used to generate the random allocation sequence, including details of any restriction (e.g. blocking, stratification).
Allocation concealment	9	Method used to implement the random allocation sequence (e.g. numbered containers or central telephone), clarifying whether the sequence was concealed until interventions were assigned.
Implementation	10	Who generated the allocation sequence, who enrolled participants, and who assigned participants to their groups.
Blinding (masking)	11	Whether or not participants, those administering the interventions, and those assessing the outcomes were blinded to group assignment. When relevant, how the success of blinding was evaluated.
Statistical methods	12	Statistical methods used to compare groups for primary outcome(s). Methods for additional analyses, such as subgroup analyses and adjusted analyses.

Table 8.1   (*Continued*)

	Item no.	Descriptor
Results		
Participant flow	13	Flow of participants through each stage (a diagram is strongly recommended). Specifically, for each group report the numbers of participants randomly assigned, receiving intended treatment, completing the study protocol, and analysed for the primary outcome. Describe protocol deviations from study as planned, together with reasons.
Recruitment	14	Dates defining the periods of recruitment and follow-up.
Baseline data	15	Baseline demographic and clinical characteristics of each group.
Numbers analysed	16	Number of participants (denominator) in each group included in each analysis and whether the analysis was by 'intention-to-treat'. State the results in absolute numbers when feasible (e.g. 10/20, not 50%).
Outcomes and estimation	17	For each primary and secondary outcome, a summary of results for each group, and the estimated effect size and its precision (e.g. 95% confidence interval).
Ancillary analyses	18	Address multiplicity by reporting any other analyses performed, including subgroup analyses and adjusted analyses, indicating those pre-specified and those exploratory.
Adverse events	19	Address multiplicity by reporting any other analyses performed, including subgroup analyses and adjusted analyses, indicating those pre-specified and those exploratory.
Discussion		
Interpretation	20	Interpretation of results, taking into account study hypotheses, sources of potential bias or imprecision and the dangers associated with multiplicity of analyses and outcomes.
Generalisability	21	Generalizability (external validity) of the trial findings.
Overall evidence	22	General interpretation of the results in the context of current evidence.

8.6   Patient flow diagram

Figure 8.1 shows a CONSORT flow diagram for an RCT of a short course of traditional acupuncture compared with usual care for persistent non-specific low back pain (Thomas *et al.*, 2006). The diagram shows that 241 eligible patients consented to be randomized. Patients were randomly allocated in the ratio of 2:1 to the acupuncture group. One hundred and sixty patients were offered acupuncture and 81 were allocated to usual care. The primary outcome was the SF-36 Bodily Pain score at 12-month follow-up. Two patients, one in each group, withdrew from the study immediately after randomization. At 12-month follow-up there were 215 patients with outcome data for analysis (147 in the acupuncture group and 68 in the usual care group). By 24-month follow-up the number of patients with data and outcomes for analysis had dropped further to 182.

The CONSORT flow diagram of Figure 8.1 enables readers quickly to understand how many eligible participants were randomly assigned to each arm of the trial and whether any imbalances are apparent regarding numbers of patients withdrawing from or failing to comply with their assigned treatment. The CONSORT statement was designed to be used to report the results of RCTs. However, only 5 of the 22 items in the checklist specifically apply to RCTs and the remaining majority of the items are applicable for most other studies that collect quantitative data. Therefore, I would recommend that the flow diagram and CONSORT checklist be used as a guideline for the reporting of the results of other studies including cross-sectional surveys and other observational studies.

8.7   Comparison of entry characteristics

Randomization is a method of removing bias in the way that treatments are allocated to patients, but it does not guarantee that the characteristics of the two groups are similar. The first table in the report of an RCT is to summarize the entry or baseline characteristics of the patients in the two groups. It is important to show that the groups are similar with respect to variables that may have an impact on the patient's response (Altman, 1991).

I do not recommend comparing the baseline characteristics of the groups by performing hypothesis tests. If the randomization is performed fairly we know that any differences between the two treatment groups must be due to chance. The key question is whether the two groups differ in a way that might affect their response to treatment, which is a question of clinical importance rather than statistical significance testing. The only use of hypothesis testing is to judge whether the randomization was performed fairly, but this will only detect major fraud since (by definition of a P-value) we expect 5% of the tests to be significant at the 5% level.

Lack of balance in a baseline variable is only potentially critical, in the sense of making a difference to the overall result of the trial, if that variable is related to the outcome variable (Altman, 1991). If there are one or more variables with known or suspected prognostic importance that are not closely balanced we can see whether those variables are related to the outcome variable, or we can simply adjust for them in the analysis as discussed later.

Table 8.2 shows the baseline characteristics of patients with non-specific back pain who were randomized to acupuncture care or usual care only. The table contains a mixture of continuous and categorical (nominal, ordinal and binary) data. Data for the intervention

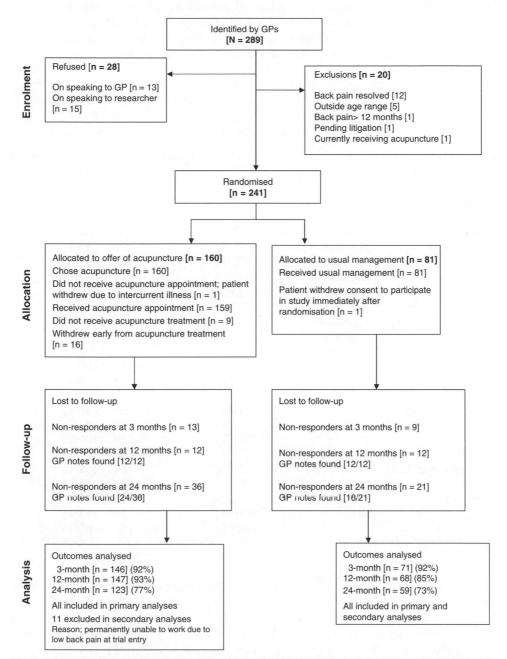

Figure 8.1 Patient progress through trial – CONSORT flow chart for acupuncture study. Reproduced from Thomas, K.J., MacPherson, H., Thorpe, L., *et al.*, 'Randomised controlled trial of a short course of traditional acupuncture compared with usual care for persistent non-specific low back pain.' *British Medical Journal*, 333(7569), 623, © 2006, with permission from the BMJ Publishing Group Limited.

Table 8.2 Baseline characteristics of patients by treatment group. Adapted by permission from BMJ Publishing Group Limited. Thomas, K.J., MacPherson, H., Thorpe, L., *et al.*, 'Randomised controlled trial of a short course of traditional acupuncture compared with usual care for persistent non-specific low back pain. *British Medical Journal*,' 333(7569), 623, © 2006.

		Treatment group					
		Usual care			Acupuncture		
Characteristic		*n*	Mean or %		*n*	Mean or %	
Age (years) (range)		80	44.0	20–64	159	41.9	26–64
Duration of back pain (weeks) (SD)		80	16.7	(14.6)	159	17.1	(13.5)
SF-36 Bodily Pain (SD)		80	30.4	(18.0)	159	30.8	(16.2)
Gender	*Male*	34/80	(43%)		60/159	(38%)	
Work status	*Full-time*	45	(56%)		82	(52%)	
	Part-time	22	(28%)		40	(25%)	
	Housewife	7	(9%)		13	(8%)	
	Retired	4	(5%)		7	(4%)	
	Student	1	(1%)		3	(2%)	
	Permanently unable to work	1	(1%)		14	(9%)	
		80	(100%)		159	(100%)	
No. of previous episodes	*None*	13	(16%)		25	(16%)	
of low back pain	*1–5*	23	(29%)		57	(36%)	
	>5	44	(55%)		77	(48%)	
		80	(100%)		159	(100%)	
Presence of leg pain	*Yes*	59/80	(74%)		106/159	(67%)	
Expectation of back pain	*Better*	30	(38%)		80	(51%)	
in six months	*Same*	37	(46%)		56	(35%)	
	Worse	12	(16%)		21	(13%)	
		79	(100%)		157	(100%)	

and control groups are reported in columns and the baseline variables are reported by row. For the categorical outcomes the percentages are also reported; this helps compare the two groups, since the 2:1 randomization schedule has resulted in twice as many patients in the acupuncture arm of the trial. For outcomes with only two categories it best to report the result as x/n (y %). For more than two categories it is best to report the total as a separate row to avoid repeating it for each category and to enable a check that all categories are present. In this way we can see that there is one missing value in 'expectation of back pain' in the control group and there are two missing values in the intervention group. The two groups appear to have similar characteristics at baseline. No hypothesis tests to compare the baseline characteristics of the two groups have been performed or reported in the table.

8.8   Incomplete data

From the CONSORT flow diagram in Figure 8.1 we see that 241 patients were randomized in the acupuncture trial but only 182 (i.e. 75% of the original cohort) had outcomes at 24 months that could be analysed. Two patients dropped out immediately after randomization and provided no data. Ideally the reasons for patients dropping out should be recorded. In the original cohort of 239 patients Table 8.2 clearly shows that the two groups were well matched. However, withdrawal may be caused by treatment-related side effects. Whatever the reason, the incomplete data, may compromise the initial baseline balance between the two treatment groups (seen in Table 8.2).

Table 8.3 compares the baseline characteristics of those patients who were randomized with those who were actually analysed. It is a useful table, rarely reported in RCTs. It helps us see if the baseline characteristics of the patients who are the basis for the analysis are now similar between the groups and also to the patients originally recruited. This table shows that in fact those subjects actually analysed were similar between the intervention and control group at baseline, and the subjects analysed were similar to those randomized.

Figure 8.2 is a graphical comparison of the mean baseline SF-36 Bodily Pain scores by treatment group and response status: whether or not the patient completed the SF-36 Bodily Pain dimension at 24-month follow-up. If the two lines are horizontal and coincide, this means the mean QoL scores at baseline are the same in both treatment groups and do not vary by response status at 24-month follow-up. From the graph it looks like there is no difference in mean baseline SF-36 Bodily Pain scores between the treatment groups and between the responders and non-responders at 24 months.

A more formal way of assessing whether or not the baseline characteristics of the responders and non-responders are the same in the two treatment groups is to fit a multiple linear regression model, with baseline QoL as the outcome and treatment group, response status and a treatment group × response status interaction term as explanatory variables:

$$QoL_{Baseline} = b_0 + b_1Group + b_2Responder + b_3Interaction. \tag{8.1}$$

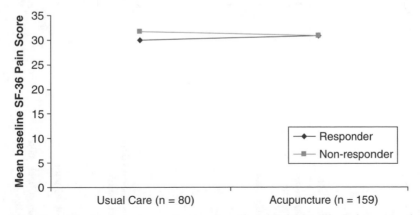

Figure 8.2   Graphical comparison of mean baseline SF-36 Bodily Pain scores by treatment group and response status at 24 months for acupuncture study (data from Thomas *et al.*, 2006).

Table 8.3 Baseline characteristics of patients of all recruited patients (n = 239) vs. those with outcomes for analysis at 24 months (n = 182) by group (data from Thomas *et al.*, 2006). Reproduced with permission from Freeman, J.V., Walters, S.J., Campbell, M.J., *How to Display Data*. BMJ Books. ©2008 Blackwell Publishing.

Characteristic	Usual care				Acupuncture			
	All patients (n = 80)		Analysed at 24 months (n = 59)		All patients (n = 159)		Analysed at 24 months (n = 123)	
	n	Mean	n	Mean	n	Mean	n	Mean
Age (years) (range)	80	44.0 20–64	59	45.5 20–64	159	41.9 26–64	123	42.5 26–64
Duration of back pain (weeks) (SD)	80	16.7 (14.6)	59	16.0 (14.1)	159	17.1 (13.5)	123	17.0 (13.3)
SF-36 Bodily Pain (SD)	80	30.4 (18.0)	59	29.9 (18.7)	159	30.8 (16.2)	123	30.8 (16.6)
Gender Male	34	(43%)	23	(39%)	60	(38%)	44	(36%)
Work status Full-time	45	(56%)	33	(56%)	82	(52%)	63	(51%)
Part-time	22	(28%)	18	(31%)	40	(25%)	33	(27%)
Housewife	7	(9%)	3	(5%)	13	(8%)	9	(7%)
Retired	4	(5%)	4	(7%)	7	(4%)	7	(6%)
Student	1	(1%)	1	(2%)	3	(2%)	2	(2%)
Permanently unable to work	1	(1%)			14	(9%)	9	(7%)
No. of previous episodes of low back pain None	13	(16%)	10	(17%)	25	(16%)	20	(16%)
1–5	23	(29%)	16	(27%)	57	(36%)	42	(34%)
>5	44	(55%)	33	(56%)	77	(48%)	61	(50%)
	80	(100%)	59	(100%)	159	(100%)	123	(100%)
Presence of leg pain Yes	59	(74%)	46	(78%)	106	(67%)	82	(67%)
Expectation of back pain in six months Better	30	(38%)	25	(42%)	80	(51%)	57	(47%)
Same	37	(46%)	23	(39%)	56	(35%)	47	(39%)
Worse	12	(16%)	10	(17%)	21	(13%)	17	(14%)
Don't know	1	(1%)	1	(2%)	1	(1%)	1	(1%)
	80	(100%)	59	(100%)	158	(100%)	122	(100%)

Table 8.4   Baseline characteristics of all recruited patients ($n = 239$) versus those with outcomes for analysis at 24 months ($n = 182$) by group (data from Thomas *et al.*, 2006).

Model*	Coefficients				95% CI for b	
	b	SE(b)	t	P-value	Lower Bound	Upper Bound
Intercept	31.75	3.68	8.630	0.000	24.50	38.99
Treatment group (0 = usual care; 1 = acupuncture)	−0.88	4.63	−0.191	0.849	−10.00	8.24
Responder at 24 months (0 = no; 1 = yes)	−1.80	4.28	−0.421	0.674	−10.24	6.64
Treatment group × responder interaction	1.74	5.34	.326	0.745	−8.78	12.27

*Dependent variable: Baseline SF-36 Bodily Pain

If treatment group is coded as 0 (usual care) and 1 (acupuncture) and response status is coded as 0 (non-responder) and 1 (responder), then the interaction term will be zero except for patients in group 1 and with a response status of 1 (i.e. randomized to acupuncture treatment and responded at 24 months).

If the regression coefficient for the interaction term is non-significant then we can say that the lines in Figure 8.2 are parallel and there is no evidence that the baseline QoL characteristics of the responders and non-responders are different between the two treatment groups. Table 8.4 shows the results of fitting such a model to the baseline SF-36 Bodily Pain data from the acupuncture study. The non-significant P-values for the interaction term and the treatment group and response status variables suggest that there is no evidence that the baseline QoL characteristics of the responders and non-responders are different between the two treatment groups.

8.9   Main analysis

The main analysis of a RCT is the comparison of the pre-specified outcome measures between the different treatment groups. If the groups are well balanced with respect to variables of known or suspected prognostic importance then we can use simple methods of analysis. For trials of two independent groups (such as the acupuncture trial) we can use the flow diagram of Figure 7.1 to decide which statistical test to use to compare outcomes. If we assume the QoL outcome is continuous then we can use the parametric two independent samples t-test or the non-parametric Mann–Whitney test to compare the outcomes as appropriate and calculate the associated confidence intervals.

Ideally, as an initial step, we should graphically display the QoL outcome data in each group to see how the data are distributed using dot plots, histograms or box-and-whisker plots as described in Chapter 6. It is likely that the QoL data will have a discrete, bounded and skewed distribution. In these circumstances Figure 7.1 would suggest that the non-parametric Mann–Whitney U-test is more appropriate for analysing the data than the parametric two independent samples t-test. However, as mentioned in Chapter 7, non-parametric tests do not easily allow for analyses such as multiple regression or the estimation of confidence intervals for treatment effects and differences. It is very important to estimate a confidence interval for the treatment effect. This is now regarded as good statistical practice (Altman et al., 2000). My own research experience suggests little difference between parametric and non-parametric methods when calculating standard errors, P-values and confidence intervals (Walters, 2003, 2004; Walters and Campbell, 2004, 2005). Therefore I tend to use standard statistical analysis methods (such as the t-test and multiple linear regression) to analyse QoL outcomes.

Table 8.5 shows the results of eight independent samples t-tests to compare the mean SF-36 dimension scores, at 12 months, between the acupuncture and usual care groups. Note that the number of observations varies considerably across the eight dimensions. The rows correspond to the eight SF-36 dimensions and are ordered by mean difference. The mean dimension scores (and their variability) are described separately for each group. A 95% confidence interval for the treatment effect, which is the difference in mean scores, is reported. Exact P-values are reported to two decimal places in the last column of the table. A footnote to the table is included describing how the SF-36 is scaled and scored, what hypothesis test has been performed and how the treatment effect (mean difference) should be interpreted. Since the SF-36 is scored on a 0–100 scale these data are reported to a precision of one decimal place.

The SF-36 is also an example of a profile QoL measure since it generates eight separate scores for each dimension of health. The scores on the eight dimensions are not independent – they are linked to the same subject. One way of graphically displaying such data is by a radar or spider plot. Figure 8.3 shows a radar plot for the overall mean SF-36 dimension scores, at 12-month follow-up, by treatment group, for the data in presented in Table 8.5. The radar plot has eight spokes corresponding to the eight QoL dimensions of the SF-36, with the centre point of the plot indicating a score of zero.

Table 8.5 Mean Bodily dimension scores at 12 months by treatment group (data from Thomas et al., 2006). Reproduced with permission from Freeman, J.V., Walters, S.J., Campbell, M.J., *How to Display Data*. BMJ Books. © 2008 Blackwell Publishing.

| | Treatment group | | | | | | | | |
| | Usual care | | | Acupuncture | | | Mean | 95% CI | |
SF-36 dimension[1]	n	Mean	SD	n	Mean	SD	difference[2]	Lower	Upper	P-value[3]
Pain	68	58.3	(22.2)	147	64.0	(25.6)	5.7	−1.4	12.8	0.12
Role Physical	57	61.8	(42.8)	134	66.0	(40.0)	4.2	−8.5	17.0	0.52
Role Emotional	57	78.4	(35.9)	133	78.2	(35.3)	−0.2	−11.2	10.9	0.98
General Health	56	65.4	(19.3)	134	64.8	(21.8)	−0.6	−7.2	6.1	0.87
Physical Functioning	57	73.4	(20.9)	133	71.7	(25.8)	−1.7	−9.4	5.9	0.65
Vitality	56	57.0	(21.6)	135	54.1	(23.3)	−2.9	−10.0	4.3	0.43
Social Functioning	68	80.7	(22.1)	147	77.8	(25.2)	−2.9	−10.0	4.1	0.41
Mental Health	56	73.3	(15.4)	135	69.0	(20.4)	−4.3	−10.3	1.6	0.15

[1]The SF-36 dimensions are scored on a 0 (poor) to 100 (good health) scale.
[2]A positive mean difference indicates the acupuncture group has the better HRQoL.
[3]P-value from two independent samples t-test.

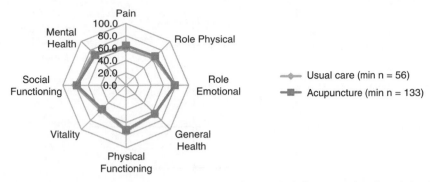

Figure 8.3   Radar plot with mean scores, at 12-month follow-up, for the eight dimensions of the SF-36 by treatment group, $n = 189$ (data from Thomas et al., 2006). Reproduced with permission from Freeman, J.V., Walters, S.J., Campbell, M.J., *How to Display Data*. BMJ Books. © 2008 Blackwell Publishing.

The spokes are linked by lines, which clearly show that the outcomes are related and are not independent. The radar plot in Figure 8.3 clearly shows that the two treatments groups, acupuncture and usual care, have similar mean QoL for all eight dimensions of the SF-36.

Figure 8.3 conceals the fact that the sample size for each dimension varies considerably. We could also report the number of subjects for each outcome. A better strategy is to report the mean scores on the spokes for subjects who have data on all the outcomes. Figure 8.4 shows the radar plot with the mean scores for 183 patients who provided data on all eight dimensions of the SF-36. Figure 8.3 is very similar to Figure 8.4. In this example it is unlikely that excluding six patients from the analysis and figure will affect the mean dimension scores to any appreciable extent.

The radar plots of Figures 8.3 and 8.4 clearly display the mean SF-36 dimension scores by treatment group. However, for an RCT or any other two-group comparison, what is required is the contrast or difference in outcomes between the groups and the

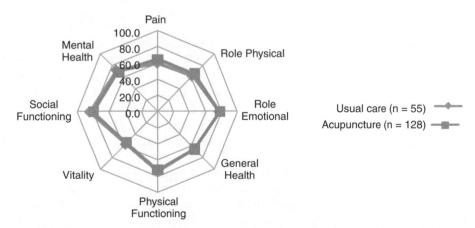

Figure 8.4   Radar plot with mean scores, at 12-month follow-up, for the eight dimensions of the SF-36 by treatment group, $n = 183$ (data from Thomas et al., 2006).

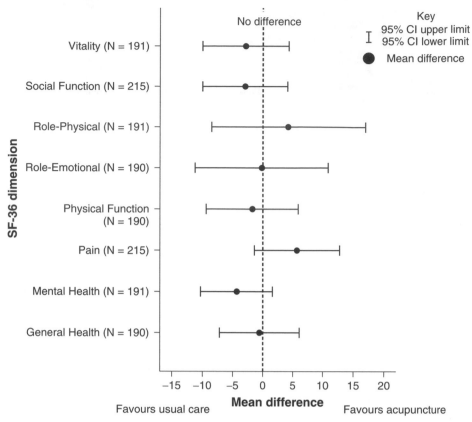

Figure 8.5 Estimated treatment effect (mean difference in SF-36 score between the acupuncture and usual care groups) and the corresponding confidence interval, at 12 months, for the eight dimensions of the SF-36 (data from Thomas *et al.*, 2006). Reproduced with permission from Freeman, J.V., Walters, S.J., Campbell, M.J., *How to Display Data*. BMJ Books. © 2008 Blackwell Publishing.

associated uncertainty or confidence interval around this estimated treatment effect. The treatment effect – the mean difference and its associated confidence interval – can be shown graphically as in Figure 8.5. Figure 8.5 shows the estimated treatment effect (mean difference in SF-36 scores between the acupuncture and usual care groups) and the corresponding confidence interval, at 12 months, for the eight dimensions of the SF-36 (Thomas *et al.*, 2006). A similar plot to this, known as a *forest* plot, is commonly used for displaying the results of systematic reviews and meta-analyses. These are discussed in Chapter 12.

Figure 8.5 is visually very impressive and the lack of any treatment effect is readily apparent. It can be useful in conference presentations. However, much of the data present in Table 8.5 is not shown. For example, the sample size per group and mean SF-36 scores (and their variability) for each group are omitted. These are important results and this information should be reported. Hence, for presentation in a scientific report or paper Table 8.5 is preferred.

Example: RCT on the effectiveness of community postnatal support workers

Morrell *et al.* (2000) used a Mann–Whitney *U*-test to compare SF-36, Edinburgh postnatal depression scale and Duke scores at 6 weeks after childbirth between a group of new mothers randomly allocated to receive extra postnatal support or usual care (control) in an RCT to establish the effectiveness of community postnatal support workers (Table 8.6). This study is unusual in that no baseline assessment of QoL was undertaken. New mothers were recruited (and randomized) just after giving birth and it was felt that it was inappropriate to assess QoL at this time. Postal follow-up questionnaires were sent to the randomized mothers at 6 weeks after childbirth. The primary outcome of the study was the SF-36 General Health dimension score at six weeks after childbirth. The authors concluded that there was no evidence of a difference between the groups in the primary outcome. There was evidence of a difference in Physical Functioning, Social Functioning and Role Physical scores, indicating better perceived health in the control group. There was some evidence of a difference in mean scores on the EPDS in favour of the control group ($P = 0.05$) There was no evidence of a difference in scores on the Duke functional social support scale. It is regarded as good statistical practice to estimate a confidence interval for treatment effect (Altman *et al.*, 2000). Unfortunately the

Table 8.6   QoL outcomes measured at 6 weeks according to allocation to extra postnatal support or control group (data from Morrell *et al.*, 2000).

	Intervention		Control			
	n	Mean (SD)	*n*	Mean (SD)	*P*-value	Mean difference (95% CI)
General Health Perception	276	75.1 (18.4)	263	76.7 (18.6)	0.22	−1.6 (−4.7, 1.4)
Physical Functioning	278	86.9 (16.0)	265	89.1 (15.4)	0.01	−2.2 (−4.6, 0.5)
Social Functioning	281	76.4 (24.1)	268	80.2 (23.8)	0.03	−3.8 (−7.7, 0.3)
Role Physical	275	65.2 (39.4)	260	73.2 (38.8)	0.008	−7.9 (−14.6, 0.9)
Role Emotional	275	77.3 (35.3)	259	77.4 (36.6)	0.77	−0.1 (−6.5, 6.1)
Mental Health	282	72.0 (17.5)	268	72.7 (17.8)	0.60	−0.7 (−3.8, 2.2)
Vitality	282	49.7 (21.3)	268	50.3 (20.9)	0.81	−0.6 (−4.1, 3.0)
Pain	282	70.7 (24.3)	268	73.8 (24.9)	0.08	−3.0 (−6.9, 1.1)
Duke Functional Social Support	260	16.7 (6.7)	253	16.6 (7.4)	0.63	0.0 (−1.3, 1.3)
Edinburgh Postnatal Depression Scale	276	7.4 (5.2)	266	6.7 (5.5)	0.05	0.7 (−0.2, 1.6)

For the SF-36, a higher score indicates better health. Conversely, for the DUFSS and EPDS, a higher score indicates poorer health.

All *P*-values from Mann–Whitney test, which compares the distribution of the two groups.

Bootstrap 95% confidence intervals calculated for characteristic of the distribution (e.g. mean difference) by the percentile method. Groups may have difference in distributions but similar characteristics (e.g. means).

Mann–Whitney U-test, unlike the t-test, will not produce confidence intervals. Therefore the authors used a non-parametric 'bootstrap' procedure to estimate confidence intervals for the mean difference. The bootstrap procedure is described in Chapter 10.   □

8.10   Interpretation of changes/differences in quality of life scores

How do you interpret the difference in QoL scores between treatment groups from a study? The thing to do is look to see what the developers of the instrument say about interpreting or understanding the QoL scores on their instrument. Ideally the developers of the QoL instrument or other users will have defined or specified the smallest difference in QoL scores on that instrument that can be regarded as clinically or practically important – the *minimum clinically important difference* (MCID). For example, the developers of the SF-36 suggested that a 5-point difference in dimension scores is the smallest difference in scores which could be considered 'clinically and socially relevant' (Ware *et al.*, 1993).

    With a statistically significant result, the confidence interval (CI) for the treatment effect will exclude zero. What is now important is whether or not the confidence limits include or exclude values for a treatment effect that can be regarded as clinically or practically important (see Figure 8.6).

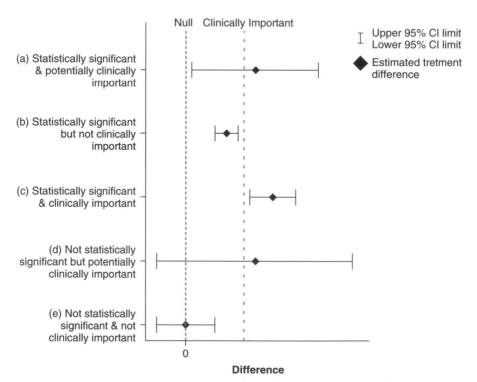

Figure 8.6   Use of confidence intervals to help distinguish statistical significance from clinical importance.

With a non-statistically significant result, the confidence interval for the treatment effect will include zero (see CIs (a), (d) and (e) in Figure 8.6). The confidence intervals may be wide and include zero and are hence consistent with no treatment effect. These wide CIs may also include values for the treatment effect that may be regarded as clinically and practically important (CIs (a) and (d)). In this case the evidence from the data is inconclusive about the treatment effect. Alternatively, the confidence intervals may be narrow and include zero and also wholly exclude values for the treatment effect which may be regarded as clinically or practically important (CI (e)). In this case the evidence from the data is conclusive as the upper and lower confidence limits do not cross any values which could be regarded as clinically and practically important. Hence, the pre-defined MCID provides a reference point to help interpret the results (and CI) for the observed treatment effect from the study data, in terms of their clinical and practical importance. There are no fixed values for the MCID. It depends on the outcome measure and may vary from study to study. This contrasts with the interpretation of the CI when trying to determine whether or not a result is statistically significant. A result is regarded as statistically significant when the confidence interval for the treatment effect excludes zero. This interpretation does not depend on the outcome measure and will not vary from study to study.

The MCID for the SF-36 dimensions is five or more points, and the Morrell *et al* (2000) study of community postnatal supported workers (Table 8.6) reported a mean difference of − 1.6 points on the General Health dimension between the intervention and control group women at 6 weeks after childbirth. This difference of −1.6 points (95% CI: −4.7 to 1.4) between the groups is neither statistically significant nor clinically important, as the confidence interval includes zero but wholly excludes a difference of five points.

8.11   Superiority and equivalence trials

The traditional RCT seeks to prove the superiority of a new treatment to an existing one. A successful conclusion from such a study is one in which such proof, of the superiority of the new treatment over the standard, is demonstrated. However, in recent years there has been an increasing interest in trials whose objective is to show that some new therapy is no worse as regards some outcome, such as QoL, than an existing treatment.

From the QoL point of view, we may wish to show that the new treatment is equivalent to the standard treatment with respect to QoL outcomes. However, it is important to be clear that failure to find a statistically significant difference between the treatment groups after completing the trial and analysing the QoL outcome data does not mean the two treatments are equivalent. It usually means the trial was too small or inadequately powered to detect the (small) actual difference in QoL between the two treatments. Indeed, with a finite number of subjects, one can never prove that two groups are exactly equivalent (Fayers and Machin, 2007).

Implicit in a comparison between two treatments is the presumption that if the null hypothesis is rejected then there is a difference in QoL between the treatments being compared. Thus one concludes that one treatment is 'superior' to the other irrespective of the magnitude of the difference observed. However, in certain situations, a new therapy may bring certain advantages over the current standard, possibly a reduced side-effects profile, easier administration or cost, but it may not be anticipated to be better with respect to the primary efficacy variable. For example, if the treatments to be compared are for an acute (but not serious) condition then perhaps a cheaper but not so efficacious (within quite wide limits) alternative to the standard treatment may be acceptable. However, if the condition is life-threatening then the limits of 'equivalence' would be narrow as any advantages of the new approach must not be offset by an unacceptable increase in (say) death rate. Under such conditions, the new approach may be required to be at least 'equivalent' to the standard in relation to efficacy if it is to replace it in future clinical use. This implies that 'equivalence' is a pre-specified maximum difference between treatments which, if observed to be less after the clinical trial is conducted, would render the two treatments equivalent (Campbell, et al., 2007)

One special form of equivalence trial is that termed a *non-inferiority* trial. Here we only wish to be sure that one treatment is 'not worse than' or is 'at least as good as' another treatment: if it is better, that is fine (even though superiority would not be required to bring it into common use). All we need is to get convincing evidence that the new treatment is not worse than the standard.

Although analysis and interpretation can be quite straightforward, the design and management of equivalence trials is often much more complex. In general, careless or inaccurate measurement, poor follow-up of patients, poor compliance with study procedures and medication all tend to bias results towards no difference between treatment groups. This implies that an intention-to-treat analysis is not likely to be appropriate since we are trying to offer evidence of equivalence. Poor study design and logistical procedures may therefore actually help hide treatment differences. In general, therefore, the quality of equivalence trials needs especially high compliance of the patients with respect to the treatment protocol.

Example: Non-inferiority trial

The results of a randomized controlled non-inferiority trial of telephone cognitive behaviour therapy (CBT) compared to face-to-face CBT in patients with obsessive compulsive disorder are reported by Lovell et al. (2006). The objectives of this study were to compare the clinical non-inferiority or equivalence of telephone CBT with conventional face-to-face CBT in patients with obsessive compulsive disorder. The primary outcome measure was the self-reported Yale Brown Obsessive Compulsive Disorder checklist (YBOCD) score post treatment. The YBOCD is a 10-item questionnaire, and responses to each question are rated on a 0 (no symptoms) to 4 (severe symptoms) scale. The total scale score range is from 0 (no symptoms) to 40 (severe symptoms). Patients were assessed at baseline, immediately after treatment and at 1-, 3- and 6-month follow-ups.

To assess non-inferiority of the two treatments the authors calculated two-sided 95% confidence intervals for the mean difference in YBOCD scores between the two treatments. Using this method, Lovell et al. (2006) stated that the experimental treatment (telephone CBT) would be regarded as not inferior to the control treatment (face-to-face CBT) at a 2.5% significance level if the upper boundary for the confidence limit (for the mean difference) was below 5 points (the range or margin of non-inferiority or equivalence). If the confidence interval covers at least some points outside this range, then differences of potential clinical importance remain a real possibility and non-inferiority cannot safely be concluded. The authors used a multiple linear regression model to adjust the mean difference (and confidence intervals) for baseline YBOCD score and site.

A total of 72 patients were randomized (36 in the telephone CBT group and 36 in the face-to-face CBT control group) across two sites. Sixty-five patients (35 intervention and

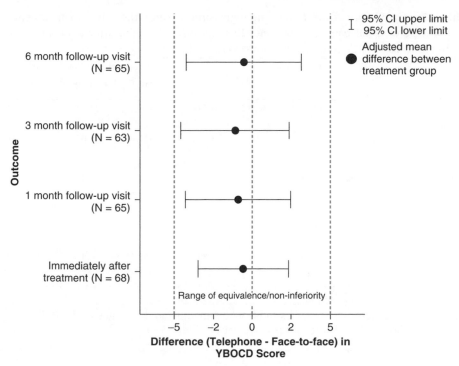

Figure 8.7 Non-inferiority of telephone versus face-to-face cognitive behaviour therapy for treatment of obsessive compulsive disorder (data from Lovell *et al.*, 2006).

30 control) had 6-month data for analysis. Figure 8.7 shows the point estimates and confidence intervals and the range of clinical non-inferiority/equivalence. The limits of all four confidence interval estimates for the outcomes are wholly within the pre-specified range of non-inferiority/equivalence. Therefore CBT delivered by telephone was equivalent to treatment delivered face-to-face in terms of YBOCD outcomes.   □

8.12   Adjusting for other variables

If we suspect that the observed differences, or imbalance, between the groups at the start of the study may have affected the outcome we can take account of the imbalance in the analysis. Adjusting a continuous outcome, such as QoL, for other variables requires the use of analysis of covariance or some form of multiple regression analysis, as described in Chapter 7. The regression model to describe this situation for two treatment groups (coded $0 =$ control, $1 =$ intervention) is

$$\text{QoL}_{\text{Followup}} = b_0 + b_1 \text{QoL}_{\text{Baseline}} + b_2 \text{Age} + b_3 \text{Sex} + b_4 \text{Group}. \tag{8.2}$$

In this model the effect of treatment on follow-up QoL can be assessed whilst adjusting for baseline QoL and other covariates such as age and sex.

Table 8.7 shows the regression coefficients when the outcome, 12-month SF-36 Bodily Pain score, was adjusted for baseline pain score and four other baseline covariates:

Table 8.7 Coefficients from a multiple regression to show the effect of treatment (acupuncture or usual care) on outcome, 12-month SF–36 pain, after adjustment for five baseline covariates (data from Thomas et al., 2006).

	Coefficients				95% confidence interval for b	
	b	SE(b)	t	P-value	Lower bound	Upper bound
Intercept	37.92	6.79	5.584	.000	24.53	51.30
SF-36 Bodily Pain baseline	.26	.10	2.572	.011	.06	.47
SF-36 Physical Functioning baseline	.24	.07	3.264	.001	.09	.38
Duration of back pain (weeks)	−.11	.12	−.955	.341	−.35	.12
How do you expect your back pain to be in 6 months time? (0 = Same/Worse ; 1= Better)	5.17	3.31	1.561	.120	−1.36	11.70
Presence of leg pain? (0 = No, 1 = Yes)	−3.70	3.52	−1.051	.294	−10.63	3.24
Treatment group (0 = usual care, 1 = acupuncture)	6.27	3.42	1.834	.068	−.47	13.02

Dependent Variable: SF-36 BodilyPain at 12 months

> The adjusted difference of 6.3 is similar to the unadjusted difference of 5.7 (95% CI: −1.4 to 12.8) although the adjusted CI is narrower (−0.5 to 13.0).

duration of current episode of pain (in weeks), expectation of back pain in six months, SF-36 Physical Functioning, and reported pain in legs.

Table 8.8 shows the recommended way of tabulating the outcomes after adjusting for other variables. The unadjusted treatment effect (with its confidence interval) should be presented alongside the adjusted treatment effect (with its confidence interval). The P-values from the two hypothesis tests can also be reported, although this is not essential. The footnote makes clear what covariates have been used to adjust the treatment comparison between the groups – again this information should be made clear in the table or the title. In this example the outcome, 12-month SF-36 Bodily Pain score, was adjusted for baseline pain score and four other baseline covariates: duration of current episode of pain (in weeks), expectation of back pain in six months (same/worse or better), SF-36 Physical Functioning, and reported pain in legs (yes or no).

It is important to make clear the sample size for both the unadjusted and adjusted analysis; ideally, they should both contain the same number of subjects. However, frequently some of the covariates used in the adjusted analysis are missing for one or two patients, even though the main outcome for these patients was recorded. Table 8.8 (and Table 8.5 for that matter) shows that 215 (147 acupuncture, 68 usual care) patients had a valid SF-36 Bodily Pain score at 12-month follow-up. However, for the adjusted analysis, three patients did not have one or more of the covariates recorded at baseline, so they are excluded from this analysis. In this example, it is unlikely that excluding three patients from the adjusted analysis will affect the comparisons between the adjusted and adjusted treatment effects.

Table 8.8 Unadjusted and adjusted differences in SF-36 Bodily Pain outcome scores between acupuncture and usual care groups at 12 months (data from Thomas *et al.*, 2006). Reproduced with permission from Freeman, J.V., Walters, S.J., Campbell, M.J., *How to Display Data*. BMJ Books. © 2008 Blackwell Publishing.

SF-36 dimension[1]	Treatment group								
	Usual care		Acupuncture			Unadjusted difference[3] (95% CI)	P-value	Adjusted[2] difference[3] (95% CI)	P-value
	n	Mean	SD	n	Mean	SD				
Bodily Pain	68	58.3	(22.2)	147	64.0	(25.6)	5.7 (−1.4 to 12.8)	0.12	6.3 (−0.5 to 13.0)	0.07

[1]The SF-36 Bodily Pain dimension is scored on a 0 to 100 (no pain) scale.
[2]n = 212 difference adjusted for baseline pain score and other baseline covariates: duration of current episode of pain (in weeks), expectation of back pain in six months (get better/stay same or get worse), SF-36 Physical Functioning, and reported pain in legs (yes/no).
[3]Improvement is indicated by a positive difference on the SF-36 Bodily Pain dimension

The result of the simple unadjusted analysis implies a difference of 5.7 (−1.4 to 12.8) in mean SF-36 Bodily Pain scores, at 12 months, between the groups, with the acupuncture group having the better outcome. The result of the adjusted analysis implies a difference of 6.3 (−0.5 to 13.0) in mean SF-36 Bodily Pain scores, at 12 months, between the groups, with the acupuncture group having the better outcome. In Table 8.8 both confidence intervals for the adjusted and unadjusted treatment effect clearly include zero (no difference) and are consistent with there being no treatment effect at 12 months.

8.13   Three methods of analysis for pre-test/post-test control group designs

Since RCTs are prospective studies they usually have a baseline or 'pre-test' measurement and at least one follow-up or 'post-test' assessment of outcome. They are an example of a *pre-test/post-test control group design*. There are some exceptions to this rule, for example the Morrell *et al.* (2000) study of new mothers only had a follow-up QoL assessment and no baseline. There are essentially three methods of analysis for such pre-test/post-test control group designs:

(1) comparison of post-treatment means (POST);

(2) comparison of mean changes (CHANGE);

(3) analysis of covariance (ANCOVA) using pre-test or baseline outcome as a covariate and treatment group as a factor.

If the pre-treatment means are the same, which is very likely in a RCT, then the estimated treatment effect from all three methods is the same (see Table 8.9). However,

Table 8.9   Mean outcome pre and post test by group.

Mean outcomes pre and post test by group			
Group	Pre-test	Post-test	Change (post-pre)
Intervention	5	10	5
Control	5	7	2
Difference (Int − Con)	0	③	③

If the pre-test (baseline) levels of the QoL out come variable are the same, which is likely in a RCT, then differences between groups, in post-test outcome or change are the same.

multiple regression or ANCOVA is the 'best' or most efficient method of analysis since it has the smallest value for the variance of the treatment effect (Frison and Pocock, 1992), which will lead to the smallest standard errors and P-values and narrowest confidence intervals. With a correlation of 0.00 between the pre and post outcomes, pre-treatment measurements are of no value. So if the correlation is less than 0.50 then POST is to be preferred to CHANGE. However, even in these circumstances ANCOVA is likely to be superior to both in most circumstances. With a correlation of 0.50 between the pre and post outcomes, then POST and CHANGE have identical variances. So if the correlation is less than 0.50 then POST is to be preferred to CHANGE. However, even in these circumstances ANCOVA is likely to be superior to both in most circumstances. CHANGE becomes less inferior to ANCOVA as the correlation between the pre- and post-test outcomes increases. With a correlation of 0.90 between the pre and post outcomes, then CHANGE and ANCOVA have similar variances. So if the correlation is more than 0.90 then CHANGE is to be preferred to ANCOVA. However, even in these circumstances ANCOVA is likely to be superior to both in most circumstances.

Table 8.10 compares the three methods of analysis for pre-test/post-test control group designs using data from the acupuncture study. Even though the correlation between baseline and 12-month follow-up SF-36 Bodily Pain was low ($r = 0.26$) the smallest P-value and narrowest confidence interval is produced by ANCOVA.

8.14 Cross-over trials

In a cross-over design the subjects receive both the test and the control treatments in a randomized order. This contrasts with the parallel group design in that each subject now provides an estimate of the difference between test and control. Situations where cross-over trials may be useful are in chronic diseases that remain stable over long periods of time, such as diabetes or arthritis, where the purpose of the treatment is palliation and not cure. The two-period cross-over design is described in Figure 8.8.

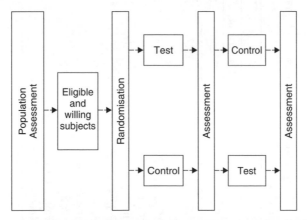

Figure 8.8 Stages of a two-group, two-period cross-over randomized controlled trial. Reproduced with permission from Campbell, M.J., Machin, D., Walters, S.J., *Medical Statistics: A Text Book for the Health Sciences*. 4th edition. John Wiley & Sons Ltd, Chichester. © 2007 John Wiley & Sons Ltd.

Table 8.10 Comparison of three methods of analysis for pre-test/post-test control group designs from the acupuncture study (data from Thomas et al., 2006).

	Treatment group						Mean difference	95% CI		P-value
	Usual care			Acupuncture				Lower	Upper	
	n	Mean	SD	n	Mean	SD				
SF-36 Bodily Pain (baseline)	68	30.7	18.1	147	31.0	16.4	0.3	−4.6	5.2	0.91
POST SF-36 Bodily Pain (12 months)	68	58.3	22.2	147	64.0	25.6	5.7	−1.4	12.8	0.12
CHANGE in SF-36 Bodily Pain score (0–12 months)	68	27.6	25.4	147	33.0	26.2	5.4	−2.1	12.9	0.16
ANCOVA regression (12 month SF-36 Bodily Pain adjusted for baseline)							5.6	−1.3	12.5	0.11

Example: Cross-over trial on faecal incontinence

Lauti *et al.* (2008) conducted a double-blind randomized cross-over trial of fibre supplement in addition to loperamide in adults with faecal incontinence. The two treatments were either 6 weeks of low-residue diet, placebo fibre supplement and loperamide followed by 6 weeks of fibre supplement, neutral diet and loperamide (Treatment A) or the reverse order (treatment B). The primary outcome was the Faecal Incontinence Severity Index (FISI). The FISI has a scale that ranges from 0 to 61, where a score of 0 would suggest no problem. Secondary outcomes included a generic QoL measure, the SF-36, and a condition-specific QoL instrument, the Faecal Incontinence Quality of Life Scale (FIQL).

Sixty-three patients were randomized, 31 to treatment schedule A and 32 to treatment schedule B. Forty-seven patients completed the study. At baseline the mean FISI score was 31 (SD 10.3). After low-residue diet, placebo fibre supplement and loperamide the FISI score was 18.4 (SD 13.2). After fibre supplementation and loperamide the FISI was 18.8 (SD 14.1). For the primary outcome, the FISI, the mean difference between treatments, from a paired t-test, was -0.8 (95% CI: -4.9 to 3.3, $P > 0.05$). Therefore no significance difference between the two diets was demonstrated. There was also no difference between the treatments for the SF-36 and FIQL. □

The two-period, two-treatment (2×2) cross-over trial has the advantage over a parallel group design testing the same hypothesis in that, because subjects act as their own controls, the number of subjects required is considerably less. There are, however, a number of problems. One difficulty with cross-over designs is the possibility that the effect of the particular treatment used in the first period will carry over to the second period. This may then interfere with how the treatment scheduled for the second period will act, and thus affect the final comparison between the two treatments (the carry-over effect). To allow for this possibility, a wash-out period, in which no treatment is given, should be included between successive treatment periods. Other difficulties are that the disease may not remain stable over the trial period, and that because of the extended treatment period, more subject drop-outs will occur than in a parallel group design.

Altman (1991) describes how to test for a period effect and a carry-over effect for a two-period, two-treatment (2×2) cross-over trial. If we have two treatments A and B, then the two treatment sequences or groups are A followed by B (group AB) or B followed by A (group BA). We first calculate for each subject the difference (d_i) and average (a_i) of the observations in the two periods, and average these for each group and denote these by $\bar{d}_{AB}, \bar{d}_{BA}, \bar{a}_{AB}$ and $\bar{a}_{BA}$ respectively.

The possibility of a period effect is tested by a two independent samples t-test to compare the difference between the periods in the two groups of patients. If there was no general tendency for patients do better in one period than the other period we would expect the mean differences between the periods in the two groups to be of the same size but having opposite signs. Therefore the test for a period effect is a two independent samples t-test comparing $\bar{d}_{AB}$ with $-\bar{d}_{BA}$.

We can investigate the possibility of a carry-over effect by noticing that in the absence of a carry-over effect, a patient's average response to the two treatments would be the same regardless of the order in which they were received. The test for a carry-over effect is therefore a two independent samples t-test comparing $\bar{a}_{AB}$ with $\bar{a}_{BA}$.

If there is no period effect and no carry-over effect the analysis of a cross-over trial is simple. A cross-over study results in a paired (or matched) analysis. Therefore one can use the methods described in Figure 7.3 such as the paired t-test or Wilcoxon matched pairs test. It is incorrect to analyse the trial ignoring this pairing, as that analysis fails to use all the information in the study design. If there is a period and/or carry-over effect then only the data from the first period should be used and the data in this period should be analysed as if we just had a two parallel group design (with no cross-over).

8.15   Factorial trials

A factorial trial is used to evaluate two or more interventions simultaneously. Note that a factorial trial is not a study which merely balances prognostic factors, such as age or gender, which are not interventions.

Example: 2 × 2 factorial design – pulmonary rehabilitation

Waterhouse *et al.* (2009) describe a randomized 2 × 2 factorial trial of community versus hospital pulmonary rehabilitation, followed by telephone or conventional follow-up and its impact on QoL, exercise capacity and use of health-care resources in patients with chronic obstructive pulmonary disease (COPD). Four different experimental conditions were evaluated. These were:

(A) hospital rehabilitation and telephone follow-up;

(B) hospital rehabilitation and no telephone follow-up;

(C) community rehabilitation and telephone follow-up;

(D) community rehabilitation and no telephone follow-up.

Here the two types of intervention or treatment are location of rehabilitation and type of follow-up. In general, the treatments in a factorial design are known as factors and usually they are applied at only one level, that is, a particular factor is either present or absent. Factorial designs are useful in two situations. The clinician may believe that the two treatments together will produce an effect that is over and above that anticipated by adding the effects of the two treatments separately (synergy), and is often expressed statistically as an interaction. Alternatively, the clinician may believe that an interaction is most unlikely. In this case, one requires fewer patients to examine the effects of the two treatments, than the combined number of patients from two separate parallel group trials, each one examining the effect of one of the treatments. The use of this 2 × 2 factorial design enabled two research questions to be asked simultaneously. Thus, groups A and B versus C and D compared hospital versus community based rehabilitation programmes, while groups A and C versus B and D measured the value of telephone versus conventional (no telephone) follow-up.

The Waterhouse *et al.* (2009) study comprised an RCT to test whether pulmonary rehabilitation undertaken in a community setting produces greater effects acutely and longer term than that undertaken in a hospital setting, as assessed by exercise capacity and health-related quality of life, and whether a simple telephone follow-up produces a greater persistence of effect of pulmonary rehabilitation compared to standard care. Two hundred and forty patients with COPD, as assessed by a respiratory physician according to GOLD criteria, with MRC 3 or greater breathlessness, were randomized to receive pulmonary rehabilitation in either a community ($n = 111$) or hospital setting ($n = 129$). Following standardized pulmonary rehabilitation for 6 weeks, patients were followed up over 18 months (with assessments post rehabilitation, approximately 8 weeks post randomization, and 6, 12 and 18 months after rehabilitation).

Evaluable QoL data were obtained post rehabilitation and 6 months post rehabilitation for 133 patients, 74/129 (57%) in the hospital group, and 59/111 (53%) in the community group. Patients were further randomized to telephone or standard follow-up, with evaluable data for $n = 41, 33, 25$, and 34 respectively in the hospital rehabilitation and telephone follow-up, hospital rehabilitation and standard follow-up, community rehabilitation and telephone follow-up, and community rehabilitation and no telephone follow-up groups. One of the QoL outcomes was the 6-month post-rehabilitation score on the Physical Components Summary (PCS) dimension of the SF-36.

The authors used a multiple regression model to analyse the data and allow for baseline QoL and the factorial design of the trial:

$$QoL_{Follow-up} = b_0 + b_1 QoL_{Baseline} + b_2 Rehabilitation$$

$$+ b_3 Follow\text{-}up + b_4 Interaction. \tag{8.3}$$

The 'Rehabilitation' variable was coded 0 for community and 1 for hospital rehabilitation; and the 'Follow-up' variable was coded 0 for no telephone follow-up and 1 for telephone follow-up. The interaction term was simply the product of these two variables (and was 0 except when a patient is in the hospital rehabilitation group with telephone follow-up, when it was 1). If the interaction term is non-significant then this can be omitted from the model and a simpler model used:

$$QoL_{Follow-up} = b_0 + b_1 QoL_{Baseline} + b_2 Rehabilitation + b_3 Follow\text{-}up. \tag{8.4}$$

In this model the effect of treatment on follow-up QoL can be assessed whilst adjusting for baseline QoL and other covariates such as age and sex and the factorial design of the trial (i.e. the other treatment group factor).

Table 8.11 shows the results of fitting models (8.3) and (8.4) to the PCS outcome in the pulmonary rehabilitation trial. The results are presented according to Montgomery *et al.*'s (2003) recommendations for factorial RCTs. The interaction term was non-significant so the results from the simpler model (8.4) are presented. At 6 months post-rehabilitation follow-up the mean difference in PCS scores between the hospital and community groups, after adjustment for baseline (post-rehabilitation) PCS score and for the factorial design, was not significant at -0.2 (95% CI: -3.0 to 2.5, $P = 0.878$). There was no significant difference in PCS scores between the telephone and standard follow-up groups, with a mean difference, after adjustment for baseline PCS score and factorial design, in 6-month post rehabilitation PCS scores of 1.8 (95% CI: -1.2 to 4.8, $P = 0.243$).   □

Table 8.11 Results for SF-36 PCS dimension from the 2 × 2 factorial pulmonary rehabilitation study (data from Waterhouse et al., 2009).

PCS score	Rehabilitation group						Follow-up group					
	Community			Hospital			No telephone follow-up			Telephone follow-up		
	n	Mean	SD	n	Mean	SD	n	Mean	SD	n	Mean	SD
Post rehabilitation (0 months)	59	33.5	7.6	74	33.2	8.4	67	32.2	7.8	66	34.5	8.1
6 months	59	32.0	7.2	74	31.3	7.7	67	30.4	7.0	66	32.8	7.7
Adjusted group difference (95% CI)[1]	−0.2	(−3.0 to 2.5)[2,4]					1.8	(−1.2 to 4.8)[3,4]				
P-value	0.878						0.243					

[1] Adjusted for post-rehabilitation PCS score and factorial design.
[2] A positive difference represents a favourable outcome for the hospital group compared to the community rehabilitation group.
[3] A positive difference represents a favourable outcome for the telephone group compared to the no telephone follow-up group.
[4] The interaction between the intervention groups was investigated as a secondary analysis and was found to be non-significant. (interaction coefficient −1.1 (95% CI: −5.0 to 2.9), P = 0.599).
The PCS score is standardized to have a mean score of 50 and a standard deviation of 10 (the same as the reference population: USA, 1998).

8.16   Cluster randomized controlled trials

In some cases, because of the nature of the intervention planned, it may be impossible to randomize on an individual subject basis in a trial. Thus an investigator may have to randomize communities to test out different types of health promotion or different types of vaccine, when problems of contamination or logistics, respectively, mean that it is better to randomize a group rather than an individual. Alternatively, one may wish to test different ways of counselling patients, and it would be impossible for a health professional, once trained in a new approach, to then switch methods for different patients following randomization. For example, the Psychological Interventions for Postnatal Depression Randomised Controlled Trial and Economic Evaluation (PONDER) RCT involved health visitors randomized to be trained or not in the new counselling techniques for detecting and treating postnatal depression (PND) in new mothers (Morrell *et al.*, 2009). The health visitors each recruit a number of new mothers who form the corresponding cluster all receiving counselling according to the training (or not) of their health professional. The simplest way to analyse these studies is 'to analyse as you randomise' (i.e. by group), rather than on an individual subject basis, by using aggregate cluster level outcomes such as the mean score per cluster. An alternative approach using individual level data is to model the outcomes with a random effect or marginal models as described in the next chapter.

Example: The PONDER cRCT

The PoNDER trial (Morrell *et al.*, 2009) was a cRCT in primary care designed to evaluate the effectiveness of new health visitor led psychological intervention in detecting and treating new mothers with PND compared to usual care. The trial randomized 100 clusters (GP practices and their associated health visitors) and collected data on 2659 new mothers with an 18-month follow-up. The participants were 1745 (in 63 clusters) women allocated to intervention, and 914 (in 37 clusters) allocated to control. The main outcome measure was the 6-month EPDS, scored on a 0–30 scale with a higher score indicating more depressive symptoms. A score greater than 12 is regarded as being 'at higher risk' of PND. Table 8.12 shows the mean EPDS score for the individual mothers and the mean EPDS score per cluster for the two treatment groups. The results of a two independent samples *t*-test on the aggregate mean EPDS score per cluster suggests that new mothers

Table 8.12   Mean 6-month postnatal EPDS scores by group from the PONDER cRCT (data from Morrell *et al.*, 2009).

	Group								
	Intervention			Control			Mean	95% CI		
6-month Outcome	n	Mean	SD	n	Mean	SD	difference	Lower	Upper	*P*-value
Aggregate mean EPDS score per cluster	63	5.4	1.2	37	6.7	2.0	−1.3	−1.9	−0.6	0.0002
EPDS score	1745	5.5	4.7	914	6.35	5.2				

P-value from two independent samples *t*-test. The EPDS is scored on a 0–30 scale. with a higher score indicating more depressive symptoms.

in the control clusters have significantly more depressive symptoms than mothers in the intervention clusters.   □

8.17   Further reading

The book by Pocock (1983) on clinical trials provides an easily readable and practical guide. Altman (1991) also has several chapters on the design and analysis of clinical trials. For more novel RCT designs such as cluster RCTs, the interested reader is referred to Donner and Klar (2000) and Murray (1998). The design and analysis of cross-over trials is described in Senn (1992).

Exercises

8.1 Table 8.13 shows the results from a fictitious pilot randomized double-blind placebo controlled trial comparing *Withania somnifera* tablets versus placebo tablets in 20 patients with knee osteoarthritis (OA knee). *Withania somnifera* is a plant and its roots and berries are used in herbal medicine. The data are the self-reported WOMAC pain dimension score, measured on a 0–20 scale with a higher score indicating increased pain, at 3 months post-randomization follow-up. One of the aims of this study was to compare QoL between OA knee patients receiving *W. somnifera* tablets with patients on placebo tablets.

(a) Write out a suitable null and alternative hypothesis for this problem and data.

(b) Do these data suggest that OA knee patients in the *W. somnifera* group have a different WOMAC pain dimension score 3 months post randomization than patients in the placebo group? Stating any assumptions you make, carry out

Table 8.13   WOMAC pain outcomes from a randomized double-blind crossover parallel group trial comparing *Withania somnifera* tablets versus placebo treatment in 20 patients with osteoarthritis of the knee.

	Placebo group ($n = 10$)	Withania somnifera group ($n = 10$)
	7	8
	2	6
	12	12
	7	11
	3	1
	7	3
	15	7
	4	10
	14	7
	1	15
Mean	7.2	8.0
SD	5.0	4.2

an appropriate hypothesis test to compare mean 3 months post-randomization WOMAC pain dimension scores between the *W. somnifera* and placebo groups of patients. Comment on the results of this hypothesis test.

(c) Calculate a 95% confidence interval for the difference in mean 3 months post-randomization WOMAC Pain dimension scores between the *W. somnifera* and placebo groups. Discuss whether the confidence interval suggests that patients in the *W. somnifera* group might have different levels of pain, at 3-month follow-up, than patients in the placebo group.

8.2 The results of a multi-centre double-blind RCT to assess the non-inferiority of duloxetine compared to paroxetine in patients with non-psychotic major depressive disorder (MDD) are shown in Table 8.14 (Lee *et al.*, 2007). Four hundred and seventy-eight patients with MDD were randomized to 8 weeks of duloxetine 60 mg ($n = 238$) or paroxetine 20 mg ($n = 240$) treatment once daily. The primary outcome was the 17-item Hamilton Rating Scale for Depression ($HAMD_{17}$) score post randomization. The $HAMD_{17}$ is scored on a $0-52$ scale with higher scores indicating more depressive symptoms. Secondary outcomes included the Hamilton Rating Scale for Anxiety (HAMA). Patients were assessed at baseline and 1, 2, 4, 6 and 8 weeks post baseline. The aim of the study was to assess the non-inferiority of duloxetine compared to paroxetine in patients with MDD using a pre-defined non-inferiority margin of 2.2 points on the $HAMD_{17}$ scale.

(a) What is the mean difference in $HAMD_{17}$ scores between the duloxetine and paroxetine groups?

(b) Calculate a 95% confidence interval for the mean difference in $HAMD_{17}$ scores between the duloxetine and paroxetine groups. Compare the 95% CI limits with the pre-defined non-inferiority margin of 2.2 points on the $HAMD_{17}$. What do you conclude? Is duloxetine non-inferior to paroxetine in patients with non-psychotic MDD with respect to the $HAMD_{17}$ outcome?

(c) What is the mean difference in HAMA scores between the duloxetine and paroxetine groups?

(d) Calculate a 95% CI for the mean difference in HAMA scores between the duloxetine and paroxetine groups. Assume that the non-inferiority margin

Table 8.14   Mean post-randomization $HAMD_{17}$ and HAMA scores by group from the duloxetine versus paroxetine non-inferiority RCT (data from Lee *et al.*, 2007).

	Duloxetine 60 mg/day ($n = 238$)		Paroxetine 20 mg/day ($n = 240$)	
	Mean	SD	Mean	SD
$HAMD_{17}$ Total	11.73	4.57	11.94	4.38
HAMA	11.17	4.54	11.25	4.34

17-item Hamilton Rating Scale for Depression ($HAMD_{17}$) total score post randomization.
Hamilton Rating Scale for Anxiety (HAMA).

for the HAMA outcome is 2.2 points. Compare the 95% CI limits with the non-inferiority margin of 2.2 points on the HAMA. What do you conclude? Is duloxetine non-inferior to paroxetine in patients with non-psychotic MDD with respect to the HAMA outcome?

8.3 Table 8.15 shows the results from a fictitious randomized double-blind cross-over trial comparing active treatment versus placebo in 20 patients with asthma. The data are the self-reported QoL measured on a 0 (poor) to 100 (good health) scale at baseline and after 2 weeks of treatment. There was a one-week wash-out period between the two treatments.

Table 8.15   QoL outcomes and results from a randomized double-blind cross-over trial comparing active versus placebo treatment in 20 patients with asthma.

Group A: active followed by placebo ($n = 10$)

	Period 1 Active	Period 2 Placebo	Period 1 −Period 2	Average $(1 + 2)/2$	Active− Placebo
	29	18	11.0	23.5	11.0
	18	4	14.0	11.0	14.0
	79	63	16.0	71.0	16.0
	88	100	−12.0	94.0	−12.0
	46	0	46.0	23.0	46.0
	48	29	19.0	38.5	19.0
	88	75	13.0	81.5	13.0
	79	21	58.0	50.0	58.0
	29	50	−21.0	39.5	−21.0
	75	4	71.0	39.5	71.0
Mean	57.9	36.4	21.5	47.2	21.5
SD	26.9	34.1	29.0	27.1	29.0

Group B: placebo followed by active ($n = 10$)

	Period 1 Placebo	Period 2 Active	Period 1 −Period 2	Average $(1 + 2)/2$	Active− Placebo
	25	18	7.0	21.5	−7.0
	43	30	13.0	36.5	−13.0
	11	32	−21.0	21.5	21.0
	63	75	−12.0	69.0	12.0
	13	41	−28.0	27.0	28.0
	70	61	9.0	65.5	−9.0
	89	61	28.0	75.0	−28.0
	14	16	−2.0	15.0	2.0
	16	32	−16.0	24.0	16.0
	50	45	5.0	47.5	−5.0
Mean	39.4	41.1	−1.7	40.3	1.7
SD	27.9	19.5	17.3	22.4	17.3

(a) Is there a tendency for asthma patients to do better in one of the two periods? Stating any assumptions you make, perform an appropriate hypothesis test to investigate the possibility of a period effect. Comment on the results of this hypothesis test.

(b) Is there a tendency for the treatment effect to carry over from one period to the next? Stating any assumptions you make, perform an appropriate hypothesis test to investigate the possibility of a treatment–period interaction. Comment on the results of this hypothesis test.

(c) Do these data suggest that asthma patients on the active treatment have a better QoL than when on placebo treatment? Depending on the results of parts (a) and (b) above, perform an appropriate hypothesis test to compare the effect of active treatment against placebo on QoL. Comment on the results of this hypothesis test. Calculate a 95% confidence interval for the difference in mean QoL scores when the patient is on active or placebo treatment. Discuss whether the confidence interval suggests that when on active treatment asthma patients have better QoL than when on placebo treatment.

8.4 Table 8.16 shows the results of a randomized, double-blind, placebo-controlled trial of nutritional supplementation during acute illness (Gariballa *et al.*, 2006). Two-hundred and twenty-five hospitalized patients (aged 65–92) were allocated at random to the supplementation group (106) or placebo (119) group. The interventions were: for the supplementation group, normal hospital diet plus 400 ml oral nutrition supplements, and for the placebo group, normal hospital diet plus placebo, both daily for 6 weeks.

One of the outcomes was the Barthel Index at baseline and 6-month follow-up. The Barthel Index consists of 10 items that measure a person's daily functioning, specifically the activities of daily living and mobility. The items include feeding, moving from wheelchair to bed and back, grooming, transferring to and from a toilet, bathing, walking on a level surface, going up and down stairs, dressing, continence of bowels and bladder. For each item the person receives a score (0, 1 or 2) based on whether they have received help while doing the task. The scores for each of the items are summed to create a total score, ranging from 0 to 20, with a higher the score indicating better functioning.

The correlation between baseline and 6-month Barthel scores was 0.45.

(a) Do these data suggest that the supplementation and placebo groups had similar mean Barthel scores at baseline? Comment on the results of the hypothesis test.

(b) Do these data suggest that the supplementation and placebo groups had similar mean Barthel scores at 6 months? Comment on the results of the hypothesis test.

(c) Discuss whether the confidence interval for the difference in 6-month follow-up Barthel scores (POST) between the supplementation and placebo groups suggests that patients in the supplementation group might have better level of QoL at 6-month follow-up than patients in the placebo group.

Table 8.16 Barthel outcomes, at baseline and 6 months, and results of three analyses (POST, CHANGE and ANCOVA) from a randomized double-blind parallel trial comparing supplementation versus placebo treatment in 225 elderly patients admitted to hospital with acute illness (data from Gariballa et al., 2006).

| | Treatment group | | | | | | Mean difference | 95% Confidence Interval | | P-value |
| | Placebo | | | Supplement | | | | | | |
	n	Mean	SD	n	Mean	SD		Lower	Upper	
Barthel Score (baseline)	119	16.5	4.4	106	16.3	4.6	0.17	−1.01	1.34	0.78
POST Barthel Score (6 months)	119	18.6	2.6	106	18.2	3.1	0.32	−0.44	1.07	0.41
CHANGE in Barthel Score (0–6 months)	119	2.1	4.0	106	1.9	4.2	0.15	−0.92	1.22	0.78
ANCOVA Regression (6 month Barthel adjusted for baseline)							0.30	−0.40	0.94	0.43

(d) Of the three types of analysis, POST, CHANGE and ANCOVA, shown in Table 8.16, which is to be preferred? Give reasons for your choice.

(e) A paper by Hsieh *et al.* (2007) suggests that the minimum clinically important difference (MCID) for the Barthel index in stroke patients is 1.85 points. Assuming the same MCID for this patient population, comment on the size of the change in Barthel scores from baseline to 6 months in the two groups and also comment on the difference in 6-month Barthel scores between the supplementation and placebo groups.

9

Exploring and modelling longitudinal quality of life data

Summary

Some studies using QoL outcomes have repeated assessments over time and are longitudinal in nature. In a randomized controlled trial and other longitudinal studies there may be a baseline QoL assessment and several follow-up assessments over time. This chapter will describe how the QoL data from such studies can be summarized, tabulated and graphically displayed. These repeated QoL measurements, on the same individual subject, are likely to be related or correlated. This means that the usual statistical methods for analysing such data, described in Chapters 7 and 8, which assume independent outcomes, may not be appropriate. This chapter will show how repeated QoL measures for each subject can be reduced to a single summary measure for statistical analysis and how standard statistical methods of analysis can then be used. Finally, the chapter will describe a more complex modelling approach, based on an extension of the linear regression model in Chapter 7, which allows for the fact that successive QoL assessments by a particular patient are likely to be correlated.

9.1 Introduction

Trials, by definition, are prospective longitudinal studies. That is, we randomly allocate patients to different treatments, follow the patients over time, observe the outcomes and then compare the treatment groups. Sometimes the RCT can have several follow-up assessments. In the acupuncture study, the patients' QoL was assessed four times – at baseline (0), 3, 12 and 24 months – using the SF-36.

With one QoL observation on each subject or experimental unit – e.g. the Community Postnatal Support Study (Morrell *et al.*, 2000) described in Chapter 8, where QoL was assessed only at 6 weeks – we are confined to modelling the population average QoL, called the *marginal* mean response; there is no other choice. However, with repeated QoL measurements, there are several different approaches that can be adopted.

Repeated measurement data must be analysed carefully. A series of hypothesis tests comparing the groups at each follow-up time point is not recommended. It is preferable to either model the data (Diggle *et al.*, 2002) or aggregate the repeated assessments into a single summary measure (such as the overall mean of the post-randomization measures or the area under the curve (AUC)). Other possible summary measures are listed in Matthews *et al.* (1990). Having identified a suitable summary measure, a simple two independent samples *t*-test or one-way analysis of variance can be applied to assess between group differences. I will split these approaches into three broad classifications (Everitt, 2002):

(1) time-by-time analysis;

(2) response feature analysis – the use of summary measures;

(3) modelling of longitudinal data.

The modelling of longitudinal data takes into account the fact that successive QoL assessments by a particular subject are likely to be correlated. The models are an extension of the linear regression model described in Chapter 7. The three alternative modelling approaches I will discuss are repeated measures ANOVA, marginal (General Estimating Equations) general linear models (GLMs), and random-effect (multi-level) GLMs. All three models require the specification of the *autocorrelation* or *serial correlation*, which is the strength of the association between successive longitudinal measurements of a single QoL variable on the same patient.

In both the marginal and random-effect approaches we model both the dependence of the QoL response on the explanatory variables and the autocorrelation among the responses. With cross-sectional data (as in Chapter 7), only the dependence of the QoL outcome Y on x need be specified; there is no correlation as the responses (Ys) are independent. If we choose to ignore the correlation that exists in longitudinal data, then Diggle *et al* (2002) mention three important consequences.

(1) incorrect inferences about regression coefficients, β;

(2) estimates of β which are inefficient, that is, less precise than is possible;

(3) suboptimal protection against biases caused by missing data.

9.2   Summarizing, tabulating and graphically displaying repeated QoL assessments

As described in Chapter 6, an important initial step, before analysing the repeated QoL assessment (using one of the three methods described above) is to tabulate and/or graphically display the data. This will give us an idea of how the QoL outcomes change over time.

In the acupuncture study, the patients' QoL was assessed at baseline (0), 3, 12 and 24 months using the SF-36 (Thomas *et al.*, 2006). Table 9.1 shows one way of presenting

Table 9.1   Mean SF-36 Bodily Pain scores over time by treatment group with all valid patients at each time point (data from Thomas et al., 2006). Reproduced with permission from Freeman, J.V., Walters, S.J., Campbell, M.J., *How to Display Data*. BMJ Books. © 2008 Blackwell Publishing.

SF-36 Bodily Pain outcome[1]	Usual care			Acupuncture			Treatment group			
							Mean	95% confidence interval		
Time (months)	n	Mean	SD	n	Mean	SD	difference[2]	Lower	Upper	P-value[3]
0	80	30.4	(18.0)	159	30.8	(16.2)				
3	71	55.4	(25.4)	146	60.9	(23.0)				
12	68	58.3	(22.2)	147	64.0	(25.6)				
24	59	59.5	(23.4)	123	67.8	(24.1)				
Mean follow-up	76	57.2	(19.8)	153	63.4	(20.9)	6.3	0.6	12.0	0.030
SF-36 Bodily Pain score										
Pain AUC	55	112.7	(36.7)	118	125.2	(39.4)	12.6	0.1	25.0	0.048

[1] The SF-36 Bodily Pain dimension is scored on a 0 (poor) to 100 (good health) scale.
[2] A positive mean difference indicates the acupuncture group has the better QoL.
[3] P-value from two independent samples t-test.

Table 9.2 Mean SF-36 Bodily Pain scores over time by treatment group with patients who completed all four QoL assessments (data from Thomas et al., 2006).

SF-36 Bodily Pain outcome[1]

				Treatment group				95% CI		
	Usual care			Acupuncture			Mean			
Time (months)	n	Mean	SD	n	Mean	SD	difference[2]	Lower	Upper	P-value[3]
0	55	29.9	(18.5)	118	31.5	(16.6)				
3	55	57.4	(26.9)	118	62.3	(22.4)				
12	55	57.8	(21.8)	118	64.1	(25.4)				
24	55	59.4	(23.7)	118	68.1	(23.8)				
Mean follow-up	55	58.2	(19.5)	118	64.8	(20.1)	6.7	0.3	13.1	0.042
SF-36 Bodily Pain score										
Pain AUC	55	112.7	(36.7)	118	125.2	(39.4)	12.6	0.1	25.0	0.048

[1] The SF-36 Bodily Pain dimension is scored on a 0 (poor) to 100 (good health) scale.
[2] A positive mean difference indicates the acupuncture group has the better QoL.
[3] P-value from two independent samples t-test.

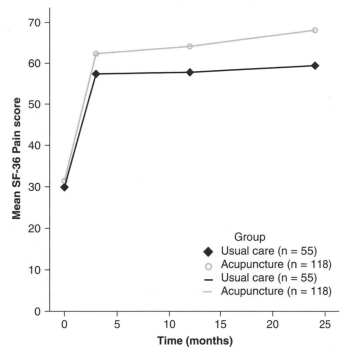

Figure 9.1 Profile of mean SF-36 Bodily Pain scores over time by treatment group – complete case analysis (data from Thomas *et al* 2006).

such data. In Table 9.1 the SF-36 Bodily Pain scores are not tested at each time point. The results of the hypothesis test and confidence intervals are only presented for the two summary measures, in the last two rows of the table. The calculation of these summary measures is described later. The sample size at each of the follow-up time points varies and therefore it is important to report the sample size for each row of the data.

Table 9.2 is in the same format as Table 9.1, but this time we report the results for only those patients who completed all four QoL assessments. This makes it easier to see how the mean Pain scores vary over time. We can plot such data as a line graph (Figure 9.1), with a separate line for each group. Figure 9.1 clearly shows how the pain outcome varies over the 2-year period. The groups have similar mean pain scores at baseline and 3 months, but by 12 and 24 months the mean scores have started to diverge, with the acupuncture group having the better outcome. Because the same numbers of subjects are included at each time point, it is legitimate to join the mean Pain scores together. However, if the data in Table 9.2 were presented in a similar figure it would be misleading to join the observed means at each time point by solid lines, since we are not measuring the same people at each time point. Figure 9.2 shows how the mean SF-36 Bodily Pain score varies over time using all available QoL data. The number of valid QoL observations per group at each assessment time point is included just below the horizontal axis. This makes clear how the number of valid QoL observations at the various follow-up assessment points declines over time and on how many subjects the calculation of each mean summary measure is based.

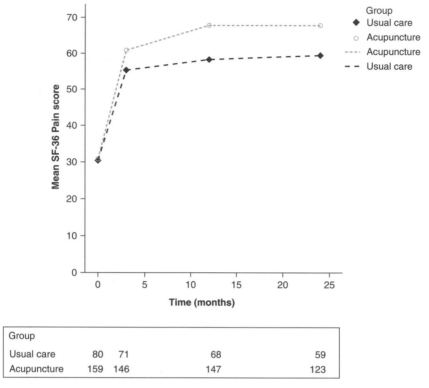

Group				
Usual care	80	71	68	59
Acupuncture	159	146	147	123

Figure 9.2   Profile of mean SF-36 Bodily Pain scores over time by treatment group – all available data (data from Thomas *et al* 2006). Reproduced with permission from Freeman, J.V., Walters, S.J., Campbell, M.J., *How to Display Data*. BMJ Books. © 2008 Blackwell Publishing.

9.3   Time-by-time analysis

A series of two independent samples *t*-tests (or the non-parametric equivalent), as described in Chapter 7, could be used to test for differences in QoL between the two groups at each time point. (In examples with more than two groups, a series of one-way ANOVAs might be used.) The procedure is straightforward but has a number of serious flaws and weaknesses (Everitt, 2001):

1. The QoL measurements in a subject from one time point to the next are not independent, so interpretation of the results is difficult.

2. The large number of hypothesis tests carried out implies that we are likely to obtain significant results purely by chance.

3. We lose information about the within-subject changes in QoL over time.

Consequently, it will not be pursued further here.

9.4   Response feature analysis – the use of summary measures

Here the repeated QoL measures for each participant are transformed into a single number considered to capture some important aspect of the participant's response. A simple and often effective strategy (Diggle *et al.*, 2002) is to:

(1) reduce the repeated QoL values into one or two summaries;

(2) analyse each summary as a function of covariates or explanatory variables, $x_1, x_2, \ldots, x_p$.

Diggle *et al.* (2002) call this strategy a *two-stage* or *derived variable* analysis, and mention that it works well when $x_{1ij} = x_{1i}$ for all i and j (i.e. the important explanatory variables do not change over time, such as baseline QoL), since the summary value which results from stage (1) can only be regressed on x_{1i} in stage (2).

Examples of summary measures include the AUC and the overall mean of post-randomization measures. Other possible summary measures are listed in Matthews *et al.* (1990) and shown in Table 9.3. Having identified a suitable summary measure, a simple *t*-test (or ANOVA) can be applied to assess between-groups differences. If the data for each patient can effectively be summarized by a pre-treatment mean and a post-treatment mean, then the analysis of covariance (ANCOVA) is the preferred method of choice (Frison and Pocock, 1992). It is superior to both the analysis of post-treatment means or analysis of mean changes. Diggle *et al.* (2002) suggested that provided the data are complete, the method of derived variables or summary measures can give a simple and easily interpretable analysis with a strong focus on particular aspects of the mean response.

9.4.1   Area under the curve

The AUC is a useful way of summarizing the information from a series of measurements on one individual (Matthews *et al.*, 1990). The AUC can also be used to summarize repeated QoL scores over time into a single measure of health for each patient.

Table 9.3   Response features suggested in Matthews *et al.* (1990).

Type of data	Property to be compared between groups	Summary measure
Peaked	Overall value of response	Mean or AUC
Peaked	Value of most extreme response	Maximum (minimum)
Peaked	Delay in response	Time to maximum or minimum
Growth	Rate of change of response	Linear regression coefficient
Growth	Final level of response	Final value or (relative) difference between first and last
Growth	Delay in response	Time to reach a particular value

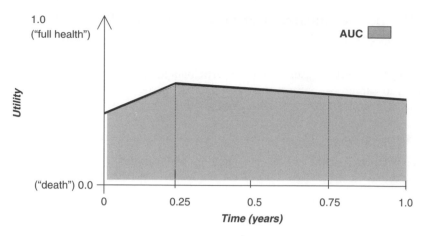

Figure 9.3   Summary measure of QoL: the AUC.

9.4.1.1   Calculating the AUC

The area (see Figure 9.3) can be split into a series of shapes called trapeziums. The areas of the individual trapeziums are calculated and then summed for each patient. The mean AUC in each group can then be calculated.

Let Y_{ij} represent the QoL response variable observed at time t_{ij} for observation $j = 1, \ldots, n_i$ on subject $i = 1, \ldots, m$. The set of repeated QoL outcomes for subject i can be collected into a single row or row vector matrix of length n_i, that is, $\mathbf{Y}_i = (Y_{i1}, Y_{i2}, \ldots, Y_{in_i})$,. The AUC for the ith subject is given by

$$\text{AUC}_i = \frac{1}{2} \sum_{j=1}^{n_i} (t_{j+1} - t_j)(Y_j + Y_{j+1}). \tag{9.1}$$

The units of the AUC are the product of the units used for Y_{ij} and t_{ij}, and may not be easy to understand, since QoL outcomes have no natural units. So it may be useful to divide the AUC by the total time to get a weighted average level of QoL over the time period. We can calculate the AUC even when there are missing data, except when the first and final observations are missing.

In the acupuncture study, the patients' QoL was assessed four times (Thomas *et al* 2006) and the AUCs calculated were based on 24 months or 2 years of follow-up. If the time t_{ij} for each QoL assessment is represented as a fraction of a year then the AUCs represent the weighted average level of QoL over the 2-year period. An AUC of 200 corresponds to 'good health' over the year, while an AUC of 0 corresponds to 'poor health'. If we divide by the total time (of 2 years) then we get back to the 0–100 scale of the original SF-36 measurement, which may make interpretation of the results easier.

Consider a patient in the acupuncture study, with SF-36 Bodily Pain scores of 33.3, 44.4, 55.6 and 77.8 at baseline (0), 3, 12 and 24 months. The AUC for this patient is

$$\text{AUC} = 0.5\{[0.25(33.3 + 44.4)] + [0.75(44.4 + 55.6)] + [1(55.6 + 77.8)]\}$$
$$= 113.9.$$

9.4.1.2   Analysis of acupuncture trial data

The aim of this randomized controlled trial with 2 years of follow-up was to determine whether a short course of traditional acupuncture improves longer-term outcomes for patients with non-specific low back pain in primary care (Thomas *et al.*, 2006). Adult patients aged 18–65 with non-specific low back pain of 4–52 weeks' duration were allocated at random to acupuncture or usual care groups. The intervention consisted of 10 individualized acupuncture treatments from one of seven qualified acupuncturists (159 patients) or usual care (80 patients). Usual care comprised a mix of interventions, including physiotherapy, drugs and back exercises. The primary outcome was the SF-36 Bodily Pain dimension at the one-year follow-up. Secondary outcomes included QoL as measured by the SF-36 at 3- and 24-month follow-up. Of the 239 patients randomized, 173/239 (72.3%) completed all four QoL assessments (55 in the usual care group and 118 in the acupuncture group). We are interested in comparing the QoL over the 2-year follow-up between the two groups.

   We will base our analysis on these 173 patients, but it should be noted that missing QoL assessments may be a serious problem with this data set and the reasons for the missing data should be thoroughly investigated. We will assume that the data are missing completely at random (see Box 13.1), that this reduced data set represents a randomly drawn subsample of the full data set and that the inferences drawn can be considered reasonable (Fayers and Machin, 2007). There is extensive discussion of the occurrence of drop-outs and missing data in a special edition of *Statistics in Medicine* (Volume 17, 1998) and both Fayers and Machin (2007) and Fairclough (2002) devote several chapters to this topic. The issue of missing data is described in Chapter 13.

   I shall use the acupuncture trial data to illustrate various simple methods for analysing longitudinal data, including ANCOVA, with mean follow-up QoL (i.e. the average of the 3-, 12- and 24-month responses) as the dependent variable and baseline QoL and treatment group as covariates, and summary measures such as the AUC. Table 8.2 shows the baseline QoL and socio-demographic characteristics of the 239 patients, with low back pain, in the acupuncture trial. The two groups were well matched at baseline for age, gender and baseline QoL.

9.4.1.3   Acupuncture trial AUC analysis

The overall QoL, as assessed by the SF-36 Bodily Pain score, of the low back pain patients over the 24-month study period (and four QoL assessments) can be summarized by the AUC. The SF-36 Bodily Pain dimension is scored on a 0–100 scale (where 100 means no pain). AUCs were calculated using the trapezium rule as described in equation (9.1). If we set the time units for the AUC calculation as a fraction of a year, then an AUC value of 200 implies the low back patient has been in 'good health' and reported no pain for the entire 24-month follow-up period; an AUC value of 0 implies the low back pain patient has been in 'poor health' with high levels of pain for the entire 24-month follow-up period. Figure 9.4 shows the histograms of the distribution of the AUC summary measure for the SF-36 Bodily Pain dimensions separately for the acupuncture and usual care groups. Although the distributions are not symmetric, the histograms are not as skewed as the raw data at each time point.

   Table 9.1 gives the results of simple comparisons of differences in mean AUC between the groups using the two independent samples *t*-test. Tables 9.1 and 9.2 suggests this

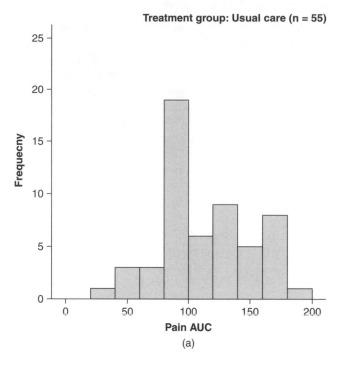

(a)

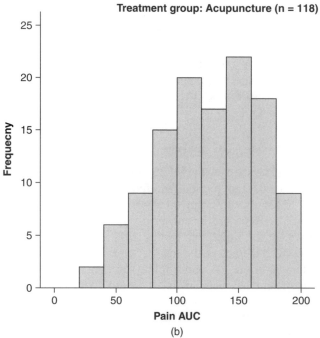

(b)

Figure 9.4   Histograms of SF-36 Bodily Pain AUC summary from acupuncture data by group (data from Thomas *et al* 2006).

difference, in areas under the curves (or lines in this graph) is of borderline statistical significance with a P-value of 0.048 and the confidence interval for the mean difference in AUCs between the groups just excluding zero at the lower limit. Therefore there is some reliable statistical evidence to suggest a difference in mean AUC pain scores between the acupuncture and usual care treated low back pain patients.

9.4.2   Acupuncture study – analysis of covariance

Figures 9.1 and 9.2 and Tables 9.1 and 9.2 suggest that SF-36 Bodily Pain scores at 3-, 12- and 24-month follow-up are fairly similar (the lines in the graph appear to be almost horizontal at these time points). Therefore another sensible summary measure would be the mean follow-up SF-36 Bodily Pain score. For this summary measure patients need only have one valid follow-up Pain score. Table 9.1 shows that 76 patients in the usual care group and 153 patients in the acupuncture group had at least one valid follow-up QoL assessment. A simple analysis would be to use the two-independent sample t-test to compare mean follow-up Pain scores between the two groups. Table 9.1 shows there is some evidence of a statistically significant difference in mean follow-up pain scores between the acupuncture and usual care groups, with acupuncture patients on average reporting mean pain scores 6.3 points higher or better than patients in the usual care group (95% CI: 0.6 to 12.0, $P = 0.03$).

The correlation between the baseline and mean follow-up pain scores is $r = 0.30$. Despite this low correlation, a more powerful statistical analysis, as described in Chapter 8, is an ANCOVA or multiple regression. This involves a multiple regression analysis with the average follow-up QoL (the mean of the 3-, 12- and 24-month assessments) as the dependent variable, $\bar{Y}_i$, and the baseline QoL (x_{Base_i}) and treatment group (x_{Group_i}, coded usual care = 0, acupuncture = 1) as covariates. Therefore the linear regression model for the ith subject is:

$$\bar{Y}_i = \beta_1 + \beta_{\mathrm{Base}} x_{\mathrm{Base}_i} + \beta_{\mathrm{Group}} x_{\mathrm{Group}_i} + \varepsilon_i, \tag{9.2}$$

where ε_i is a random error term with $\varepsilon_i \sim N(0, \sigma^2)$ and β_1 is a constant.

The regression coefficient estimate, $\hat{\beta}_{\mathrm{Group}}$, for group represents the difference in mean follow-up QoL between the usual care and acupuncture groups after adjustment for baseline QoL. A positive value for the regression coefficient for $\hat{\beta}_{\mathrm{Group}}$ indicates that the acupuncture group has a better mean SF-36 Bodily Pain score at follow-up than the usual care group after adjustment for baseline SF-36 Bodily Pain score.

The regression analysis shown in Table 9.4 suggests that there is reliable statistical evidence of a difference in average (3-, 12-, 24-month) follow-up SF-36 Bodily Pain scores between the acupuncture and usual care treated back pain patients after adjustment for baseline SF-36 Bodily Pain score.

Instead of reducing the repeated QoL responses to summary statistics, we can model the individual QoL responses, y_{ij}, for subject i for observation j at time t_{ij}, in terms of the p explanatory variables $x_{1ij}, x_{2ij}, \ldots, x_{pij}$. The next section will discuss three distinct strategies for analysing the repeated QoL responses.

Table 9.4 Unadjusted and adjusted differences in mean follow-up SF-36 Bodily Pain outcome scores between acupuncture and usual care groups (data from Thomas et al 2006).

SF-36 dimension[1]	Usual care		Acupuncture			Unadjusted difference[3] 95% CI	P-value	Adjusted[2] difference[3] (95% CI)	P-value
	n	Mean	SD	n	Mean	SD				
Mean follow-up Pain score	76	57.2	(19.8)	153	63.4	(20.9)	6.3 (0.6 to 12.0)	0.030	6.1 (0.7 to 11.6)	0.027

[1]The SF-36 Bodily Pain dimension is scored on a 0 to 100 (no pain) scale.
[2]N = 229 difference adjusted for baseline Pain score.
[3]Improvement is indicated by a positive difference on the SF-36 Bodily Pain dimension

9.5   Modelling of longitudinal data

Both Diggle *et al.* (2002) and Fayers and Machin (2007) emphasize the importance of graphical presentation of longitudinal data prior to modelling. Figures 9.1 and 9.2 show the mean levels of QoL in patients with low-back pain, before and during treatment, for the Pain dimension of the SF-36. The curves do not overlap and there is some evidence to suggest that for later QoL measurements the curves are parallel and that the mean difference between treatments is now fairly constant.

Figure 9.5 shows some simple example profiles of the possible treatment effects on the QoL outcome over time. These five graphs lead to the specification of five possible statistical models for the QoL outcome:

(a) QoL Outcome = constant;

(b) QoL Outcome = baseline + time;

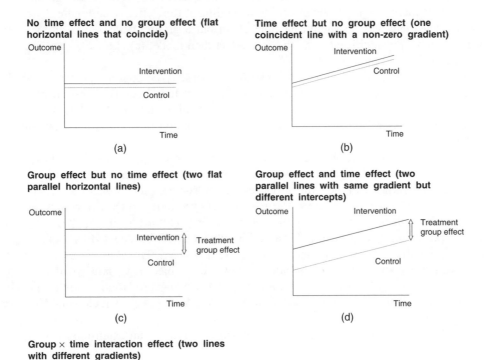

Figure 9.5 Modelling of longitudinal outcome data and interpreting the coefficients from the model.

(c) QoL Outcome = baseline + group;

(d) QoL Outcome = baseline + time + group;

(e) QoL Outcome = baseline + time + group + group × time interaction.

Ideally these models should be investigated in reverse order, that is, starting with model (e). If there is a significant group × time interaction term in model (e), then Figure 9.5(e) shows an example of the possible pattern of the outcome over time by group. The group by time interaction term in the model represents the additional effect of the intervention (compared to the control) on the QoL outcome over time. If there is no significant group × time interaction then we can fit a simpler model (d) to the QoL outcome data to see if there is both a significant group and time effect in this model. Figure 9.5(d) shows an example of the possible pattern for the QoL outcome over time by group. If only the group or time effect was statistically significant, but not both, we would then go on to fit model (b) or (c). Depending on the results of model (d), we would either go on to fit model (b) if there was no group effect but a significant time effect (see Figure 9.5(b)) or model (c) if there was no significant time effect but a group effect (see Figure 9.5(c)). In the event of no significant group or time effect then model (a) is most appropriate for the outcome data (Figure 9.5(a)).

Figures 9.1 and 9.2 suggest that model (d) or (b) may be appropriate for the SF-36 Bodily Pain outcome in the acupuncture trial. The next few sections of this chapter will describe two ways in which we can fit such longitudinal models to QoL data. Before we do so, it is necessary to introduce some statistical notation to describe the longitudinal models.

Let y_{ij} represent the QoL response variable and let $x_{1ij}, x_{2ij}, \ldots, x_{pij}$ be p explanatory variables observed at time t_{ij}, for observation $j = 1, \ldots, n_i$ on subject $i = 1, \ldots, m$. The mean and variance of the QoL responses y_{ij}, for subject i and observation j, are represented by $E(y_{ij}) = \mu_{ij}$ and $Var(y_{ij}) = \upsilon_{ij}$. The set of n_i repeated QoL outcomes for subject i can be gathered together into a list or vector of length n_i, $\mathbf{Y}_i = (y_{i1}, y_{i2}, \ldots, y_{in_i})$. The overall mean or expected QoL value for subject i will be denoted by $E(\mathbf{Y}_i) = \mu_i$. We shall let the $n_i \times n_i$ covariance matrix $Var(\mathbf{Y}_i) = V_i$. The jkth element of V_i is the covariance between QoL observation j and k for subject i, y_{ij} and y_{ik}, denoted by $Cov(y_{ij}, y_{ik}) = \upsilon_{ijk}$. We shall use R_i for the $n_i \times n_i$ (auto-)correlation matrix of $\mathbf{Y}_i$. The responses for all subjects are referred to as $\mathbf{Y} = (\mathbf{Y}_1, \mathbf{Y}_2, \ldots, \mathbf{Y}_m)$, which is an N-vector of length $N = \sum_{i=1}^{m} n_i$.

The longitudinal model we will consider will be based on an extension of the linear regression model (7.1),

$$y_{ij} = \beta_1 x_{ij1} + \beta_2 x_{ij2} + \ldots + \beta_p x_{ijp} + \varepsilon_{ij}, \qquad (9.3)$$

where $(\beta_1, \beta_2, \ldots, \beta_p)$ is a list of unknown regression coefficients and ε_{ij} is a Normally distributed random error term with variance σ_ε^2 and $\varepsilon_{ij} \sim N(0, \sigma_\varepsilon^2)$. However, unlike the simple linear regression model used in Chapters 7 and 8, the residuals ε_{ij} are now assumed to be correlated, that is, $Corr(\varepsilon_{ij}, \varepsilon_{ik}) = \rho(x_{ij}, x_{ik}; \mathfrak{R})$. The correlation matrix, $\mathfrak{R}$, is estimated by a working correlation matrix, R_i, that usually assumes the repeated QoL outcomes for a subject are correlated. Typically, $x_{ij1} = 1$ for all i and j, and β_1 is then the intercept term in the linear model.

9.5.1   Autocorrelation

Let y_{i1} and y_{i2} represent the values of two successive QoL assessments by the same (ith) patient and m represent the total number of patients completing both assessments in the sample. Then the strength of association or *autocorrelation* between successive longitudinal measurements of QoL on the same patient is given by

$$r_T(1, 2) = \frac{\sum_{i=1}^{m} (y_{i1} - \bar{Y}_1)(y_{i2} - \bar{Y}_2)}{\sqrt{\sum_{i=1}^{m} (y_{i1} - \bar{Y}_1)^2 \sum_{i=1}^{m} (y_{i2} - \bar{Y}_2)^2}}, \tag{9.4}$$

where $\bar{Y}_1$ and $\bar{Y}_2$ are the sample mean QoL scores at times t_1 and t_2, respectively. (This is equivalent to Pearson's product moment correlation coefficient.)

Suppose that QoL is assessed on numerous occasions and the measurements at different times are $y_{i0}, y_{i1}, \ldots, y_{iT}$ for patient i at time T in the study. Then equation (9.4) can be used, one pair at a time, with the respective y_{ij} replacing the y-values. If there are assessments at $T + 1$ time points, there will be $(T + 1)T/2$ pairs of assessments, leading to separate autocorrelation coefficients. For example, for $T = 4$ there are $(5 \times 4)/2 = 10$ autocorrelation coefficients that may be calculated.

In the acupuncture trial QoL assessment was carried out at 0, 3, 12 and 24 months (i.e. $3 + 1$ time points). Table 9.5 summarizes the resulting 10 auto-correlations for the assessments up to 24 months. The pattern of the observed autocorrelation matrix R gives a guide to the so-called error structure associated with the successive QoL measurements. Table 9.5 shows that the autocorrelation coefficients range between 0.19 and 0.57. The pattern of values suggests decreasing correlation as the observations become further apart.

Several underlying patterns of the autocorrelation matrix R are used in the modelling of QoL data. The error structure is *independent* (sometimes termed *random*) if the off-diagonal terms of the autocorrelation matrix R are zero. The repeated QoL observations on the same subject are then independent of each other, and can be regarded as though they were observations from different individuals.

On the other hand, if all the correlations are approximately equal or *uniform* then the matrix of correlation coefficients is termed *exchangeable*, or *compound symmetric*. This means that we can reorder (exchange) the successive observations in any way we choose in our data file without affecting the pattern in the correlation matrix.

Frequently, as the time or lag between successive observations increases, the autocorrelation between the observations decreases. Thus, we would expect a higher

Table 9.5   Autocorrelation matrices for the Pain dimension of the SF-36 from back pain patients in the acupuncture study assessed at four time points.

Bodily Pain ($n = 173$)				
Time (months)	0	3	12	24
0	1.00			
3	0.24	1.00		
12	0.27	0.56	1.00	
24	0.19	0.47	0.57	1.00

autocorrelation between QoL assessments made only two days apart than between two QoL assessments made one month apart. This is in contrast to the uniform correlation model above. In such a situation one may postulate that the relationship between the size of the correlation and the 'lag' (i.e. the time from t_j to t_k) may be of the form

$$\rho_T(t_j, t_k) = \rho^{\phi|t_j - t_k|}. \tag{9.5}$$

The $|t_j - t_k|$ implies that if the difference between t_j and t_k is negative the sign should be ignored and ϕ takes a constant value that is usually less than 1. A correlation matrix of this form is said to have an *autoregressive structure* (sometimes called *multiplicative* or *time series*). Diggle *et al.* (2002) refer to this as the *exponential correlation model*.

The autocorrelation pattern affects the way in which computer packages estimate the regression coefficients in the corresponding statistical model, and so it should be chosen with care. We will now concentrate on longitudinal data analysis problems where the regression of y on x is the scientific focus and the number of experimental units (m) – patients in our case – is much greater than the number of observations per unit (n).

9.5.2   Repeated measures analysis of variance

In some situations QoL assessments may be made over a limited period rather than over an extended time span. In this case in may be reasonable to assume that all the subjects complete all the assessments. Thus instead of having a fragmented data file with the number of observations for each subject varying from subject to subject, the file has a regular or rectangular shape. This enables the repeated measures ANOVA approach to be considered (Fayers and Machin, 2007).

Diggle *et al.* (2002) say that ANOVA has limitations that prevent its recommendation as a general approach for longitudinal data. The first is that it fails to exploit the potential gains in efficiency from modelling the covariance among repeated observations. The second limitation is that ANOVA methods usually require a complete balanced array of data. As Fayers and Machin (2007) point out, this is the main difficulty with repeated measures ANOVA in QoL research, since there are seldom equal numbers of QoL assessments recorded per patient. Diggle *et al.* (2002) point out that the use of repeated measures ANOVA implies an exchangeable autocorrelation between any two observations on the same patient. This may not always be appropriate for QoL assessments. It is therefore better to use a regression modelling approach rather than repeated measures ANOVA for analysing longitudinal QoL data.

9.5.3   Marginal general linear models – generalized estimating equations

The second strategy is to model the marginal mean as in a cross-sectional study. Since repeated values are not likely to be independent, this marginal analysis must also include assumptions about the form of the correlation. For example, in the linear model we can assume that mean QoL life response for subject i is

$$E(\mathbf{Y}_i) = \beta_1 \mathbf{X}_{1i} + \beta_2 \mathbf{X}_{2i} \ldots + \beta_p \mathbf{X}_{pi}, \tag{9.6}$$

with variance $\mathrm{Var}(\mathbf{Y}_i) = V_i(\alpha)$. The β_ps and α must be estimated. The marginal model approach has the advantage of separately modelling the mean and covariance. Valid inferences about β_ps can sometimes be made even when an incorrect form for the $V(\alpha)$ is assumed.

Marginal models are appropriate when inferences about the population average are the focus. For example, in a clinical trial the average difference between control and treatment is most important, not the difference for any one individual. In a marginal model, the regression of the response on explanatory variables is modelled separately from the within-person correlation. In regression, we model the marginal expectation, $E(y_{ij})$, as a function of explanatory variables. By marginal expectation, we mean the average response over the subpopulation that shares a common value of x. The marginal expectation is what we modelled in the analysis of the cross-sectional studies in the Chapter 7.

A marginal model has the following assumptions (Diggle *et al.*, 2002):

1. The marginal expectation of the response, $E(y_{ij}) = \mu_{ij}$, depends on explanatory variables $x_{1ij}, x_{2ij}, \ldots, x_{pij}$, by

$$h(\mu_{ij}) = \beta_1 x_{ij1} + \beta_2 x_{ij2} + \cdots + \beta_p x_{ijp}, \tag{9.7}$$

   where h is a known *link function* such as the identity link for continuous responses or the logit for binary responses or log for counts.

2. The marginal variance depends on the marginal mean according to $\text{Var}(y_{ij}) = v(\mu_{ij})\phi$, where v is a known variance function and ϕ is a scale parameter which may need to be estimated.

3. The correlation between y_{ij} and y_{ik} is a function of the marginal means and perhaps of additional parameters α, that is, $\text{Corr}(y_{ij}, y_{ik}) = \rho(\mu_{ij}, \mu_{ik}; \alpha)$ where $\rho(.)$ is a known function.

The marginal regression coefficients, β, have the same interpretation as the coefficients from a cross-sectional analysis. Consider a simple linear regression model for QoL over time for a group of hospital patients following surgery say,

$$y_{ij} = \beta_1 + \beta_2 t_{ij} + \varepsilon_{ij}, \tag{9.8}$$

where t_{ij} is the time of the QoL assessment, say in months post surgery, of patient i at visit j, y_{ij} is the QoL at time t_{ij} post surgery and ε_{ij} is a mean-zero residual. Since patients' QoL will not all improve (or deteriorate) at the same rate, the residuals $\varepsilon_{i1}, \varepsilon_{i2}, \ldots, \varepsilon_{in_i}$, for patient i are likely to be correlated with one another. The marginal modelling approach is to assume

(1) $E(y_{ij}) = \beta_1 + \beta_2 t_{ij}$,

(2) $\text{Corr}(\varepsilon_{ij}, \varepsilon_{ik}) = \rho(t_{ij}, t_{ik}; \alpha)$.

Assumption (1) is that the average QoL for all patients in the population at any time t is $\beta_1 + \beta_2 t_{ij}$. The parameter β_2 is therefore the change per month in the population average QoL. Assumption (2) specifies the nature of the autocorrelation; a specific simple example might be that

$$\text{Corr}(\varepsilon_{ij}, \varepsilon_{ik}) = \rho(t_{ij}, t_{ik}; \alpha) = \alpha_0, \tag{9.9}$$

a constant, so that the autocorrelation matrix is exchangeable or compound symmetric. This constant common correlation, $\rho = \alpha_0$, is also the intra-cluster correlation coefficient (ICC).

In the marginal approach, we separate the modelling of the regression and the correlation; either can be changed without necessarily changing the other (Diggle *et al.*, 2002). A more complex example would be to consider the same linear regression but this time let the errors follow an autoregressive structure as introduced in (9.5). Again the mean response is $E(y_{ij}) = \beta_1 + \beta_2 t_{ij}$. The covariance structure is now given by $\text{Cov}(Y_{ij}, Y_{ik}) = \sigma^2 \exp(-\phi|t_j - t_k|)$ and the variance is assumed to be independent of the mean.

The marginal generalized linear modelling approach uses *generalized estimating equations* (GEEs) to estimate the regression coefficients (Liang and Zeger, 1986). In the GEE approach any required covariance structure and any link function may be assumed and the parameters estimated without specifying the joint distribution of the repeated observations. Estimation is via a multivariate analogue of the *quasi-likelihood* approach (Wedderburn, 1974). In the marginal modelling approach, we only need to specify the first two moments of the responses for each person (i.e. the mean and variance). With continuous Normally distributed data, the first two moments fully determine the likelihood, but this is not the case for other members of the *generalized linear model* family (Diggle *et al.*, 2002).

Since the parameters specifying the structure of the correlation matrix are rarely of great practical interest (they are what is known as *nuisance parameters*), simple structures (e.g. exchangeable or first-order autoregressive) are used for the within-subject correlations, giving rise to the so-called *working correlation matrix*. Liang and Zeger 1986 show that the estimates of the parameters of most interest (i.e. those that determine the mean profiles over time) are still valid even when the correlation structure is incorrectly specified.

Diggle *et al.* (2002) conclude that the GEE method of estimation enjoys two useful and important properties:

(1) $\hat{\beta}$ is nearly efficient relative to the maximum likelihood estimates of β in many practical situations provided that $\text{Var}(Y_i)$ has been reasonably approximated.

(2) $\hat{\beta}$ is consistent as the sample size gets larger (i.e. $m \to \infty$), even if the covariance of Y_i is incorrectly specified.

When the regression coefficients are the scientific focus, as in the examples in this chapter, one should invest the lion's share of time in modelling the mean structure, while using a reasonable approximation to the covariance. The robustness of the inferences about β can be checked by fitting a final model using different covariance assumptions and comparing the two sets of estimates and their robust standard errors. If they differ substantially, a more careful treatment of the covariance model may be necessary (Diggle *et al.*, 2002).

The process of fitting marginal models using GEEs begins by assuming the simple independence form for the autocorrelation matrix R, and fitting the model as if each assessment were from a different patient. Once this model is obtained the corresponding residuals are calculated and these are then used to estimate the autocorrelation matrix assuming it is of the exchangeable (or autoregressive) type. This matrix is then used to fit the model again, the residuals are calculated once more, and the autocorrelation matrix obtained. The iteration process is repeated until the corresponding regression coefficients that are obtained in the successive models converge or differ little on successive occasions (Fayers and Machin, 2007).

9.5.3.1 Analysis of acupuncture trial data using marginal models

The non-overlapping lines in Figure 9.1 imply there is unlikely to be a 'treatment $\times$ time' interaction. However, it is still important to test for any such interaction in any regression model. Fortunately, with the marginal model approach this is relatively easy to do and simply involves the addition of an extra regression coefficient to the model. If treatment is coded as a 0–1 variable (i.e. $0 =$ usual care and $1 =$ acupuncture) and assessment time as a continuous variable, then the additional interaction term is simply the product of these two variables (which will be 0 for all the usual care group patients and equal to the QoL assessment time in the acupuncture group patients).

The marginal model we used for the acupuncture trial data for analysing the three QoL assessments over time was

$$\text{Pain}_{ij} = \beta_1 + \beta_{\text{Base}} x_{\text{Base}\_i} + \beta_{\text{Time}} t_{ij} + \beta_{\text{Group}} x_{\text{Group}\_i} + \varepsilon_{ij}, \tag{9.10}$$

where Pain_{ij} is the QoL at time t_{ij} post baseline; t_{ij} is the time of the QoL assessment, in months post baseline, of patient i at visit j; x_{Base_i} is the baseline QoL assessment for subject i; x_{Group_i} is the treatment group ($0 =$ usual care, $1 =$ acupuncture) for subject i; β_1 is a constant and ε_{ij} is the residual error. The marginal modelling approach is to assume

(1) $E(\text{Pain}_{ij}) = \beta_1 + \beta_{\text{Base}} x_{\text{Base}\_i} + \ldots + \beta_{\text{Time}} t_{ij} + \beta_{\text{Group}} x_{\text{Group}\_i}.$ (9.11)

(2) $\text{Corr}(\varepsilon_{ij}, \varepsilon_{ik}) = \rho(t_{ij}, t_{ik}; \alpha).$ (9.12)

The marginal regression models were fitted in STATA version 10 (StataCorp, 2008) using the $\texttt{xtgee}$ command with an identity link function ($\texttt{link(iden)}$) and the $\texttt{robust}$ standard errors option. We used an exchangeable autocorrelation structure $\text{Corr}(\varepsilon_{ij}, \varepsilon_{ik}) = \rho(t_{ij}, t_{ik}; \alpha)$ for the marginal model, using the STATA command $\texttt{corr(exc)}$. This is equivalent to saying that the correlation between the repeated QoL assessments for each subject is constant, that is, $Corr(\varepsilon_{ij}, \varepsilon_{ik}) = \rho(t_{ij}, t_{ik}; \alpha) = \alpha_0$. The exchangeable autocorrelation structure assumed a working correlation matrix with

$$R_{s,t} = \begin{cases} 1, & s = t, \\ \alpha_0, & \text{otherwise}, \end{cases}$$

between outcomes at times s and t.

The observed correlation matrices in Table 9.5 clearly show that the off-diagonal terms are non-zero and that the assumption of an independent autocorrelation matrix for the marginal model is unrealistic. The observed correlation matrix suggests the correlations between the three post-baseline QoL assessments at 3, 12 and 24 months are of similar magnitude and range between 0.47 and 0.57. This suggests the assumption of an exchangeable correlation structure for the repeated QoL assessment for this data in not unrealistic.

According to the STATA reference manual (StataCorp, 2008), the $\texttt{robust}$ option specifies that the Huber–White sandwich estimator of variance is to be used in place of

Table 9.6 Estimated regression coefficients from a marginal model (model (e)) with interaction to show the effect of treatment (acupuncture or usual care) on outcome (SF-36 Bodily Pain score) over time after adjustment for baseline pain, assuming an exchangeable correlation ($n = 229$).

Pain*	b	Semi-robust SE(b)	z	P-value	95% CI Lower	Upper
Pain (baseline)	0.4	0.07	4.85	<0.001	0.2	0.5
Time (months)	0.1	0.16	0.77	0.441	−0.2	0.4
Group	4.0	3.61	1.12	0.265	−3.1	11.1
Interaction	0.2	0.19	0.92	0.360	−0.2	0.5
Constant	44.8	4.02	11.16	<0.001	37.0	52.7

*The outcome variable is SF-36 Bodily Pain score with a higher score indicating less pain.

the default iteratively reweighted least squares (IRLS) variance estimator. This produces valid standard errors even if the within-subject correlations are not as hypothesized by the specified correlation structure. It does, however require that the model correctly specifies the mean. As such, the resulting standard errors are labelled 'semi-robust' instead of 'robust'.

9.5.3.2 Treatment by time interactions

In a previous section we mentioned the importance of looking for a 'treatment × time' interaction. This can easily be done by creating a new variable x_{Int_ij}, which is the product of the treatment group and time variables, and adding the extra term β_{Int} to model (9.10) and fitting this new model,

$$Pain_{ij} = \beta_1 + \beta_{Base}x_{Base\_i} + \beta_{Time}t_{ij} + \beta_{Group}x_{Group\_i} + \beta_{Int}x_{Int\_ij} + \varepsilon_{ij}. \quad (9.13)$$

Table 9.6 shows the results of fitting this marginal model. The interaction term was not statistically significant (from zero). Thus there was no reliable evidence of a treatment × time interaction. Therefore we can now use the simpler model (9.10) without the interaction term to test for a group and time effect on QoL.

Table 9.7 shows the estimated regression coefficients for the group and time variables. There is some evidence that SF-36 Bodily Pain scores increase over time. However, we are interested in the effect of treatment and comparing Pain over time across the usual

Table 9.7 Estimated regression coefficients from a marginal model (model (d)) to show the effect of treatment (acupuncture or usual care) on outcome (SF-36 Bodily Pain score) over time after adjustment for baseline pain assuming a exchangeable correlation ($n = 229$).

Pain*	b	Semi-robust SE(b)	z	P-value	95% CI Lower	Upper
Pain (baseline)	0.4	0.07	4.86	<0.001	0.2	0.5
Time (months)	0.2	0.09	2.79	0.005	0.1	0.4
Group	6.1	2.66	2.29	0.022	0.9	11.3
Constant	43.5	3.57	12.18	<0.001	36.5	50.4

*The outcome variable is SF-36 Bodily Pain score.

Table 9.8 Observed and estimated within-patient autocorrelation matrices (exchangeable model) from the low back pain patients in the acupuncture trial. The upper diagonal gives the observed matrix before model fitting whilst the lower gives the exchangeable form after model fitting* .

Time (months)	3	12	24
3	1.00	*0.56*	*0.47*
12	0.49	1.00	*0.57*
24	0.49	0.49	1.00

*The model contains time, baseline QoL and group as covariates.

care and acupuncture treated groups. Since there is no reliable evidence of a group $\times$ time interaction the interpretation of the treatment group coefficient is relatively straightforward. The P-value, 0.022, for the treatment group regression coefficient in Table 9.7 suggests a significant difference in Pain scores between the usual care and acupuncture treated groups. Since the SF-36 Bodily Pain dimension is scored on a 0 to 100 (no pain) scale, the regression coefficient suggests that acupuncture treated patients have, at all follow-up assessments, on average a 6.1 point (95% CI: 0.9 to 11.3) better or improved Pain score than patients in the usual care group after adjusting for baseline Pain score.

Table 9.8 shows the estimated within subject correlation matrices for the SF-36 Bodily Pain outcome if we fit model (9.10) and assume a compound symmetric or exchangeable correlation structure for the repeated QoL assessments. The upper diagonal gives the observed matrix before the model fitting. The fitted autocorrelation was 0.49. The observed deviations between the fitted model and observed autocorrelations are not too great, suggesting that the assumption of compound symmetry is not unreasonable.

9.5.4 Random effects models

A third approach, the random effects model, assumes that the correlation arises among repeated responses because the regression coefficients vary across individuals. Here we model the conditional expectation of y_{ij} given the person-specific coefficients, β_i, for subject i, by,

$$E(y_{ij}|\beta_i) = \beta_{1i}x_{ij1} + \beta_{2i}x_{ij2} + \cdots + \beta_{pi}x_{ijp}. \tag{9.14}$$

Since there are too few data on a single person to estimate β_i from $(\mathbf{Y}_i, \mathbf{X}_i)$ alone, we further assume that the β_i are independent realizations from some distribution with mean β. If we write $\beta_i' = \beta_i + \mathbf{U}_i$, where β is fixed and $\mathbf{U}_i$ is a zero-mean random variable, then the basic heterogeneity assumption can be restated in terms of the latent variables $\mathbf{U}_i$. That is, there are unobserved factors represented by the $\mathbf{U}_i$ that are common to all QoL responses for a given person but vary across people, thus indicating the correlation.

The advantage of the random effects model is that there are fewer regression parameters to estimate. It is based on the assumption that the subjects in the study are chosen at random from some wider patient population. This will seldom be true, at least in the context of a clinical trial for which trial patients are screened for eligibility and entered only after giving informed consent. However, it is usually reasonable to assume that trial patients have been chosen at random from a large number of potentially eligible patients, and that they represent a random selection from this artificial population. Thus, a random effects model is frequently applied whenever a study includes a large numbers of patients (Fayers and Machin, 2007).

The random effects model is most useful when the objective is to make inference about individuals rather than the population average. Thus a random effects approach will allow us to estimate the QoL status of an individual patient. The regression coefficients, β, represent the effect of the explanatory variables on an individual patient's QoL. This is in contrast to the marginal model coefficients, which describe the effect of the explanatory variables on the population average.

The random effects model to estimate the QoL, y_{ij}, as a function of p explanatory variables, $x_{1ij}, x_{2ij}, \ldots, x_{pij}$, observed at time t_{ij}, for observation $j = 1, \ldots, n_i$ on subject $i = 1, \ldots, m$, is

$$y_{ij} = \underbrace{\beta_1 x_{ij1} + \beta_2 x_{ij2} + \ldots + \beta_p x_{ijp}}_{\text{Fixed portion}} + \underbrace{\omega_i + \varepsilon_{ij}}_{\text{Random}} . \tag{9.15}$$

Here ε_{ij} is a Normally distributed random error term with variance σ_ε^2 and $\varepsilon_{ij} \sim N(0, \sigma_\varepsilon^2)$; ω_i is a random effect of subject i across all subjects with $\omega_i \sim N(0, \sigma_\omega^2)$. Variation in ω_j induces variation in the mean outcome across all subjects, represented by σ_ω^2, the between-subjects variance. This model assumes that the effect of the explanatory variables is homogenous across the subjects. This is sometimes known as the *random intercept* model.

The fixed portion of the model, $\beta_1 x_{ij1} + \beta_2 x_{ij2} + \cdots + \beta_p x_{ijp}$, simply states that we want one overall regression line representing the population average QoL. The random effect ω_i serves to shift this regression line up or down according to each individual subject.

The ICC estimate $\hat{\rho}$ is given by

$$\hat{\rho} = \frac{\hat{\sigma}_\varepsilon^2}{\hat{\sigma}_\varepsilon^2 + \hat{\sigma}_\omega^2}, \tag{9.16}$$

where σ_ε^2 is the individual measurement variability of the outcome and σ_ω^2 is the between-subjects variation.

Random effects generalized linear models are sometimes referred to as generalized linear mixed models, because they have a mixed (fixed and random) composition. If we assume that a random effects model is appropriate, such models can be fitted using multi-level modelling statistical software such as MLwiN (Goldstein *et al.*, 1998). Use of multi-level modelling as opposed to marginal modelling allows examination of the 'error' parts of the model in more detail. For the analysis of the continuous QoL outcomes the STATA function xtmixed was used to fit the random effects model (9.15) using restricted maximum likelihood estimation (REML).

We earlier mentioned the importance of looking for a treatment × time interaction. The interaction term from the random effects model was not statistically significant. So we can use the following random effects model for the acupuncture data:

$$\text{Pain}_{ij} = \beta_1 + \beta_{\text{Base}} x_{\text{Base\_}i} + \beta_{\text{Time}} t_{ij} + \beta_{\text{Group}} x_{\text{Group\_}i} + \varepsilon_{ij} + \omega_i. \tag{9.17}$$

Table 9.9 Estimated regression coefficients from a random effects model (model (d)) to show the effect of treatment (acupuncture or usual care) on outcome (SF-36 Bodily Pain score) over time after adjustment for baseline pain ($n = 229$).

Pain*	b	SE(b)	z	P-value	95% CI Lower	Upper
Pain (baseline)	0.4	0.08	4.76	<0.001	0.2	0.5
Time (months)	0.2	0.08	2.93	0.003	0.1	0.4
Group	6.1	2.74	2.23	0.026	0.7	11.5
Constant	43.5	3.38	12.85	<0.001	36.8	50.1

*The outcome variable is SF-36 Bodily Pain score.

The P-value, 0.026, for the treatment group regression coefficient in Table 9.9 suggests a significant difference in Pain scores between the usual care and acupuncture treated groups. Since the SF-36 Bodily Pain dimension is scored on a 0 to 100 (no pain) scale, the regression coefficient suggests that acupuncture treated patients have, at all follow-up assessments, on average a 6.1 point (95% CI: 0.7 to 11.5) better or improved Pain score than patients in the usual care group after adjusting for baseline Pain score. The estimated treatment effect is the same as the marginal model although the standard error is larger for the random effects model (which means the confidence intervals are wider and the P-value larger).

The estimated individual measurement variability of the outcome $\hat{\sigma}_\varepsilon^2$ is 16.63^2 and the between subject variation σ_ω^2 is 16.39^2. The ICC estimate, $\hat{\rho}$, from equation 9.16, is

$$\hat{\rho} = \frac{16.63^2}{16.63^2 + 16.39^2} = 0.49$$

which is the same as the exchangeable autocorrelation estimate from the marginal model.

9.5.5   Random effects versus marginal modelling

The two approaches of random effects and marginal modelling lead to different interpretations of between-subjects effects. In random effects models, a between-subjects effect represents the difference between subjects conditional on having the same random effect, whereas the parameters of marginal models represent the average difference between subjects.

Diggle et al. (2002) demonstrate that, in the linear case, it is possible to formulate the two regression approaches to have coefficients with the same interpretation. That is, coefficients from linear random effects models can have marginal interpretations as well. With non-linear link functions, such as the logit, this is not the case. So in practice, for continuous QoL outcomes, it does not really matter whether or not you use a marginal or random effects model.

In practice when it comes to choosing between a random effects and a marginal model, the important thing is to choose the model which best answers the scientific research question being asked in the study (Diggle et al., 2002). In a clinical trial we are clearly interested in the average difference in QoL outcomes between the intervention and control groups, not the difference in QoL for any one individual. For this research question a marginal model appears to be appropriate as the treatment effect of a marginal model represents the average difference in QoL between the treatment and control groups across the whole population without being specific to the individuals used in the trial. However, in a clinical trial we may also be interested in the effect of the intervention or control treatment on an individual subject. In these circumstances, the random effects model would give the effect of the intervention or control treatment on an individual subject. There is a continuing debate on this subject; see Lee and Nelder (2004) for more details.

Table 9.8 shows that there is the reasonable agreement between the fitted model and observed autocorrelations. This suggests that the assumption of an exchangeable autocorrelation structure is reasonable for this data set. In practice it is often difficult to choose whether an exchangeable or autoregressive autocorrelation structure is appropriate (Fayers and Machin, 2007). My experience and empirical evidence seem to suggest that the simpler exchangeable autocorrelation model is a reasonable approximation for the underlying correlation structure.

Example: 2 × 2 factorial design – pulmonary rehabilitation

Waterhouse et al. (2009) describe a randomized 2×2 factorial trial of community versus hospital pulmonary rehabilitation, followed by telephone or conventional follow-up and its impact on QoL, exercise capacity and use of health-care resources in patients with chronic obstructive pulmonary disease. Four different experimental conditions were evaluated. These were:

(A) hospital rehabilitation and telephone follow-up;

(B) hospital rehabilitation and no telephone follow-up;

(C) community rehabilitation and telephone follow-up;

(D) community rehabilitation and no telephone follow-up.

The use of this 2×2 factorial design enabled two research questions to be asked simultaneously. Thus, groups A and B versus C and D compared hospital-versus community-based rehabilitation programmes, while groups A and C versus B and D measured the value of telephone versus conventional (no telephone) follow-up.

The main aim of the analysis was to establish whether long-term QoL outcomes post rehabilitation changed differently over time after hospital or community rehabilitation and telephone versus conventional follow-up. The QoL outcome data were longitudinal and consisted of five repeated observations over time: baseline (pre-rehabilitation), post rehabilitation, 6 months post rehabilitation, 12 months and 18 months) on each of the patients.

Since the four post-rehabilitation follow-up visits were approximately 6 months apart, time was reclassified as 1 (post rehabilitation), 2 (6 months post rehabilitation), 3 (12 months), 4 (18 months). The rehabilitation group variable Rehab was coded as $0 =$ community rehabilitation, $1 =$ hospital rehabilitation; and the follow-up variable Follow was coded as telephone versus conventional ($0 =$ conventional follow-up (no telephone) and $1 =$ telephone follow-up). One of the QoL outcomes was the post-rehabilitation scores on the SF-6D QoL measure.

The authors used a marginal generalized linear model for longitudinal data,

$$\text{QoL}_{ij} = \beta_1 + \beta_{\text{Base}} QoL_{\text{Base}\_i} + \beta_{\text{Time}} t_{ij} + \beta_{\text{Rehab}} \text{Rehab}_i + \beta_{\text{Follow}} \text{Follow}_i + \varepsilon_{ij},$$

$$(9.18)$$

with coefficients estimated using generalized estimating equations with robust standard errors and an exchangeable autocorrelation matrix to analyse the SF-6D outcome and allow for the longitudinal nature of the data, baseline QoL and the factorial design of the trial. An interaction term, the product of Rehab and Follow (which was 0 except when a patient was in the hospital rehabilitation group with telephone follow-up, when it had a value of 1), was non-significant ($P = 0.608$) so it was omitted and the simpler model (9.18) used. In this model the effect of treatment on follow-up QoL can be assessed whilst adjusting for baseline QoL and other covariates such as time and the factorial design of the trial (i.e. the other treatment group factor).

Table 9.10 shows the results of fitting model (9.18) to the SF-6D outcome in the pulmonary rehabilitation trial. The SF-6D is scored on a 0.29 to 1.00 (good health) scale. The results are presented according to Montgomery's recommendations for factorial RCTs (Montgomery et al., 2003). The interaction term was non-significant so the results from the simpler model (9.18) are presented. On average the mean difference in post-rehabilitation SF-6D scores between the hospital and community groups, after adjustment for baseline SF-6D score, time (follow-up visit) and the factorial design, was not significantly different at 0.01 (95% CI: -0.01 to 0.02, $P = 0.222$). There was no significant difference in SF-6D scores between the telephone and standard follow-up groups, with a mean difference, after adjustment for baseline SF-6D score, time (follow-up visit) and factorial design, of 0.02 (95% CI: -0.00 to 0.04, $P = 0.071$). $\qquad\square$

9.5.6   Use of marginal and random effects models to analyse data from a cluster RCT

Chapter 8 described a simple way to analyse data from a cluster RCT (cRCT) by analysing by group, rather than on an individual subject basis, by using aggregate cluster level outcomes such as the mean score per cluster. An alternative approach using individual level data is to model the outcomes with a random effect or marginal model.

With a slight change of notation, random effects or marginal models can also be used to analyse individual subject level outcomes from a cRCT. Suppose that we have a continuous QoL outcome, y_{ij}, for the ith patient in the jth cluster in the cRCT. Then a model assuming independent outcomes is

$$y_{ij} = \beta_1 + \beta_2 x_{ij} + \varepsilon_{ij}, \qquad (9.19)$$

where x_{ij} is an indicator variable for the experimental group ($1 = $ intervention, $0 = $ control); $\varepsilon_{ij} \sim N(0, \sigma_\varepsilon^2)$ and $\text{Corr}(\varepsilon_{ij}, \varepsilon_{kj}) = 0$; β_1 is the mean outcome in the control group and β_2 is the intervention effect.

A random effects model to account for clustering is

$$y_{ij} = \beta_1 + \beta_2 x_{ij} + \mu_{aj} + \varepsilon_{ij}, \qquad (9.20)$$

where μ_{aj} is a random effect of cluster j across all patients with $\mu_{aj} \sim N(0, \sigma_a^2)$.

The marginal model takes the same form as equation (9.19):

$$y_{ij} = \beta_1 + \beta_2 x_{ij} + \varepsilon_{ij}, \qquad (9.21)$$

but assumes that the residuals ε_{ij} are correlated, $\text{Corr}(\varepsilon_{ij}, \varepsilon_{kj}) = \rho(x_{ij}, x_{kj}; \mathfrak{R})$. The correlation matrix, $\mathfrak{R}$, is estimated by an exchangeable correlation matrix, R, that assumes

Table 9.10 Estimated regression coefficients from a marginal model to show the effect of rehabilitation group or follow-up group on outcome (SF-6D utility score) over time after adjustment for baseline SF-6D score, time and the factorial design ($n = 167$).

SF-6D score	Rehabilitation Group						Follow-up Group					
	Community			Hospital			No telephone follow-up			Telephone follow-up		
	n	Mean	SD	n	Mean	SD	n	Mean	SD	n	Mean	SD
Baseline	103	0.59	(0.11)	124	0.59	(0.11)	115	0.59	(0.11)	112	0.59	(0.11)
Post rehabilitation (0 months)	78	0.63	(0.12)	89	0.64	(0.11)	81	0.63	(0.11)	86	0.63	(0.12)
6 months	68	0.58	(0.11)	88	0.61	(0.11)	80	0.59	(0.11)	76	0.60	(0.12)
12 months	70	0.60	(0.12)	78	0.59	(0.10)	78	0.58	(0.11)	70	0.62	(0.12)
18 months	65	0.58	(0.11)	88	0.58	(0.10)	78	0.57	(0.11)	75	0.59	(0.09)
Adjusted group difference (95% CI)[1]	0.01	(−0.01 to 0.03)[2,4]					0.02	(−0.00 to 0.04)[3,4]				
P-value	0.222						0.071					

The SF-6D is scored on a 0.29 to 1.00 (good health) scale.

[1] Adjusted for baseline SF-6D score, time (follow-up visit) and factorial design.

[2] A positive difference represents a favourable outcome for the hospital group compared to the community rehabilitation group.

[3] A positive difference represents a favourable outcome for the telephone group compared to the no telephone follow-up group.

[4] The interaction between the intervention groups was investigated as a secondary analysis and was found to be non-significant. (interaction coefficient = −0.01 (95% CI: −0.05 to 0.03, $P = 0.608$).

Table 9.11 Estimated regression coefficients from a marginal model to show the effect of group on outcome, 6-month EPDS score, after adjustment for 6-week EPDS and other covariates from the PONDER cRCT, $n = 2624$ (data from Morrell *et al.*, 2009).

Outcome: 6-month EPDS	b	Semi-robust SE(b)	z	P-value	95% CI Lower	Upper
EPDS (6 weeks)	0.5	0.02	20.86	<0.001	0.4	0.5
Lives alone	1.3	0.42	3.23	0.001	0.5	2.2
(0 = no, 1 = yes)						
History of PND	1.0	0.30	3.32	<0.001	0.4	1.6
(0 = no, 1 = yes)						
Life event	0.8	0.16	5.22	<0.001	0.5	1.1
(0 = no, 1 = yes)						
Group (0 = control, 1 = intervention)	−0.8	0.21	−3.79	<0.001	−1.2	−0.4
Constant	2.6	0.21	12.35	<0.001	2.2	3.0

The EPDS is scored on a 0–30 scale, with a higher score indicating more depressive symptoms.

the outcomes for a patient within a cluster are equally correlated with the outcome of every other patient within that cluster and this common correlation, ρ, is the ICC, $R'_{ii} = 1\, if\, i = i'$ or $R'_{ii} = \rho$ otherwise.

Example: The PONDER cRCT

The PONDER trial (Morrell *et al.*, 2009) was a cRCT in primary care designed to evaluate the effectiveness of new health visitor led psychological intervention in detecting and treating new mothers with postnatal depression (PND) compared to usual care. The PONDER trial randomized 100 clusters (GP practices and their associated health visitors) and collected data on 2659 new mothers with an 18-month follow-up. The participants were 1745 (in 63 clusters) women allocated to intervention and 914 women (in 37 clusters) allocated to control. The main outcome measure was the 6-month EPDS score. The EPDS is scored on a 0–30 scale, with a higher score indicating more depressive symptoms. A score greater than 12 is regarded as being 'at higher risk' of PND. Table 9.11 shows the regression coefficients from fitting a marginal generalized linear model, (9.21) with coefficients estimated using generalized estimating equations with robust standard errors and an exchangeable autocorrelation matrix to analyze the 6-month EPDS outcome and allow for the clustered nature of the data. The results of the marginal model suggests that new mothers in the intervention clusters have significantly lower 6-month EPDS scores (i.e. less depressive symptoms), −0.8 (95% CI: −1.2 to −0.4, P= 0.001) than mothers in the intervention clusters after allowing for 6-week EPDS score, lives alone, history of PND, any life events. The estimated ICC was 0.081 from the model implying a small effect of clustering. A random-effects model produced similar regression estimates. □

9.6   Conclusions

This chapter has described two main methods for analysing QoL data from studies that have repeated QoL assessments over time and are longitudinal in nature: summary measures and longitudinal models. The initial analysis should be to summarize, tabulate and graphically display the repeated QoL assessments. With a limited number of individual subjects, say less than 20, the individual data values can be plotted over time. For studies with larger samples we can only plot summary measures such as the mean QoL at each time point. These graphical displays will give us an idea of the pattern or profile of QoL over time. Typically these graphs usually show an initial increase or decrease in QoL post baseline followed by a levelling off over time. In these circumstances summary measures such as the AUC or the overall post-randomization mean QoL provide a valid and simple method of analysis without the need for a more complex longitudinal model. The book by Diggle *et al.* (2002) provides a comprehensive and practical guide to the analysis of longitudinal data.

Exercises

9.1 The NAMEIT trial was a 48-week, randomized double-blind RCT to compare Neoral with methotrexate versus placebo plus methotrexate in patients with early severe rheumatoid arthritis (Allard *et al.*, 2000). In order to assess the impact of the treatments on patients' QoL, the SF-36 was completed by subjects at seven time points, weeks 0 (baseline), 8, 16, 24, 32, 40, 48. Of the 306 subjects randomized, 223 (72.9%) completed the study, 111 in the placebo group and 112 in the Neoral group. Figure 9.6 shows the mean levels of QoL in patients with rheumatoid arthritis, before and during treatment, for the Pain dimension of the SF-36.

(a) Describe the pattern of QoL over time.

(b) From the graph what do you think would be suitable summary measures for this outcome and data?

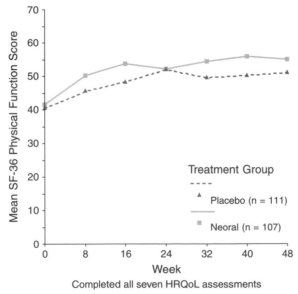

Figure 9.6 Profile of mean SF-36 Bodily Pain scores over time by treatment group for the NAMEIT data (Allard *et al.*, 2000).

9.2 Table 9.12 shows the mean SF-36 Bodily Pain scores over time by treatment group from the NAMEIT trial. It also shows the results of time-by-time analysis and a series of eight independent samples t-tests to test for differences between the two groups at each time point.

(a) Do these data suggest that the Neoral and placebo groups had similar mean SF-36 Bodily Pain scores at baseline? Comment on the results of the hypothesis test.

(b) Do these data suggest that the Neoral and placebo groups had similar mean SF-36 Bodily Pain scores at 8 weeks? Comment on the results of the hypothesis test.

(c) Do these data suggest that the Neoral and placebo groups had similar mean SF-36 Bodily Pain scores at 16 weeks? Comment on the results of the hypothesis test.

(d) Discuss whether the confidence interval for the difference in mean follow-up SF-36 Bodily Pain scores between the Neoral and placebo groups suggests that patients in the Neoral group might have better level of QoL at follow-up than patients in the placebo group.

(e) Of the three types of analysis, time-by-time, mean follow-up and AUC, shown in Table 9.12, which is to be preferred? Give reasons for your choice.

(f) Assume that the minimum clinically important difference for the SF-36 Bodily Pain dimension in rheumatoid arthritis patients is 5 points. Comment on the size of the difference in mean AUC scores between the two groups and also comment on the difference in mean follow-up SF-36 Bodily Pain scores between the Neoral and placebo groups.

9.3 Table 9.13 shows the result of fitting a marginal general linear model to the SF-36 Bodily Pain outcome data from the NAMEIT study.

(a) What is meant by an exchangeable autocorrelation?

(b) Do these data suggest that the Neoral and placebo groups have similar mean follow-up (post-randomization) SF-36 Bodily Pain scores? Discuss whether the confidence interval for the difference in mean follow-up SF-36 Bodily Pain scores between the Neoral and placebo groups suggests that patients in the Neoral group might have better level of QoL at follow-up than patients in the placebo group.

(c) Do these data suggest that the SF-36 Bodily Pain scores change over time?

(d) Assume the minimum clinically important difference for the SF-36 Bodily Pain dimension in rheumatoid arthritis patients is 5 points. Comment on the size of the difference in mean Pain scores between the two groups.

(e) Comment on the regression coefficients for baseline pain, age and gender in the model in Table 9.13. Is follow-up SF-36 Bodily Pain score significantly associated with baseline pain, age and gender?

Table 9.12 Mean SF-36 Bodily Pain scores over time by treatment group with all valid patients at each time point.

SF-36 Bodily Pain outcome[1]

| | Treatment group | | | | | | | | |
| Time (weeks) | Placebo | | | Neoral | | | Mean difference[2] | 95% CI | | P-value[3] |
	n	Mean	SD	n	Mean	SD		Lower	Upper	
0	152	38.3	(19.4)	152	39.0	(19.2)	0.7	−3.6	5.1	0.742
8	144	45.1	(20.3)	145	47.9	(20.5)	2.8	−1.9	7.5	0.238
16	133	49.2	(22.1)	132	55.6	(20.7)	6.3	1.2	11.5	0.016
24	124	51.2	(21.2)	123	56.7	(22.8)	5.6	0.0	11.1	0.049
32	117	52.2	(20.3)	118	57.1	(22.5)	4.8	−0.7	10.3	0.086
40	115	52.5	(21.7)	114	59.6	(21.6)	7.1	1.5	12.7	0.014
48	130	51.1	(23.6)	128	57.6	(22.3)	6.4	0.8	12.1	0.025
Mean follow-up	148	48.6	(17.9)	146	54.3	(18.7)	5.7	1.5	9.9	0.008
SF-36 Bodily Pain score										
Pain AUC	113	50.4	(16.1)	111	55.3	(17.0)	5.0	0.6	9.3	0.026

[1] The SF-36 Bodily Pain dimension is scored on a 0 (poor) to 100 (good health) scale.
[2] A positive mean difference indicates the Neoral group has the better QoL.
[3] P-value from two independent samples t-test.

Table 9.13 Estimated regression coefficients from a marginal model to show the effect of treatment (Neoral or placebo) on outcome (SF-36 Bodily Pain score) over time after adjustment for baseline pain, age and sex, assuming an exchangeable autocorrelation in rheumatoid arthritis patients ($n = 293$).

SF-36 Bodily Pain*	b	Semi-robust SE (b)	z	P-value	95% CI Lower	Upper
Pain (baseline)	0.49	0.05	9.12	<0.001	0.38	0.59
Age (years)	−0.03	0.09	−0.3	0.767	−0.20	0.15
Sex (0 = female, 1 = male)	2.02	2.01	1.01	0.315	−1.92	5.95
Time (weeks)	0.15	0.03	4.8	<0.001	0.09	0.22
Group (0 = placebo, 1 = Neoral)	5.01	1.81	2.76	0.006	1.45	8.56
Constant	26.99	4.76	5.67	<0.001	17.67	36.32

*The outcome variable is the SF-36 Bodily Pain score; a higher score indicates less pain.

Table 9.14 Estimated regression coefficients from a marginal model to show the effect of group on outcome, 6-month SF-36 Mental Component Summary score, after adjustment for 6-week MCS and other covariates from the PONDER cRCT, $n = 2499$ (Morrell *et al.*, 2009).

Outcome: 6-month MCS score	b	Semi-robust SE (b)	z	P-value	95% CI Lower	Upper
MCS (6 weeks)	0.4	0.0	15.89	<0.001	0.39	0.49
Lives alone (0 = no, 1 = yes)	−1.7	1.1	−1.64	0.100	−3.82	0.34
History of PND (0 = no, 1 = yes)	−3.1	0.7	−4.42	<0.001	−4.48	−1.73
Life event (0 = no, 1 = yes)	−1.4	0.4	−3.98	<0.001	−2.12	−0.72
Group (0 = control, 1 = intervention)	1.4	0.5	2.96	0.003	0.46	2.28
Constant	29.6	1.4	21.24	<0.001	26.88	32.34

The SF-36 Mental Component Summary Scale is scored so that a higher score indicates better mental health.

9.4 The PONDER trial was a cRCT in primary care designed to evaluate the effectiveness of a new health visitor led psychological intervention in detecting and treating new mothers with postnatal depression compared to usual care. The PONDER trial randomized 100 clusters (GP practices and their associated health visitors) and collected data on 2659 new mothers with an 18-month follow-up. The participants were 1745 women (in 63 clusters) allocated to intervention and 914 women (in 37 clusters) allocated to control. Secondary outcomes included the SF-36 Mental Component Summary (MCS) scale measure. Table 9.14 shows the regression coefficients from fitting a marginal generalized linear model, with coefficients estimated using generalized estimating equations with robust standard errors and an exchangeable autocorrelation matrix to analyse the 6-month MCS outcome and allow for the clustered nature of the data. The estimated ICC from the model was 0.016.

(a) Comment on the estimated ICC. Does this suggest that within a health visitor cluster the individual mothers' MCS scores are strongly correlated with each other?

(b) Do these data suggest that the intervention and control group mothers have similar mean 6-month MCS scores? Discuss whether the confidence interval for the difference in mean follow-up SF-36 MCS scores between the intervention and control groups suggests that mothers in the intervention group might have better level of mental health at follow-up than mothers in the control group.

(c) Assume that the minimum clinically important difference for the SF-36 MCS is 5 points. Comment on the size of the difference in mean MCS scores between the two groups.

(d) Comment on the regression coefficients for 6-week MCS score, history of PND, living alone and history of PND in the model in Table 9.14. Is 6-month follow-up SF-36 MCS score significantly associated with 6-week MCS score, history of PND, living alone and history of PND?

10

Advanced methods for analysing quality of life outcomes

Summary

The majority of items on individual QoL instruments are usually measured or scored on an ordered categorical scale. These responses across similar questions are then summed to generate a QoL measurement. These 'summated scores' tend to generate QoL data with skewed, discrete and bounded distributions. This may mean that standard statistical methods for analysing QoL data (described in Chapters 6–9), such as the t-test and linear regression, may not be appropriate. This chapter describes more advanced statistical methods for analysing QoL data. The bootstrap method for estimating confidence intervals is described, as are several methods for analysing ordinal outcomes such as proportional odds and stereotype models.

10.1 Introduction

QoL is usually measured or scored on an ordered categorical (ordinal) scale. This means that responses to individual questions or items are usually classified into a small number of response categories which can be ordered (e.g. poor, moderate, good). In planning and analysis, the question responses are often analysed by assigning equally spaced numerical scores to the ordinal categories (e.g. 0 = poor, 1 = moderate, 2 = good). The scores across similar questions are then summed to generate a QoL measurement. These 'summated scores' gives the appearance that the QoL instruments are continuous measurements. However the skewed, discrete and bounded distribution of QoL measures may lead to several problems in determining sample size and analysing the data (Walters *et al.*, 2001b; see Box 6.1).

Figure 10.1 shows histograms of the SF-36 Bodily Pain dimension at 12 month for 215 patients with low back pain in the RCT of acupuncture versus usual care (Thomas *et al.*,

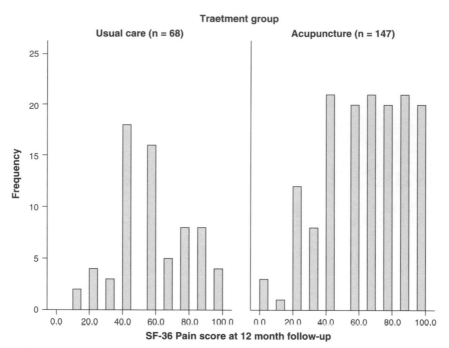

Figure 10.1 Histogram of 12 month SF-36 Bodily Pain score by treatment group from the acupuncture RCT (data from Thomas *et al.*, 2006).

2006). The histograms clearly illustrate the skewed, discrete and bounded distribution of the QoL outcome. This suggests that standard methods such as the *t*-test and linear regression which assume that the data are Normally distributed and have similar variances may not be appropriate.

Conventional statistical advice implies that the method of analysis should be chosen on the basis of the shape of the distribution of the data. The method of analysis used also has important implications for the interpretation of the results, since different methods compare different aspects of the distributions.

The *parametric* two independent sample *t*-test compares arithmetic means. The *non-parametric Mann–Whitney U* -test is often interpreted as a comparison of medians, although it is in fact an overall comparison of distributions in terms of both shape and location.

Methods based on the *t*-test are strictly valid only if the QoL data are Normally distributed. However, a *t*-test, and the confidence interval derived from it, will be reliable if either the skewness is not too extreme or the sample sizes are moderately large. Although the *t*-test is very robust to non-Normality, this cannot be guaranteed, so the results may have to be treated cautiously.

Medical journals such as the *British Medical Journal* and *Lancet* now expect scientific papers submitted to them to contain confidence intervals when appropriate. To compensate for the important advantage of being free of assumptions about the distribution of the data there is the disadvantage that non-parametric methods tend to be more suited to hypothesis testing than estimation. So how do we estimate non-parametric confidence intervals?

There is a non-parametric method for constructing a CI for the difference between the medians of two groups of observations. It requires the restrictive assumption that the samples are from populations with distributions that are identical in shape, and differ only by a shift in location. (It is also a non-parametric CI for the difference between two means.) The method is described in Altman *et al.* (2000). It is not widely used, but another more popular non-parametric method is the *bootstrap* (Efron and Tibshirani, 1993).

10.2   Bootstrap methods

The bootstrap is a computer-intensive method for statistical analysis (Efron and Tibshirani, 1993). It involves repeatedly drawing random samples from the original data, with replacement. It seeks to mimic in an appropriate manner the way the sample is collected from the population in the bootstrap samples from the observed data. The phrase 'with replacement' means that any observation can be sampled more than once. Bootstrap methods can be used for hypothesis tests, calculating confidence intervals and regression analyses.

According to Everitt (1995):

> The bootstrap is a data-based simulation method for statistical inference, which can be used to study the variability of estimated characteristics of the probability distribution of a set of observations, and provide confidence intervals for parameters in situations where these are difficult or impossible to derive in the usual way.

The term 'bootstrap' derives from the phrase 'to pull oneself up by one's bootstraps'. Efron and Tibshirani (1993) mention that the phrase is thought to be based on one of the eighteenth-century adventures of Baron Munchausen by Rudolph Erich Raspe. The Baron had fallen to the bottom of a deep lake. Just when it looked like all was lost, he thought to pick himself up by his own bootstraps!

The basic idea of the bootstrap involves repeated random sampling with replacement from the original data, $\mathbf{x} - (x_1, x_2, \ldots, x_n)$, to produce random samples of the same size n as the original sample, each of which is known as a *bootstrap sample*, $\mathbf{x}^*$, and each of which provides an estimate, $\hat{\theta}^*$, of the parameter of interest, θ. It is important that sampling is done with replacement, because sampling without replacement would simply give a random permutation of the original data, with many statistics such as the mean being exactly the same (Campbell, 2006).

Repeating the process a larger number of times provides the required information on the variability of the estimator, since the standard error is estimated from the standard deviation of the statistics derived from the bootstrap samples. The point about the bootstrap is that it produces a variety of values, whose variability reflects the standard error that would be obtained if samples were repeatedly taken from the whole population.

10.3   Bootstrap methods for confidence interval estimation

For the example in Box 10.1, the best estimate of the statistic of interest (mean QoL) is the observed mean QoL from the original data – not the mean of the bootstrap means,

Box 10.1 A simple example of the bootstrap

Consider a data set with five patients and associated QoL outcomes (measured on a 1–10 scale).

A	B	C	D	E
1	5	10	2	2

We take 1000 bootstrap random samples. The first bootstrap sample of size 5 is:

B	C	A	B	C	
5	10	1	5	10	$\text{mean}_1 = 6.20$

The second bootstrap sample of size 5 is:

E	C	B	B	B	
2	10	5	5	5	$\text{mean}_2 = 5.40$

The 1000th bootstrap random sample of size 5 is:

D	D	D	D	D	
2	2	2	2	2	$\text{mean}_{1000} = 2.00$

Our 1000 samples yield the following sample statistics:

Observed mean	4.00
Observed standard deviation	3.67
Observed standard error	1.64

The observed means are summarized in the histogram in Figure 10.2.

which is biased. The standard deviation (SD) of the 1000 or so bootstrap means is the bootstrap standard error (SE). In Figure 10.2 the standard deviation of the means or standard error is 1.47. This SE can be used to calculate CIs using standard methods: estimate $\pm 1.96 \times$ SE(estimate). These bootstrap CIs are called Normal. Alternatively, non-parametric bootstrap CIs based on the percentiles of the cumulative distribution of the 1000 bootstrap means can be calculated. For example, a percentile-based 95% CI is given by the 2.5th and 97.5th percentiles of the distribution of the bootstrap means.

Suppose that we wish to calculate a 95% confidence interval for the mean from a sample $\mathbf{x} = (x_1, x_2, \ldots, x_n)$. We take a random sample $\mathbf{x}^*$, with replacement, from the data, of the same size as the original sample, and calculate the mean of the data, $\hat{\theta}^*$, in this bootstrap random sample. We do this repeatedly, say B times. So we now have B bootstrap samples $\mathbf{x}_1^*, \mathbf{x}_2^*, \ldots, \mathbf{x}_B^*$, and B estimates of the sample mean, one from each bootstrap sample $(\hat{\theta}_1^*, \hat{\theta}_2^*, \ldots, \hat{\theta}_B^*)$. If these are ordered in increasing value,

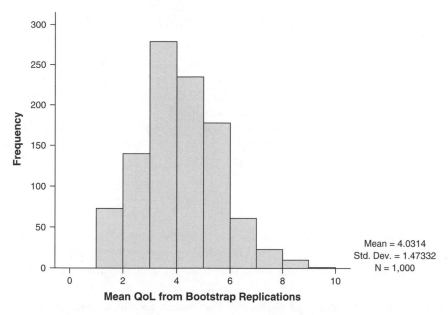

Figure 10.2 Histogram of mean QoL from 1000 bootstrap samples of size 5.

$(\hat{\theta}^*_{(1)}, \hat{\theta}^*_{(2)}, \ldots, \hat{\theta}^*_{(B)})$, a bootstrap 95% CI for the mean would be from the $0.025B$th to the $0.975B$th largest values. For a $100(1 - \alpha)\%$ interval the limits would the $(\alpha/2)B$th and $(1 - \alpha/2)B$th largest values. This is known as the *percentile method* and, although it is an obvious choice, it is not the best method for bootstrapping confidence intervals, because it can have a bias, which one can estimate and correct for. This leads to methods such as the *bias-corrected method* and the *bias-corrected and accelerated* (BC_a) method, the latter being the preferred option (Davison and Hinckley, 1997; Efron and Tibshirani, 1993). The paper by Carpenter and Bithell (2000) provides a useful practical guide for medical statisticians on bootstrap confidence intervals.

The bootstrap can be applied to data with a more complex structure than the simple single sample example considered above. For comparing QoL outcomes in two groups, say one with QoL data with a distribution F and the other with an independent distribution G, a bootstrap approach would proceed from separate estimates $\hat{F}$ and $\hat{G}$, with bootstrap samples chosen independently from each estimated distribution.

Using the bootstrap method, valid bootstrap confidence intervals can be constructed for all common estimators such as the sample mean, median, proportion, difference in means, and difference in proportions. The bootstrap can also be used for other statistics (such as ratios) and more complex data sets. With a two-group RCT, we should randomly sample with replacement separately for each group. In economic evaluations alongside clinical trials both cost and effect data are measured for each individual patient. Therefore we randomly sample with replacement each patient and their paired cost and effect data. This takes into account the correlations between cost and effect outcomes.

The current versions of STATA and S-PLUS now have built-in procedures for bootstrapping and estimating bootstrap CIs. Unfortunately SAS and SPSS do not have built-in bootstrap procedures so you will have to write your own. RESAMPLING STATS is another software package than can perform simple bootstrapping. Simple bootstrapping can also be performed in EXCEL or any other stats package with a random number generator.

Table 10.1 shows the mean 12-month SF-36 Bodily Pain score for the acupuncture and usual care group and the mean difference and associated 95% confidence interval based on the t-distribution. Table 10.2 shows various bootstrap confidence intervals, for the mean difference in 12-month SF-36 Bodily Pain scores between the acupuncture and usual care groups, based on 1000 bootstrap samples.

The confidence intervals were estimated using the `bootstrap` procedure in STATA version 10 (StataCorp, 2008). According to Efron and Tibshirani (1993) each interval $(\hat{\theta}_{lo}, \hat{\theta}_{up})$ can be described by its *length* and *shape*,

$$\text{length} = \hat{\theta}_{up} - \hat{\theta}_{lo}, \text{ and shape} = \frac{\hat{\theta}_{up} - \hat{\theta}}{\hat{\theta} - \hat{\theta}_{lo}}. \tag{10.1}$$

'Shape' measures the symmetry of the interval about the point estimate $\hat{\theta}$. A shape >1.00 indicates greater distance from $\hat{\theta}_{up}$ to $\hat{\theta}$ than from $\hat{\theta}$ to $\hat{\theta}_{lo}$. Conversely, a shape <1.00 indicates a greater distance from $\hat{\theta}$ to $\hat{\theta}_{lo}$ than from $\hat{\theta}_{up}$ to $\hat{\theta}$. The bootstrap Normal (and

Table 10.1 Mean 12-month SF-36 Bodily Pain scores for the acupuncture and usual care group and the mean difference and 95% confidence interval (data from Thomas *et al.*, 2006).

| | Treatment group | | | | | | 95% CI | | |
| | Usual care | | | Acupuncture | | Mean | | | |
	n	Mean	SD	n	Mean	SD	Difference	Lower	Upper	P-value
SF-36 Bodily Pain score	68	58.3	22.2	147	64.0	25.6	5.69	−1.42	12.80	0.116

Table 10.2 Bootstrap 95% confidence intervals for the mean difference in 12 month SF-36 Bodily Pain score between the acupuncture and usual care group (data from Thomas *et al.*, 2006).

Variable	No. of bootstrap resamples	Observed mean difference	Bias	SE	95% CI Lower	Upper	Length	Shape	Method
SF-36 Bodily Pain	1000	5.69	0.05	3.33	−0.84	12.22	13.06	1.00	(N)
					−0.90	11.70	12.60	0.91	(P)
					−0.93	11.69	12.62	0.91	(BC)
					−0.93	11.67	12.61	0.90	(BC$_a$)
					−1.42	12.80	14.22	1.00	(t)

(t) t-distribution based confidence interval
(N) Normal confidence interval
(P) percentile confidence interval
(BC) bias-corrected confidence interval
(BC$_a$)) bias-corrected and accelerated confidence interval

t-distribution based) intervals are symmetrical about $\hat{\theta}$, having shape $= 1.00$ by definition. Therefore shape is a measure of skewness of the CI about the point estimate. A shape >1.00 implies the CI is 'positively' skewed, with a long tail to the right, while a shape <1.00 implies the CI is 'negatively' skewed.

Table 10.2 shows that the estimates and lengths of the CIs are similar, with the bootstrap BC_a interval producing the narrowest interval. Table 10.2 also shows that the percentile, BC and BC_a intervals are non-symmetric about the point estimate of the mean difference. So in this example dataset there appears little advantage in using the bootstrap confidence intervals compared to conventional methods of confidence interval estimation. My own research (Walters, 2003, 2004; Walters and Campbell, 2004, 2005), using a variety of data sets, with the SF-36 outcome, found that using the bootstrap to estimate confidence intervals produced results similar to conventional statistical methods. These results suggest that bootstrap methods are not more appropriate for analysing QoL outcome data than standard methods.

Example: Bootstrap confidence intervals

Morrell *et al* (2000) calculated bootstrap percentile based confidence intervals for the mean difference in SF-36, Edinburgh Postnatal Depression Scale and Duke scores at 6 weeks after childbirth between a group of new mothers randomly allocated to receive extra postnatal support or usual care (control) in an RCT to establish the effectiveness of community postnatal support workers (Table 8.6). □

10.4   Ordinal regression

Throughout this book I have assumed that the various QoL scales are continuous for statistical analysis purposes. This is because I fundamentally believe there is an underlying latent continuous QoL scale and we are simply measuring discrete values of this scale with our QoL instrument (see Chapter 6). Most researchers (and authors) tend to do this. However, if you fundamentally believe there is *not* an underlying latent continuous QoL scale, then the only alternative is to treat the data as ordinal.

Figure 10.3 shows the histograms of the SF-36 Role Physical (RP) dimension scores at 6 weeks after childbirth for intervention and control groups for 494 new mothers from the community postnatal support workers (CPSW) study (Morrell *et al.*, 2000). The graphs clearly show the skewed and discrete nature of the outcome data for the SF-36 RP dimension from this study. The RP dimension is scored on a $0-100$ scale but actually has only five possible scores: 0, 25, 50, 75 and 100.

Suppose that the QoL measure has a large number of ordered categories, most of which should be occupied if the underlying scale really is continuous, but the scale is measured imperfectly by an instrument with a limited number of discrete values. It is often worth treating this discrete scale as if it were continuous. An informal rule of thumb (Walters *et al.*, 2001c) is that this discrete scale should be treated as continuous if it has seven or more categories and as ordinal otherwise. So, for example, of the eight SF-36 dimensions six have more than seven discrete categories and only two (the Role Physical and Role Emotional scales) have less than seven discrete categories.

Walters *et al.* (2001c) base this informal rule of thumb on Whitehead's (1993) sample size formula for ordinal data (see Chapter 4). Whitehead illustrates the dependence of

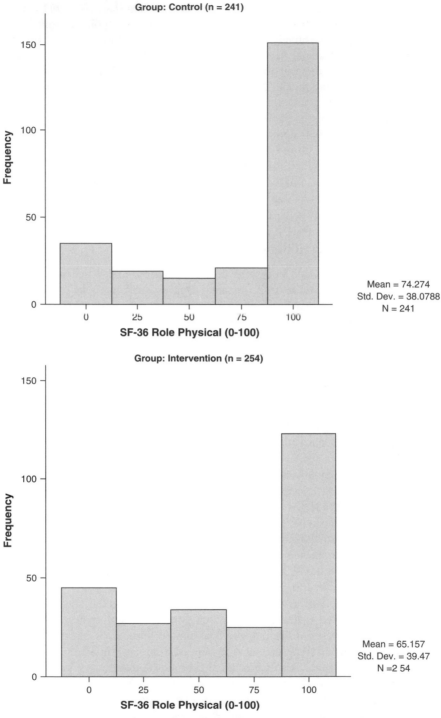

Figure 10.3 Distribution of the SF-36 Role Physical dimension at 6 weeks after childbirth for 495 new mothers from the CPSW study by group (data from Morrell *et al.*, 2000).

sample size n on the number of categories k. It is assumed that all categories are equally probable ($\bar{\pi}_1 = \bar{\pi}_2 = \cdots = \bar{\pi}_k$). Whitehead shows that the sample size calculated from equation (4.10) (denoted by $n(k)$) when there are k equally probably categories, keeping OR, α and β constant, is

$$n(k) = \frac{0.75}{1 - 1/k^2} n(2).$$ (10.2)

In the limit as $k \to \infty$, $n(k) \to 0.75n$.

The limiting case is approached in large samples in which a full ranking of patient outcomes is achieved. A full ranking is equivalent to a categorization with one patient in each category. So for continuous data the sample size using equation (4.10) tends to be 75% of the binary outcome case. Equation (10.2) says that little is gained by using more than five categories, since $n(5) = 0.78n(2)$, and the hypothesis test will be $(0.75/0.78) \times 100 = 96\%$ efficient relative to the use of a full ranking (with more than five categories). When the data truly are Normally distributed with equal variances the Mann–Whitney test for untied data is 96% efficient relative to the t-test (Armitage et al., 2002). Thus with five equally probable categories the test is 92% efficient relative to the t-test, when the data are truly Normally distributed. These relative efficiencies are all asymptotic, and are only valid for moderate to large sample sizes, so it is reasonable to require more than five categories in the assumption. Note that occasionally it will be obvious that the assumption of a continuous scale does not hold, such as when one of the categories is death.

Heeren and D'Agostino (1987) demonstrated the robustness of the two-independent samples t-test when applied to ordinal data (with three, four or five categories) and samples of size 20 or less, although they assumed the scales were equally spaced and cautioned on generalising the results to scales with more than five values. However, the Central Limit Theorem is likely to ensure the robustness of the t-test if the sample size is large and there are seven or more occupied categories.

10.5   Comparing two independent groups: Ordinal quality of life measures (with less than 7 categories)

If the QoL outcomes are measured on an ordinal scale, with less than seven categories, then the statistical hypothesis test used in this instance (to compare two independent groups) is the Mann–Whitney U-test with allowance for ties or chi-squared test for trend. In general the MW test gives very similar P-values to the chi-squared test for trend (Altman, 1991). The difficulty with this method is that it does not allow covariates, and does not provide estimates of population parameters.

The simplest approach to analysing ordinal data is to dichotomize the data and use logistic regression. However, this method ignores useful information in the data, may not be very powerful (Armstrong and Sloan, 1989) and introduces the problem of where to choose the cut point. If one were to keep the ordinal structure then there are number of models possible (Ananth and Kleinbaum, 1997; Manor et al., 2000; Walters et al., 2001c; Lall et al., 2002). These include proportional odds, continuation ratio, polytomous and stereotype. We will illustrate these various models using the CPSW data and the five-category RP dimension of the SF-36. Table 10.3 shows the frequency distribution

Table 10.3 Descriptive statistics for SF-36 Role Physical dimension at 6 weeks for control and intervention group mothers from the CPSW trial.

	Control $n = 241$			Intervention $n = 254$			Odds ratio Int/Con
	n	(%)	Cumulative %	n	(%)	Cumulative %	
RP Score							
0.0	35	(14.5)	14.5	45	(17.7)	17.7	0.79
25.0	19	(7.9)	22.4	27	(10.6)	28.3	0.73
50.0	15	(6.2)	28.6	34	(13.4)	41.7	0.56
75.0	21	(8.7)	37.3	25	(9.8)	51.6	0.56
100.0	151	(62.7)	100.0	123	(48.4)	100.0	
Total	241	100.0		254	100.0		
Mean	74.3			65.2			
SD	38.1			39.5			
Median	100.0			75.0			
25th percentile	50.0			25.0			
75th percentile	100.0			100.0			
Age (years)							
Mean	28.1			28.0			
SD	5.6			5.7			
Parity	n	(%)		n	(%)		
First child	119	(49.4)		133	(52.4)		
Second or more	122	(50.6)		121	(47.6)		
Normal delivery							
No	76	(31.5)		81	(31.9)		
Yes	165	(68.5)		173	(68.1)		

of the RP dimension at 6 weeks after childbirth for new mothers in the control and intervention groups, respectively. Table 10.3 also summarizes three potential confounding variables or covariates, age at delivery, parity and type of delivery.

10.6 Proportional odds or cumulative logit model

The *proportional odds* or *cumulative logit* model is based on the cumulative response probabilities rather than the category probabilities (McCullagh and Nelder, 1989). Consider, for example, a QoL outcome variable Y with k categorical outcomes y_i denoted by $i = 1, \ldots, k$ and suppose that we have a set of p covariates $(x_1, x_2, \ldots, x_p)$. The cumulative logit or proportional odds model is

$$\gamma_i = \Pr(Y \le y_i | x_1, x_2, \ldots, x_p) = \frac{\exp(\alpha_i + \beta_1 x_1 + \beta_2 x_2 + \cdots + \beta_p x_p)}{1 + \exp(\alpha_i + \beta_1 x_1 + \beta_2 x_2 + \cdots + \beta_p x_p)},$$
$$i = 1, \ldots, k - 1. \tag{10.3}$$

This can be expressed equivalently in logit(γ_i) form as

$$\text{logit}(\gamma_i) = \log\left[\frac{\gamma_i}{1 - \gamma_i}\right] = \log\left[\frac{\Pr(Y \le y_i | x_1, \ldots, x_p)}{\Pr(Y > y_i | x_1, \ldots, x_p)}\right]$$

$$= \alpha_i + \beta_1 x_1 + \beta_2 x_2 + \cdots + \beta_p x_p \qquad i = 1, \ldots, k-1, \qquad (10.4)$$

where $\gamma_i = \Pr(Y \le y_i | x_1, x_2, \ldots, x_p)$ is the cumulative probability of being in category i or lower given the set of covariates (note that for $i = k$, $\Pr(Y \le y_i | x_1, x_2, \ldots, x_p) = 1$). The $\alpha_1, \alpha_2, \ldots, \alpha_{k-1}$ and $\beta_1, \beta_2, \ldots, \beta_p$ parameters are treated as unknown and the intercept parameters α_i must satisfy the condition $\alpha_1 \le \alpha_2 \le \ldots \le \alpha_{k-1}$ (McCullagh and Nelder, 1989). The regression coefficient β_p for a binary explanatory variable x_p (e.g. control or intervention group) is the log odds ratio for the Y by x_p association, controlling for the other covariates in the model, that is, the treatment effect on QoL after adjusting for prognostic factors such as age, parity and type of delivery.

The $\beta_1, \beta_2, \ldots, \beta_p$ regression parameters do not depend on the category i, so that the model (10.4) assumes that the relationship between each of the covariates and Y (QoL) is independent of i (the response category). This assumption of identical log odds ratios across the k categories is the proportional odds assumption.

The proportional odds model is useful when one believes that QoL is a continuum, which is measured imperfectly by an instrument with a limited number of values. The proportional odds model is invariant when the codes for the response Y are reversed (i.e. y_1 recoded as y_k, y_2 recoded as y_{k-1}, and so on). Also the proportional odds model is invariant under the collapsibility of adjacent categories of the ordinal response, implying that when y_1 and y_2 are combined, the estimate of the odds ratio remains essentially the same as the odds ratios obtained for the individual categories (Greenland, 1994).

10.7   Continuation ratio model

An alternative to the proportional odds model is the *continuation ratio model*. This may be relevant when an ordinal QoL scale may be thought of as a progression through various stages, so that people start with 'excellent' and deteriorate to 'poor' and are unlikely to reverse this trend. The cumulative probabilities $\gamma_i = \Pr(Y \le y_i | x_1, x_2, \ldots, x_p)$ of being in category i or lower in the cumulative logit model (10.4) are replaced by the probability of being in category i (i.e. $\pi_i = \Pr(Y = y_i)$) divided by the probability of being in a category higher than i (i.e. $\Pr(Y > y_i)$):

$$\text{logit}\left(\frac{\pi_i}{1 - \gamma_i}\right) = \log\left[\frac{\left(\frac{\pi_i}{1-\gamma_i}\right)}{\left(1 - \frac{\pi_i}{1-\gamma_i}\right)}\right] = \log\left[\frac{\Pr(Y = y_i | x_1, \ldots, x_p)}{\Pr(Y > y_i | x_1, \ldots, x_p)}\right]$$

$$= \alpha_i + (\beta_1 x_1 + \beta_2 x_2 + \cdots + \beta_p x_p), \qquad i = 1, \ldots, k-1. \quad (10.5)$$

When the 'logit' expansion is replaced by the 'complementary log-log' link function in model (10.5), the resulting model (10.6) is

$$\log\left[-\log\left(\frac{\pi_i}{1 - \gamma_i}\right)\right] = \alpha_i + (\beta_1 x_1 + \beta_2 x_2 + \cdots + \beta_p x_p) \qquad i = 1, \ldots, k-1.$$

$$(10.6)$$

The continuation ratio model is not invariant under the collapsing or reversal of categories. It is best suited to circumstances where the individual categories of the QoL scale are of interest and a monotonic progression through the individual categories is expected. Armstrong and Sloan (1989) have given a useful comparison of the proportional odds and continuation ratio models.

Chi-squared (χ^2) score tests are available for tests of the proportional odds assumption, but these lack power (Brant, 1990; Peterson and Harrell, 1990). Also the model is robust to mild departures from the assumption of proportional odds. A crude test would be to examine the odds ratios and, if they are all greater than unity or all less than unity, then a proportional odds model will suffice (Walters et al., 2001c), although with increasing numbers of categories it is less likely that proportional odds assumption remains true.

The ordinal regression method also allows us to adjust the treatment effect for other prognostic factors and covariates (such as centre, sex and age). The regression coefficients and their standard errors also enable confidence intervals to be calculated. The statistical packages SPSS, SAS and STATA have procedures for fitting proportional odds or continuation ratio models.

10.8   Stereotype logistic model

For the cumulative logit model (10.4), the QoL outcome variable Y is assumed to have an unobserved underlying variable (say Z), which takes on a continuous form. For example, 'Age' may be represented by ordered categories 'young', 'middle-aged', 'old' and 'very old'. In this case, there is an underlying variable, calendar age.

QoL scales are sometimes constructed in such a way that there is no underlying variable that directly links to the ordered y-response categories. (Although, as mentioned, this is one of my key assumptions, that there actually is an underlying latent continuous QoL variable.) For instance, when assessing 'pain' one may use a rating scale of the form 'none', 'mild', 'moderate' and 'severe'. Here pain is rated depending on other factors such as its severity and type of pain. Although the rating scale is in principle ordered, there may be no underlying variable (continuous or otherwise) that directly relates the factors and links these up with the categories on the scale. Anderson (1984) recognized these types of ordered categories as being truly discrete and referred to the response as a *judged* or *assessed* variable. As the cumulative logit model would be inappropriate for analysing such variables, Anderson introduced another model known as the *stereotype* model. One of the main advantages of the stereotype model over other regression models is that it does not assume an a priori ordering of the y-response categories.

The stereotype model is based on the polytomous regression model (Anderson, 1984), which does not impose any restrictions on the ordering of the categories. The ordinality is built into it by imposing a structure on the regression coefficients. Consider a QoL outcome variable Y with k ordered categorical outcomes y_i denoted by $i = 1, 2, \ldots, k$, and let $x_1, x_2, \ldots, x_p$ denote a set of p covariates. The ordinary polytomous regression model can be written as

$$\Pr(Y = y_i | x_1, x_2, \ldots, x_p) = \frac{\exp(\alpha_i + \beta_{i1}x_1 + \beta_{i2}x_2 + \cdots + \beta_{ip}x_p)}{\sum_{i=1}^{k} \exp(\alpha_i + \beta_{i1}x_1 + \beta_{i2}x_2 + \cdots + \beta_{ip}x_p)}, \quad (10.7)$$

where $\alpha_k = 0$ and $\beta_{kj} = 0 (j = 1, \ldots, p)$ to ensure identifiability. The log probability ratios are formed for model (10.7) by comparing each response category (y_i) with a reference category (y_k). The choice of the reference category is arbitrary, but we shall use the first category. Thus, the log probability ratio can be represented by a linear model of the form

$$\log\left[\frac{\Pr(Y = y_i | x_1, x_2, \ldots, x_p)}{\Pr(Y = y_1 | x_1, x_2, \ldots, x_p)}\right] = \alpha_i + \beta_{i1}x_1 + \beta_{i2}x_2 + \cdots + \beta_{ip}x_p, \qquad i = 2, \ldots, k.$$

$$(10.8)$$

The regression coefficient β_{ip} for the pth covariate x_p corresponds to the log-probability ratio comparing $(Y = y_i)$ versus $(Y = y_1)$ for a unit increase in x_p.

From model (10.8) it is clear that the ordinal nature is not accounted for in any way. The ordinality can be built into this model by imposing a structure on the regression coefficients $\beta_{ij}(j = 1, \ldots, p)$. Anderson (1984) proposed modelling the regression coefficients, β_{ij}, by imposing the relationship

$$\beta_{ij} = \phi_i \beta_j, \qquad i = 2, \ldots, k; j = 1, \ldots, p, \qquad (10.9)$$

where β_j is a list of new parameters and the ϕ_i can be thought of as the scores attached to the response y_i. Note that since $\beta_{1j} = 0$, we have $\phi_1 = 0$, and a further constraint, $\phi_k = 1$ (in order to uniquely identify the parameters when using estimated scores). Substituting (10.9) into (10.8) yields the stereotype model

$$\log\left[\frac{\Pr(Y = y_i | x_1, x_2, \ldots, x_p)}{\Pr(Y = y_1 | x_1, x_2, \ldots, x_p)}\right] = \alpha_i + \phi_i(\beta_1 x_1 + \beta_2 x_2 + \cdots + \beta_p x_p), \qquad i = 2, \ldots, k.$$

$$(10.10)$$

Thus, it can be seen that the stereotype model determines a set of parameters $\{\phi_i\}$ for the dependent variable and a single parameter β_j for each covariate. The ϕ_i are decided upon for the response variable and are directly tied up with the effect of the explanatory variables. Thus, with a positive β_j, when the log probability ratios $\{\phi_i \beta_j\}$ form a decreasing trend, the ϕ_i parameters also become ordered such that

$$\phi_k \beta_j \geq, \ldots, \phi_2 \beta_j \geq \phi_1 \beta_j = 0 \text{ then } 1 = \phi_k \geq, \ldots, \phi_2 \geq \phi_1 = 0. \qquad (10.11)$$

Here we can say that the effect of the covariates upon the first log probability ratio is greater than their effect upon the second and so on (or the effect is the same upon the consecutive log probability ratios), and that, provided (10.11) holds, model (10.10) is an ordered regression model.

The model fitted does not necessarily require the ϕ_i to be ordered; whether there is ordering or not is purely determined by the empirical evidence provided by the data. Two categories denoted by k_1 and k_2 are indistinguishable with respect to the covariates if $\phi_{k1} = \phi_{k2}$, that is, the effect of the covariates is the same in the two categories. The product $\phi_i \beta_p$ for the pth covariate x_p corresponds to the log probability ratio comparing $(Y = y_i)$ versus $(Y = y_1)$ for a unit increase in x_p.

Greenland (1994) argues strongly in favour of the stereotype model when there is no underlying continuum that is directly related to the response categories, but where each state is assessed. The STATA statistical package has a procedure for performing stereotype regression via constrained polytomous logistic regression (Hendrickx, 2000).

The stereotype model can also be fitted in SAS using PROC CATMOD. Further details of the stereotype model when applied to QoL outcomes are given in Lall *et al.* (2002).

Table 10.4 shows the results of fitting a binary logistic model, cumulative logit model, continuation ratio model, polytomous model and stereotype model to the RP data with group, delivery and parity as factors and age as a covariate. For the logistic model the outcome variable is dichotomized into a score of 100 (good health) and less than 100 (less than good health). The OR of 0.54 (95% CI: 0.37 to 0.78) for the binary logistic model implies that the odds of new mothers in the intervention group having 'good' health are 0.54 times those of mothers in the control group after allowing for age, parity and delivery. That is, new mothers in the intervention group are significantly less likely to report good health than control group mothers.

Similarly, the proportional odds model implies that having been randomized to the intervention group carried with it an odds ratio of 0.56 (95% CI: 0.40 to 0.80) compared to women randomized to the control group for being in a given category or below (i.e. better QoL) after allowing for age, parity and delivery. As the proportional odds model assumes a constant OR for all categories, Table 10.4 and Figure 10.4 show how the four $(k-1)$ observed ORs compare with the estimated common OR of 0.56 from the model. All observed ORs are less than 1 and seem similar to the model estimate. However, a chi-squared score test of proportional odds was $\chi^2 = 112.1$ on 12 degrees of freedom, $P = 0.0001$. Thus, there is strong statistical evidence to reject the assumption of proportional odds. So the proportional odds model may not be appropriate, although the model is robust to mild departures from the assumptions.

Again similarly, the continuation ratio model OR estimate implies that being randomized to the intervention group carried with it an odds ratio of 0.60 (95% CI: 0.44 to 0.80) compared to new mothers randomized to the control group for better QoL after allowing for age, parity and delivery.

The polytomous logistic model implies that, for women in the intervention group, the probability of having an RP score of 25 compared to 0 is 1.04 times the probability for

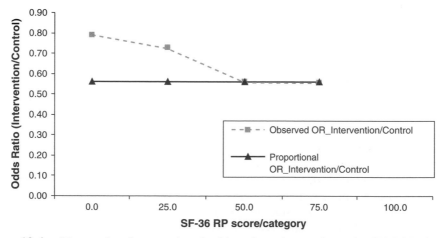

Figure 10.4   Observed and proportional odds ratio estimates from the SF-36 Role Physical dimension at 6 weeks after childbirth for control and intervention group mothers from the CPSW trial.

Table 10.4 Results of fitting various binary and ordinal models to the SF-36 Role Physical dimension score at 6 weeks after childbirth for the intervention and control group mothers from the CPSW study.

Model[1]	$\hat{\beta}$	$SE(\hat{\beta})$	P-value	OR[6]	95% CI for OR		χ^2 Goodness of fit[7]
Logistic regression (binary)[2]	−0.623	0.19	0.001	0.54	0.37	0.78	40.6 on 4 df, $P = 0.0001$
Proportional odds[3]	−0.576	0.18	0.001	0.56	0.40	0.80	59.7 on 4 df, $P = 0.0001$
Continuation ratio	−0.518	0.15	0.001	0.60	0.44	0.80	52.0 on 4 df, $P = 0.0001$
Polytomous model[4]							
25 vs 0	0.039	0.387	0.919	1.04	0.49	2.22	90.9 on 16 df, $P = 0.0001$
50 vs 0	0.5	0.4	0.213	1.64	0.75	3.60	
75 vs 0	−0.136	0.383	0.723	0.87	0.41	1.85	
100 vs 0	−0.528	0.2805	0.06	0.59	0.34	1.02	
Stereotype[5]							
$\hat{\beta}$							
25 vs 0 ($\phi_2\hat{\beta}$)	−0.469	0.28	0.093	0.63	0.36	1.10	
50 vs 0 ($\phi_3\hat{\beta}$)	−0.361			0.70	0.65		
75 vs 0 ($\phi_4\hat{\beta}$)	−0.424			0.65	0.71		
100 vs 0 ($\phi_5\hat{\beta}$)	−0.342			0.71			
	−0.469			0.63			

[1] All models include age, parity and delivery as covariates.
[2] The response variable was dichotomized into (0, 25, 50, 75) versus 100.
[3] The response variable is RP score, i.e. 0, 25, 50, 75, 100.
[4] The response variable is the RP score with 0 as the reference category.
[5] With $\phi_1 = 0$, $\phi_2 = 0.77$, $\phi_3 = 0.90$, $\phi_4 = 0.73$, $\phi_5 = 1.00$
[6] Odds ratio except for the polytomous and stereotype models where it is the ratio of probability ratios.
[7] Likelihood ratio statistics for testing null model (no covariates) against the extended model (with covariates).

women in the control group; the corresponding ratios for an RP score of 50 as opposed to 0, 75 as opposed to 0, and 100 as opposed to 0 are 1.64, 0.87 and 0.59, respectively. For the last three categories the trend in the probability ratios is monotonic as the health status goes from the 'poor' stage (i.e. an RP score of 50) through to the better stages (i.e. RP scores of 75 or 100).

Attaching a set of scores to the beta parameters in the polytomous model leads to the formation of the stereotype model (Table 10.4). The ϕ_i are decided upon for the response variable and are directly tied up with the effect of the explanatory variables (age, delivery, parity and group). The model does not necessarily require the ϕ_i to be ordered, and indeed the empirical evidence provided by the data suggests the ϕ_i are not ordered.

In this model the probability, for subjects in the intervention group, of having an RP score of 25 compared to a score of 0 is 0.70 times the probability for subjects in the control group; the corresponding ratios for an RP score of 50 as opposed to 0, 75 as opposed to 0, and 100 as opposed to 0 are 0.65, 0.71 and 0.63, respectively.

10.9   Conclusions and further reading

This chapter has described two types of advanced methods for analysing QoL data: the bootstrap method for estimating confidence intervals, and several models for analysing ordinal outcomes such as proportional odds and stereotype. If you fundamentally believe there is an underlying latent continuous QoL scale and you are measuring discrete values of this scale with your QoL instrument, then my recommendation is to treat the data as continuous and use linear regression models. This is what most researchers tend to do. However, if you fundamentally believe there is *not* an underlying latent continuous QoL scale then the only alternative is to treat the QoL data as ordinal and use regression models for ordinal data. My own research experience suggests little difference between parametric and non-parametric methods when calculating standard errors, P-values and confidence intervals (Walters, 2003, 2004; Walters and Campbell, 2005). Therefore I tend to use standard statistical analysis methods (such as the t-test and multiple linear regression) to analyse QoL outcomes.

Carpenter and Bithell (2000) provide a practical introduction to bootstrap confidence intervals. The books by Efron and Tibshirani (1993) and Davison and Hinckley (1997) provide a comprehensive and practical guide to the bootstrap. For the reader who is interested in ordinal regression models, the papers by Ananth and Kleinbaum (1997) and Lall *et al.* (2002) provide a good introduction. A fuller and more comprehensive description is given in the books by McCullagh and Nelder (1989) and Agresti (1984, 2002, 2007).

11

Economic evaluations

Summary

With the rapid advances in modern medicine, most people accept that no publicly funded health-care system can possibly pay for every new medical treatment that becomes available. The enormous costs involved (and the finite or limited health-care resources available) mean that choices on treatments have to be made. This has led to the development of health economic evaluation techniques to assess the costs and benefits of alternative treatments to help decide which treatment to use. This chapter describes utility- or preference-based QoL measures and how these can be combined with time spent in a particular health state to produce a measure in terms of quality-adjusted life years. It shows how an incremental cost–effectiveness ratio can be used to combine cost and effects from economic evaluations alongside clinical trials and how this estimate can be displayed on the cost–effectiveness plane. The chapter ends with a discussion of the use of cost-effectiveness acceptability curves to allow for the sampling variability or uncertainty in cost and effects.

11.1 Introduction

With the rapid advances in modern medicine, most people accept that no publicly funded health-care system can possibly pay for every new medical treatment that becomes available. The enormous costs involved (and the finite or limited health-care resources available) mean that choices have to be made on different treatments. Therefore it makes sense to concentrate on treatments that improve the quality and/or length of someone's life and, at the same time, are an effective use of limited health-care resources. The United Kingdom's National Institute for Health and Clinical Excellence (NICE) takes all these factors into account when it carries out technology appraisals and economic evaluations of new treatments to assess their clinical and cost effectiveness. NICE Technology Appraisal panels or expert review groups (comprising both health professionals and patients) examine independently verified evidence on how well a treatment works and

Quality of Life Outcomes in Clinical Trials and Health-Care Evaluation   Stephen J. Walters
© 2009 John Wiley & Sons, Ltd

whether it provides good value for money. To ensure NICE's judgements are fair, they use a standard and internationally recognized method to compare different treatments and measure their clinical effectiveness: the quality-adjusted life years measurement (QALY).

11.2   Economic evaluations

Economic evaluation is a series of techniques developed to assess the costs and benefits of alternative health-care interventions to provide a decision-making framework for which intervention to adopt. Economic evaluation is now playing an increasing role in the allocation of scarce health-care resources. There is now an expectation from health-care policy- and decision-makers that evidence supporting the cost-effectiveness of new health-care interventions is provided along with the usual data on clinical efficacy and safety (National Institute for Clinical Excellence, 2004). There are two general approaches to performing an economic evaluation of a health-care intervention (Willan and Briggs, 2006). One approach combines the clinical efficacy and safety data from RCTs with cost data from secondary non-trial sources in a decision analysis model. The second approach uses health-care resource utilization data, efficacy and safety data collected on individual patients prospectively as part of an RCT. The purpose of the next few sections is to provide an illustrated summary of the key statistical issues related to the cost-effectiveness comparison of two groups. We shall assume that patients are randomized to a new experimental treatment or standard control treatment in a two-group RCT and the measures of cost and effectiveness are observed at the subject level.

11.3   Utilities and QALYs

Some QoL instruments have been designed to measure the utility of, preference for, or desirability of a specific level of health status or a specific outcome. Utilities can be measured or valued for various possible health states. This can be done by asking patients who are in that particular health state at the time of measurement to value or express a preference for the particular health state. Alternatively, it can be done by describing the health state to subjects who may or may not have had personal experience of the health state being measured and asking them to value or express a preference for the particular health state. The health state utility or preference value is usually a number between 0.0 (death) and 1.0 (full health or functioning with no adverse symptoms). There are three main methods for valuing or assessing the preferences of subjects for health states: the visual analogue rating scale, the time trade-off and the standard gamble method. These methods are beyond the scope of this book and are described in Brazier et al. (2007). Examples of preference-based QoL instruments include the Quality of Well-Being scale, Health Utilities Index, EQ-5D and SF-6D.

The conventional way of using these utilities is to combine them with the length of time in that particular health state to produce a single index number called the quality-adjusted life year (QALY). This is done by multiplying the utility value by the time (in years) spent in that health state. For example, 2 years in a health state with a utility value of 0.5 would result in 1 QALY (equivalent to 1 year of perfect health). An important point to note is that health state utility values do not have any natural units. However, if the utilities are multiplied by the amount of time spent in that particular health state, then they become QALYs (and are measured in units of time).

QALYs allow for varying times spent in different health states by calculating an overall score for each patient. Hence, if a patient progresses through four health states that have estimated utilities U_1, U_2, U_3 and U_4, spending time t_i $(i = 1, \ldots, 4)$ in each state, then

$$QALY = U_1 t_1 + U_2 t_2 + U_3 t_3 + U_4 t_4. \tag{11.1}$$

This is analogous to the area under the curve (AUC) which was described in Chapter 9 (see Figure 9.3).

In the acupuncture study (Thomas *et al.*, 2006) QoL was measured at four time points (0, 3, 12 and 24 months) over a 2-year period using the SF-6D preference-based utility measure. Consider a patient with SF-6D utility scores of 0.70, 0.80, 0.85, 0.85 at baseline $(t_1 = 0$ years), 3 months $(t_2 = 0.25)$, 12 months $(t_3 = 1)$ and 24 months $(t_4 = 2)$, respectively. The patient has a QALY of

$$0.5\{(0.25 - 0)(0.70 + 0.80) + (1 - 0.25)(0.80 + 0.85) + (2 - 1)(0.85 + 0.85)\} = 1.66.$$

Individual QALYs can then be averaged across each group and compared using standard methods (as described in previous chapters).

Most people place greater value upon QoL benefits that are immediate rather than those that may arise a year or two in the future. Therefore it may be relevant to discount future QoL gains by converting or reducing the future value of the utility score to their present-day value.

11.4   Economic evaluations alongside a controlled trial

It is becoming increasingly common to carry out economic evaluations alongside pragmatic randomized controlled trials (EEACTs) in order to assess both the costs and benefits of alternative treatments. Since health care tends to be expensive and most societies have limited or constrained resources to devote to it, it is important to assess costs and cost-effectiveness as well as clinical outcomes. Costs are usually derived from information about the quantity of health-care resources used by each patient in the trial. The quantities of each resource used are multiplied by fixed unit cost values and are then summed over the separate types of resource use to give a total cost per patient.

11.5   Cost-effectiveness analysis

Cost-effectiveness analysis (CEA) is one form of full economic evaluation, where both the costs and consequences of heath programmes or treatments are examined. The aim of CEA is to compare the costs and effects of one new experimental treatment compared to another relevant alternative treatment. If we know the population mean or expected costs of the standard control treatment (μ_{CostC}) and the new experimental treatment (μ_{CostT}), and similarly their expected effectiveness $(\mu_{EffectC}$ and $\mu_{EffectT})$, then differences in costs and effects can be defined as

$$\Delta C = \mu_{CostT} - \mu_{CostC}, \Delta E = \mu_{EffectT} - \mu_{EffectC}. \tag{11.2}$$

These differences in costs, and effects can be displayed graphically on the so-called cost–effectiveness (CE) plane, with differences in costs on the vertical axis and differences in effects on the horizontal axis (Figure 11.1).

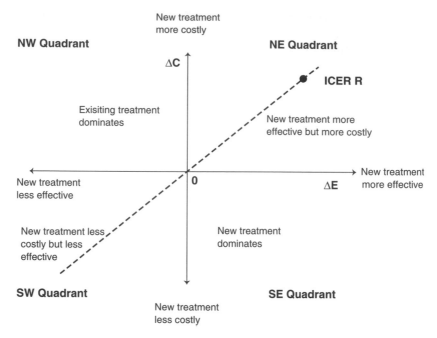

Figure 11.1   The cost–effectiveness (CE) plane.

11.6   Cost–effectiveness ratios

Figure 11.1 shows the four quadrants of the CE plane. If $\Delta C < 0$ and $\Delta E > 0$ then the experimental treatment is dominant, being both cheaper and more effective (i.e. we are in the southeast quadrant of the CE plane). If $\Delta C > 0$ and $\Delta E < 0$, then we are in the northwest quadrant of the CE plane. In these circumstances the existing treatment dominates, being both cheaper and more effective. When $\Delta C > 0$ and $\Delta E > 0$ or $\Delta C < 0$ and $\Delta E < 0$, neither the experimental nor standard treatment is dominant (i.e. we are in the northeast or southwest quadrants of the CE plane). The *incremental cost–effectiveness ratio* (ICER), R, is defined in these two quadrants as

$$R = \frac{\mu_{CostT} - \mu_{CostC}}{\mu_{EffectT} - \mu_{EffectC}} = \frac{\Delta C}{\Delta E}. \tag{11.3}$$

The ICER measures the extra cost for achieving an extra unit of effectiveness by adopting the experimental treatment over the standard. When comparing a new treatment with a control treatment in an EEACT the true population mean values (μ_{CostC}, μ_{CostT}, $\mu_{EffectC}$ and $\mu_{EffectT}$) are unknown and we have to use the sample estimates to calculate the ICER. The estimated ICER, $\hat{R}$, is thus given by

$$\hat{R} = \frac{\bar{x}_{CostT} - \bar{x}_{CostC}}{\bar{x}_{EffectT} - \bar{x}_{EffectC}}, \tag{11.4}$$

where $\bar{x}_{CostT}$, $\bar{x}_{CostC}$, $\bar{x}_{EffectT}$ and $\bar{x}_{EffectC}$ are the estimated sample mean costs and effects for the two treatments, respectively.

Table 11.1 Example sample statistics from the acupuncture data. Reproduced from Ratcliffe, J., Thomas, K.J. MacPherson, H., *et al.*, 'A randomised controlled trial of acupuncture care for persistent low back pain: cost effectiveness analysis.' *British Medical Journal*, 333, 623, ©2006, with permission from BMJ Publishing Group Ltd.

Outcome	Group Acupuncture			Usual care			Mean difference	95% CI		P-value*
	n	Mean	SD	n	Mean	SD		Lower	Upper	
NHS cost, discounted (£)	105	459.70	376.39	44	345.21	550.44	114.50	−39.74	268.73	0.14
QALY gain (SF-6D)	105	1.453	0.248	44	1.426	0.191	0.027	−0.056	0.110	0.52
ICER (£)							4225			

*P-value from two independent samples *t*-test.

Example: Acupuncture study

Ratcliffe *et al.* (2006) report the results of an economic evaluation conducted alongside the acupuncture trial (described previously in Chapter 8) to evaluate the cost-effectiveness of acupuncture compared to usual care in the treatment and management of persistent non-specific low back pain. The main outcome measure was the incremental cost per QALY gained over 2 years.

Health-care resource use data over a 24-month period were collected from general practice patient notes and a patient self-completed questionnaire on the use of resources. The data collected included: acupuncture visits; various NHS visits (including hospital inpatient stays, hospital outpatient visits, general practitioner consultation, physiotherapy and other NHS practitioner consultations); private health-care visits; use of over-the-counter and prescription medicines; and time off work.

Effectiveness data were measured using the SF-6D preference- or utility-based measure of QoL at baseline, 3, 12 and 24 months. The SF-6D generates a single index value where 0 represents death and 1 perfect health with intermediate values for all remaining health states. The utilities or valuations were based on the preference weights obtained for a series of health states defined by the SF-6D from a sample of 611 members of the UK general population (Brazier *et al.*, 2002). The authors then calculated the AUC to measure the QALY gain over the 2-year period for each patient. Table 11.1 shows that 149 low back pain patients (105 in the acupuncture group and 44 in the usual care group) provided valid cost and QALY data (valid SF-6D scores at 4 time points). □

11.7   Cost–utility analysis and cost–utility ratios

If benefit or effectiveness is measured using utilities and QALYs, then a specific form of economic evaluation called *cost–utility analysis* can be performed. In these circumstances the estimated incremental cost–utility ratio (ICUR) can be calculated using the sample mean costs ($\bar{x}_{CostT}$, $\bar{x}_{CostC}$) and QALYs ($\bar{x}_{QALYT}$ and $\bar{x}_{QALYC}$) for the two treatments, respectively. The estimated ICUR, $\hat{R}$, is given by

$$\hat{R} = \frac{\bar{x}_{CostT} - \bar{x}_{CostC}}{\bar{x}_{QALYT} - \bar{x}_{QALYC}}, \tag{11.5}$$

expressed in terms of '£ per QALY'. This ICUR can be used to assign the most efficient use of health-care funds.

In the United Kingdom, guidance from NICE (2004) states that the cost-effectiveness of new treatments is considered on a case-by-case basis. Generally, however, if a treatment costs more than £20, 000–£30, 000 per QALY, then it would not be considered cost-effective.

11.8   Incremental cost per QALY

Table 11.1 shows the mean costs and mean QALY gains for acupuncture treatment compared to usual care for treatment of low back pain. The estimated ICER (or utility ratio) for acupuncture compared to usual care for treatment of low back pain, based on these data, is

$$\hat{R} = \frac{\bar{x}_{\text{CostT}} - \bar{x}_{\text{CostC}}}{\bar{x}_{\text{QALYT}} - \bar{x}_{\text{QALYC}}} = \frac{459.70 - 376.38}{1.453 - 1.426} = \frac{114.50}{0.027} = £4225 \text{ per QALY}.$$

As I have suggested throughout this book, it is good statistical practice to report confidence intervals for estimates. Unfortunately, there is a problem with estimating confidence intervals for ratio estimates: the variance (and hence the standard error) of a ratio estimator

---

Box 11.1 Bootstrap process for estimating confidence intervals for ICER

Assume that we have paired cost and effect data for n_C pairs of patients in the control group and n_T pairs of patients in the treatment group.

1. Sample with replacement n_C cost and effect pairs from the patients in the control group and calculate the bootstrap estimates for the mean cost $\bar{x}^*_{\text{CostC}}$ and effect $\bar{x}^*_{\text{EffectC}}$ for the bootstrap sample.

2. Sample with replacement n_T cost and effect pairs from the patients in the treatment group and calculate the bootstrap estimates for the mean cost $\bar{x}^*_{\text{CostT}}$ and effect $\bar{x}^*_{\text{EffectT}}$ for the bootstrap sample.

3. Calculate the bootstrap estimate of the ICER:

$$\hat{R}^* = \frac{\bar{x}^*_{\text{CostT}} - \bar{x}^*_{\text{CostC}}}{\bar{x}^*_{\text{EffectT}} - \bar{x}_{\text{EffectC}^*}}.$$

4. Repeat this resampling process B times, to get B bootstrap estimates of the ICER. B is typically of the order of 1000 or more.

5. Order these B estimates of the sample ICER in increasing value.

6. A percentile-based bootstrap $100(1 - \alpha)\%$ confidence interval for the ICER is from the $(\alpha/2)B$th to the $(1 - \alpha/2)B$th largest values. A 95% CI would be from the $0.025B$th to $0.975B$th largest values.

does not exist. Briggs *et al.* (1999), Briggs and Gray (1999) and Briggs (2001) describe several methods for calculating CIs for cost–effectiveness ratios, including: Taylor series, Fieller's method and the bootstrap.

The first two methods are parametric methods and assume that the sampling distribution of the ICER follows a Normal distribution. Theory and practical experience suggest that the sampling distribution of the ICER is likely to be non-Normal, and the Taylor series and Fieller's method will provide poor estimates of the variance (and standard error) of the ICER estimate. Alternatively, the non-parametric approach of bootstrapping (described previously in Chapter 10) may provide a method of estimating confidence limits for the ICER. The bootstrap method does not depend on parametric assumptions for the sampling distribution of the ICER. The bootstrap involves creating an empirical estimate of the sampling distribution of the ICER by repeated resampling with replacement from the original data. In EEACTs both cost and effect data are measured for each individual patient. Therefore we randomly sample with replacement each patient and their paired cost and effect data. This takes into account the correlations between cost and effect outcomes. Box 11.1 describes the bootstrap algorithm for estimating confidence intervals for the ICER.

Figure 11.2 shows the estimated sampling distribution for the ICER from the acupuncture data in Table 11.1. The percentile-based 95% confidence limits for the

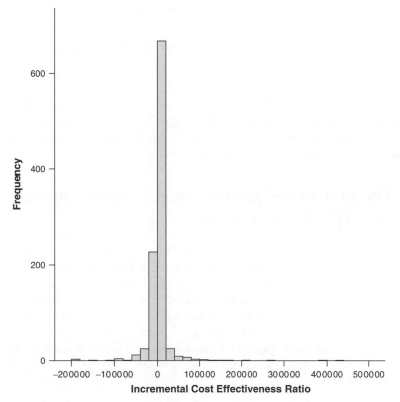

Figure 11.2 Bootstrap estimate of the ICER sampling distribution from the acupuncture study (data from Ratcliffe *et al.*, 2006).

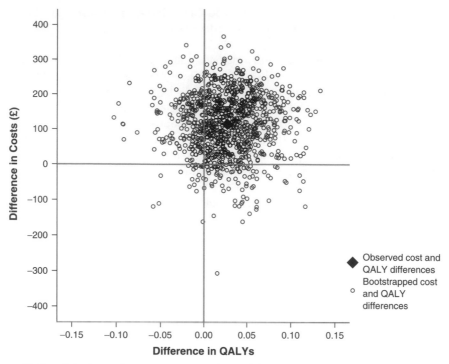

Figure 11.3   CE plane for acupuncture data with 1000 bootstrap samples (data from Ratcliffe *et al.*, 2006).

ICER were – £39 964 to £46 248 per QALY, with the best estimate of the statistic (ICER) being the observed ICER of £4225 per QALY from the original data.

The bootstrap resampling approach can be displayed on the CE plane by plotting the simulated individual cost–effect pairs in Figure 11.3.

11.9   The problem of negative (and positive) incremental cost–effectiveness ratios

The ICER is only calculated for the northeast and southwest quadrants where the ICER is *positive*. In the northwest and southwest quadrants the ICER is *negative* and its magnitude conveys no useful meaning. Furthermore, negative ICERs in the northwest quadrant (favouring the existing treatment) are qualitatively different from negative ICERs in the southeast quadrant (favouring new treatment), yet will be grouped together in any rank-ordering exercise to estimate bootstrap confidence intervals.

For the acupuncture data, Table 11.2 and Figure 11.3 show that the bootstrap replicates, whilst mainly falling in the northeast quadrant (around 70%), cover all four quadrants of the CE plane.

Table 11.2 Bootstrapped acupuncture data: which quadrant of the CE plane?

Quadrant	Frequency	Percent
NE quadrant – new treatment more effective but more costly	701	70.1%
SE quadrant – new treatment dominates	79	7.9%
SW quadrant – new treatment cheaper but less effective	22	2.2%
NW quadrant – existing treatment dominates	198	19.8%
Total	1000	100%

11.10 Cost-effectiveness acceptability curves

When the bootstrap replications cover all four quadrants (as they do in Figure 11.3), it turns out the bootstrap approach to estimating confidence intervals fails to distinguish between those ICERs (both positive and negative) that favour the new treatment and those that favour the existing treatment. One solution to this problem is the cost-effectiveness acceptability curve (CEAC).

If the estimated ICER lies below some shadow price or ceiling ratio ($R_{Ceiling}$) reflecting the maximum that decision-makers are willing to invest to achieve a unit of effectiveness, then it should be implemented. In the UK guidance from NICE indicates that a ceiling ratio of £20000 per QALY represents the threshold of what the NHS can afford to pay for additional QALYs, unless other arguments exist for adopting the new technology.

Therefore, in terms of the bootstrap replications on the CE plane in Figure 11.4, uncertainty could be summarized by considering how many of the bootstrap replications fall below and/or to the right of the line with slope equal to $R_{Ceiling}$, lending support to the cost-effectiveness of the intervention. Of course, the appropriate value of $R_{Ceiling}$ is itself unknown. However, $R_{Ceiling}$ can be varied in order to show how the evidence in favour of the cost-effectiveness of the intervention varies with $R_{Ceiling}$. In Figure 11.4, $R_{Ceiling}$ is £1000 per QALY and about 12% of the bootstrap replicates are below and/or to the right of this line. The resulting CEAC for the acupuncture data is shown in Figure 11.5. Assuming an implicit threshold of a maximum willingness to pay of £20000 for a QALY, then the CEAC of Figure 11.5 suggests that the probability of the cost per QALY of acupuncture for low back pain falling below this threshold value was around 73%.

Example: Acupuncture trial

Ratcliffe *et al.* (2006) imputed missing cost and SF-6D data and reported an overall ICER for the treatment of low back pain of £4241 per QALY at 24 months. Assuming an implicit threshold of a maximum willingness to pay of £20000 for a QALY, then the probability of the cost per QALY of acupuncture for low back pain falling below this threshold value was over 90%. The authors concluded: 'If £20,000 is taken as the maximum acceptable cost effectiveness ratio, then acupuncture for the treatment of low back pain seems cost effective.' □

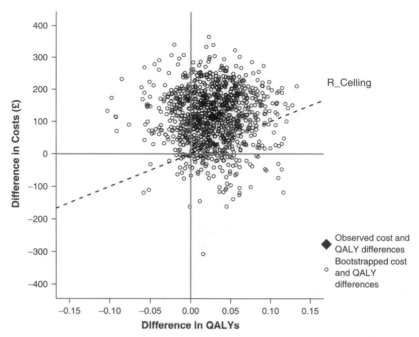

Figure 11.4   CE plane for acupuncture data with 1000 bootstrap resamples and ceiling ratio, R_{Ceiling}, of £1000 per QALY (data from Ratcliffe *et al.*, 2006).

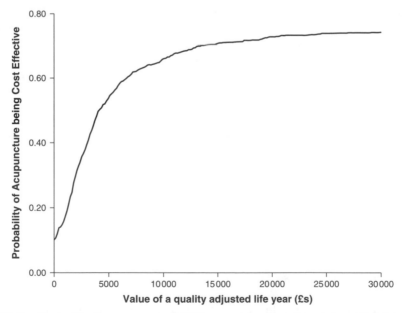

Figure 11.5   Cost-effectiveness acceptability curve for the acupuncture trial data. Reproduced from Ratcliffe, J., Thomas, K.J. MacPherson, H., *et al.*, 'A randomised controlled trial of acupuncture care for persistent low back pain: cost effectiveness analysis.' *British Medical Journal*, 333, 623, ©2006, with permission from BMJ Publishing Group Ltd.

11.11 Further reading

This chapter has described economic evaluations alongside clinical trials. The book by Drummond *et al* (2005) provides a good general introduction to methods for the economic evaluation of health-care interventions. The partner book by Drummond and McGuire (2001) shows how to apply the theory of economic evaluation in practice. For readers interested in the different methods of measuring and valuing health, the book by Brazier *et al.* (2007) provides a comprehensive description. The statistical methods used in the analysis of cost-effectiveness data are more fully discussed in Willan and Briggs (2006).

Exercises

11.1 Consider two patients, A and B, whose QoL was assessed at four time points, 0 , 6, 12 and 24 months with a utility-based QoL measure. Patient A had utility scores of 0.80, 0.70, 0.60 and 0.60 at 0, 6, 12 and 24 months, respectively. Patient B had utility scores of 0.50, 0.50, 0.70 and 0.80 at 0, 6, 12 and 24 months, respectively.

(a) Calculate the QALY for patient A.

(b) Calculate the QALY for patient B.

(c) Compare the QALYs for patients A and B. What do you notice?

(d) Plot the utility scores as a scatter/line graph, similar to Figures 9.1 and 9.2, with a separate line for each patient and time (in years) on the horizontal axis and utility score on the vertical axis. Comment on the shape of the QoL/utility profiles over time.

11.2 Table 11.3 shows the mean QALYs and mean costs for 233 patients with venous leg ulcers. Patients with venous leg ulcers were randomized to a new intervention which involved treatment at a specialist clinic by nurses trained to use compression bandaging or usual care/treatment by district nurses in the patient's own home. Patients were followed up from 12 months from randomization and NHS resource use data (and costs) and QALY data were collected (Morrell *et al.*, 1998).

(a) Calculate the mean difference in QALYs between the clinic and home groups and its associated 95% confidence interval. Comment on the results.

Table 11.3 Mean QALYs and costs for venous leg ulcer patients by treatment group.

	Clinic			Home			Mean difference	95 CI Lower	Upper
	n	Mean	SD	*n*	Mean	SD			
QALY	120	0.386	0.356	113	0.2731	0.3377			
Cost £	120	877.60	674.30	113	863.09	865.32			
ICER									

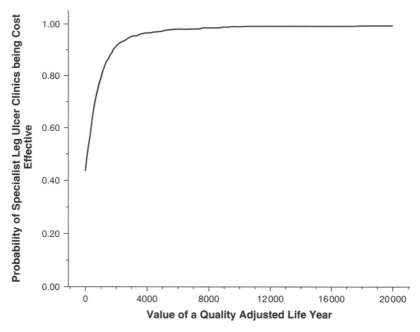

Figure 11.6 Cost-effectiveness acceptability curve for the leg ulcer trial data.

(b) Calculate the mean difference in costs between the clinic and home groups and its associated 95% confidence interval. Comment on the results.

(c) Calculate the ICER (cost per QALY) to compare the cost-effectiveness of specialist leg ulcer clinics with usual care at home or patients with venous leg ulcers.

(d) In which quadrant of the cost-effectiveness plane does the estimated ICER from (c) lie?

Figure 11.6 shows the CEAC for the data from the leg ulcer trial based on 1000 bootstrap replications.

(e) Assume a threshold of a maximum willingness to pay of £20 000 for QALY. What is the probability of specialist clinics for venous leg ulcers falling below this value?

(f) Do you think specialist clinics for venous leg ulcers are cost-effective compared to usual treatment?

12

Meta-analysis

Summary

Quality of life measures are becoming more frequently used in clinical trials and health services research, both as primary and secondary endpoints. Hence, it is now also more common to combine the QoL results from several similar studies to produce an overall estimate of the treatment effect. Meta-analysis is the statistical analysis of the data from a collection of studies in order to synthesize the results. The rationale for meta-analysis is to increase the power and precision of estimates of treatment effects and exposure risks. This chapter will describe how the treatment effect from studies which have used different QoL instruments can be summarized as a standardized effect size called the standardized mean difference (SMD). It will show how these standardized outcomes can then be combined using a fixed or random effects statistical model to produce an overall summary measure of the treatment effect, pooled across all the studies. The chapter will also show how these effect sizes can be graphically displayed as forest plots and funnel plots.

12.1 Introduction

Meta-analysis is the statistical analysis of the data from a collection of studies in order to synthesize the results. The rationale for meta-analysis is to increase the power and precision of estimates of treatment effects and exposure risks. Thus, the reason for adding a meta-analysis to a systematic review is to obtain the best overall estimate of the effect of an intervention or treatment. By combining the results of all the studies available we increase the power to detect important treatment effects.

Traditionally, when seeking advice in controversial or novel areas, clinicians and scientists have relied heavily on 'informed' editorials or narrative reviews. Spector and Thompson (1991) say that there is now good evidence to suggest that these methods are subject to bias and inaccuracy. Reviewers using traditional methods are less likely to detect a small but significant effect or difference than reviewers using formal statistical

Quality of Life Outcomes in Clinical Trials and Health-Care Evaluation   Stephen J. Walters
© 2009 John Wiley & Sons, Ltd

techniques. As most current medical reviews do not use scientific methods to assess and present data, different reviewers often reach different conclusions based on the same data. For these reasons some formal statistical process of review should replace the informal approach. Meta-analysis can be used to resolve uncertainty when reports, editorials or reviews disagree.

The major limitation of meta-analysis is that it can only work with what is available. A meta-analysis can only include studies that are published or in some other way retrievable. The available studies may be incomparable or give inadequate data. They may vary in design, quality, outcome measure or population studied. Publication bias is the main concern regarding the availability of studies. Authors are more likely to submit, and editors more likely to publish, studies with significant results. This is also called the 'file drawer problem'; those doing a meta-analysis wonder about the influence that studies tucked away in file drawers might have on their results. A meta-analysis must be updated as more studies become available, in order to maintain its usefulness.

12.2   Planning a meta-analysis

The four steps common to the planning of a meta-analysis (Petitti, 1999) are:

1. *Defining the problem.* The problem definition is a general statement of the broad issue that the study addresses.

2. *Developing a study protocol.* The protocol is the blueprint for the conduct of the study. It also serves as a permanent record of the original study objectives and of the study methods and procedures. A study protocol should be prepared before the study begins. The protocol should have sections on: objectives; background; information retrieval; data collection and analysis (see Table 12.1).

3. *Acquiring resources.* Planning a study that uses meta-analysis should include a realistic assessment of the resource needs for the study. A meta-analysis can

Table 12.1   Elements of a study protocol for meta-analysis (based upon Petitti, 1999).

Section	Meta-analysis
Objectives	State main objectives
	Specify secondary objectives
Background	Brief review
Information	Describe overall strategy
Retrieval	Specify MEDLINE search terms
	Explain approach to unpublished reports
Data Collection	Describe procedures for abstracting data from publications (blinding, reliability checks, handling of missing data)
	Describe quality rating scheme and procedures for assessing quality
Analysis	State methods for estimating variance for individual studies
	State model to be used and explain choice
	Specify approach to missing data
	Describe how quality rating scheme will be used in the analysis
Appendices	Copies of data collection forms

require a substantial investment in personnel resources, article retrieval, information abstraction, computer resources and specialist software.

4. *Procuring administrative procedures.* Fewer administrative approvals are necessary for a meta-analysis, but approval to use unpublished data may be necessary.

Having developed a protocol for the meta-analysis the next steps are to (Petitti, 1999):

1. identify studies with relevant data;

2. check eligibility criteria for inclusion and exclusion of the studies;

3. abstract the data;

4. analyse the abstracted data statistically.

After abstracting the data and before proceeding to stage 4 it is important to ask whether a meta-analysis is appropriate.

12.2.1   Is a meta-analysis appropriate?

In answering this question, two points are raised:

1. Can the results of the studies be expressed as an 'effect measure' (such as an odds ratio, rate difference or mean difference) which has a numerical value and can be combined into a single estimate?

2. More importantly, does it make sense to combine the results of the different studies into a single estimate?

The answer to the latter question should only be 'yes' if the following are sufficiently similar across all studies:

- the populations receiving the interventions (P);
- the intervention (I);
- the comparison intervention (C);
- the outcomes being measured (O).

These are known as the four elements of the PICO model to formulate a search question for a systematic review.

12.2.2   Combining the results of different studies

Meta-analysis is the final and perhaps not the most important stage of the following process. Much of the benefit can be obtained simply by graphically representing the results of different studies. After a systematic review of the literature to identify relevant studies, the effect measure to be combined is chosen. The quality of the studies should then be assessed and where possible ranked or graded. The results of the individual studies are then represented on a graph which shows a point estimate of each study's effect size, with its confidence interval indicated by a horizontal line on either side of the point. An example of this type of graph is shown in Figure 12.1.

Example: Treating osteoarthritis

Towheed *et al.* (2005) reviewed the use of glucosamine for treating osteoarthritis and identified 20 RCTs, with 2750 patients overall, suitable for inclusion. Of these, 15 trials were placebo controlled and reported pain QoL outcomes post randomization. Figure 12.1 shows of the results for the 15 studies. Each study is listed with its sample size, mean pain scale score, and its variability separately for the glucosamine and placebo groups. The mean treatment differences are plotted, with horizontal lines indicating the lower and upper 95% confidence limits. The calculation and interpretation of these results is described later in this chapter. □

The studies can be placed on the graph in chronological order (as above) but can also be ranked in other ways, for example by quality, to show visually whether the results of the better studies are similar to the others. At this point the decision about whether to proceed to a formal meta-analysis (statistical synthesis) can be made. The graph will help in deciding whether the results of the individual studies are sufficiently similar for it to make sense to combine them into a single estimate. Figure 12.1 suggests the outcomes of the studies are broadly similar, although the results of the D'Ambrosio study appear to be somewhat different from the rest in strongly favouring glucosamine treatment.

12.2.3   Choosing the appropriate statistical method

There are two key questions:

1. What outcome measures am I combining?

2. Which 'model' should I use?

There are two main models used for meta-analysis: the fixed effects and the random effects models (Table 12.2). There is considerable debate about which of these should be used. A decision will be based partly on the data and partly on philosophy.

Table 12.2   Methods that can be used in meta-analysis according to the underlying model assumption and the type of effect measure.

Model Assumption	Methods	Effect Measures
Fixed Effects	Mantel–Haenszel	Ratio (typically odds ratio; can be applied to rate ratio and risk ratio (relative risk))
	Peto	Ratio (approximates the odds ratio)
	General variance based	Ratio (all types) and difference
Random effects	DerSimonian–Laird	Ratio (all types) and Difference

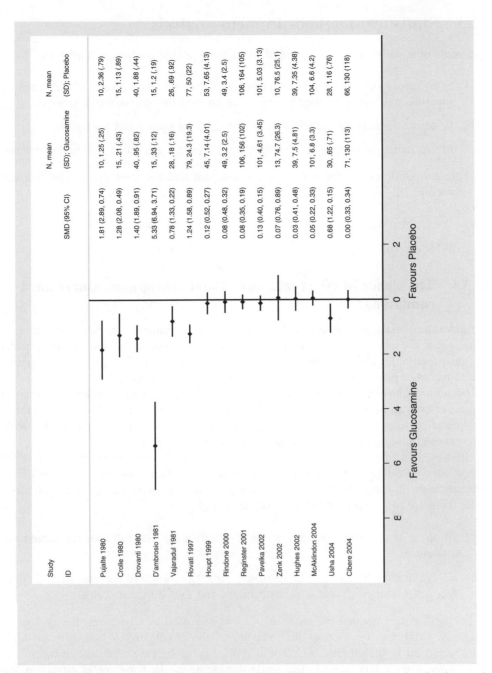

Figure 12.1 Forest plot of standardized mean difference in post-randomization pain score in 15 RCTs comparing glucosamine and placebo treatment for osteoarthritis. From Towheed, T.E., Maxwell, L., Anastassiades, *et al.*, Glucosamine therapy for treating osteoarthritis. *Cochrane Database of Systematic Reviews* 2005, Issue 2. Art. No.: CD002946. DOI: 10.1002/14651858.CD002946.pub2. © 2005 Cochrane Collaboration, reproduced with permission.

12.3   Statistical methods in meta-analysis

The goals of a statistical analysis of QoL data from several studies are threefold:

1. to estimate a summary measure of effect size, estimate the variance of the summary measure, and then calculate a confidence interval for the summary measure;

2. to derive a summary statistic that can be used for hypothesis testing;

3. to use statistical methods to test the hypothesis that the effects are homogeneous.

This section describes the statistical methods that address these goals. The two key questions are:

1. What effect measure?

2. What model?

12.3.1   The choice of effect measure: What outcome measures am I combining?

In randomized trials and cohort studies the effect of treatment can be estimated as a difference in the rates of disease between the treatment (or exposed) group and the control (or unexposed) group, as the ratio of disease rates measured as incidence density (i.e. with denominators of person-time), as the ratio of rates measured as cumulative incidence (i.e. with denominators of person), or as an odds ratio (OR). In population-based case–control studies, effect can be estimated as an odds ratio or as an attributable risk. It is usual to measure effect using either the odds ratio or a rate ratio in non-experimental studies. Rate differences are more often used to measure effect in randomized trials.

Studies that measure effect on a continuous scale are often the subject of meta-analysis. Throughout this book, I have regarded QoL outcomes as continuous measurements. In meta-analysis of studies where effect size is measured on a continuous scale, there are two situations to be considered:

(i) all of the studies used the same measure of effect (i.e. they all used the same QoL instrument);

(ii) all of the eligible studies addressed the same question, but the measure of effect was made using different QoL instruments and thus different scales.

For QoL data, provided the same instrument was used in all studies, the raw *mean difference* (MD) can be used as the measure of the effect size. When different QoL scales are used in the studies, which will typically be the case, then the *standardized mean difference* (SMD) is used. The SMD represents the QoL treatment effects as the number of standard deviations between the two mean QoL treatment scores. To calculate the SMD and its variance (and standard error) for each study we require an estimate of the mean treatment effect in each group, the corresponding standard deviation and the number of patients in each group.

There are two common formulations of the SMD: Cohen's *d* and Hedges' adjusted *g*. The Cochrane Reviews Group recommends the use of Hedges' adjusted *g*, which is

Table 12.3 Formula for calculating standardized mean difference effect sizes and their standard errors for continuous outcomes with two independent groups.

Name	SMD effect size	Standard error of SMD
Cohen's d	$SMD_d = \dfrac{\bar{x}_1 - \bar{x}_2}{SD_{Pooled}}$ Where $SD_{Pooled} = \sqrt{\dfrac{(n_1-1)sd_1^2 + (n_2-1)sd_2^2}{(n_1-1)+(n_2-1)}}$	$SE(SMD_d) = \sqrt{\dfrac{N}{n_1 n_2} + \dfrac{SMD_d^2}{2(N-2)}}$
Hedges' adjusted g	$SMD_d = \dfrac{\bar{x}_1 - \bar{x}_2}{SD_{Pooled}}\left(1 - \dfrac{3}{4N-9}\right)$	$SE(SMD_g) = \sqrt{\dfrac{N}{n_1 n_2} + \dfrac{SMD_g^2}{2(N-3.94)}}$

Where $N = n_1 + n_2$ is the total number of participants in group 1 (n_1) and group 2 (n_2) respectively, and $\bar{x}_1$ and sd_1 and $\bar{x}_2$ and sd_2 are the estimated mean treatment effects (and their associated standard deviations) in Group 1 and Group 2 respectively.

very similar to Cohen's d, but includes an adjustment for small-sample bias. Table 12.3 shows the equations for calculating these two SMDs and their associated standard errors.

Table 12.4 shows the SMD in post-randomization pain scores and their associated standard errors for the 15 RCTs comparing glucosamine and placebo treatment for osteoarthritis (Towheed *et al.*, 2005).

12.3.2   Model choice: fixed or random?

The previous section described how to summarize each study by calculating a standardized mean effect size and its corresponding standard error. The next stage is to combine these estimated standardized treatment effects to provide an overall average treatment effect. There are two ways of doing this, using either a fixed or random effects model. Both models use what is a called an *inverse variance* (IV) method to combine the results across the studies. The IV method weights the individual study effect sizes according to the reciprocal of their variance, hence the name. The statistical methods used to combine study results when fixed effects are assumed differ from the methods used when random effects are assumed.

In an analysis based on a fixed effects model, inference is conditional on the studies actually done. In an analysis based on the random effects model, inference is based on the assumption that the studies are a random sample of some hypothetical population of studies. The question of the appropriate model for a meta-analysis is not just theoretical and the model choice can have important consequences for conclusions based on the meta-analysis (Petitti, 1999). There are strong opinions about the appropriateness of both models. Several statisticians have expressed a preference for the fixed effects approach (Peto, 1987; Thompson & Pocock, 1991); others favour the random effects approach (Meier, 1987; Fleiss and Gross, 1991). Examples of results that seem counterintuitive for one method but not the other can be developed for both the fixed effects model and the random effects model.

Table 12.4 Standardized mean differences in post-randomization pain scores and their associated standard errors for the 15 randomized controlled trials comparing glucosamine and placebo treatment for osteoarthritis (data from Towheed et al., 2005).

Study i	Study	Glucosamine			Placebo			SD_{Pooled}	Cohen's d SMD_d	Hedges' adjusted g SMD_g	$SE(SMD_d)$	$SE(SMD_g)$
		n_1	$Mean_1$	sd_1	n_2	$Mean_2$	sd_2					
1	Cibere 2004	71	129.72	113.23	66	129.62	118.02	115.56	0.001	0.001	0.17	0.17
2	Crolle 1980	15	0.21	0.43	15	1.13	0.89	0.70	−1.316	−1.281	0.41	0.41
3	D'ambrosio 1981	15	0.33	0.12	15	1.20	0.19	0.16	−5.475	−5.327	0.82	0.82
4	Drovanti 1980	40	0.95	0.82	40	1.88	0.44	0.66	−1.413	−1.400	0.25	0.25
5	Houpt 1999	45	7.14	4.01	53	7.65	4.13	4.08	−0.125	−0.124	0.20	0.20
6	Hughes 2002	39	7.50	4.81	39	7.35	4.38	4.60	0.033	0.032	0.23	0.23
7	McAklindon 2004	101	6.80	3.30	104	6.60	4.20	3.78	0.053	0.053	0.14	0.14
8	Pavelka 2002	101	4.61	3.45	101	5.03	3.13	3.29	−0.128	−0.127	0.14	0.14
9	Pujalte 1980	10	1.25	0.25	10	2.36	0.79	0.59	−1.894	−1.814	0.55	0.55
10	Reginster 2001	106	156.10	101.90	106	164.20	104.50	103.21	−0.078	−0.078	0.14	0.14
11	Rindone 2000	49	3.20	2.50	49	3.40	2.50	2.50	−0.080	−0.079	0.20	0.20
12	Rovati 1997	79	24.30	19.30	77	50.00	22.00	20.68	−1.243	−1.237	0.18	0.18
13	Usha 2004	30	0.65	0.71	28	1.16	0.76	0.73	−0.694	−0.685	0.27	0.27
14	Vajaradul 1981	28	0.18	0.16	26	0.69	0.92	0.65	−0.787	−0.775	0.28	0.28
15	Zenk 2002	13	−74.70	26.30	10	−76.50	25.10	25.79	0.070	0.067	0.42	0.42

The random effects assumption means that the analysis addresses the question, 'Will the treatment produce benefit on average?', whereas the fixed effects assumption means that the analysis addresses the question, 'Did the treatment produce benefit on average in the studies at hand?' (Bailey, 1987). The random effects model is appropriate if the question is whether the treatment or the risk factor will have an effect. If the question is whether the treatment has caused an effect in the studies that have been done, then the fixed effects model is appropriate.

Peto (1987) states that analysis using the random effects model is 'wrong' because it answers a question that is 'obtuse and uninteresting.' Thompson and Pocock (1991) describe as 'peculiar' the premise of the random effects model that studies are representative of some hypothetical population of studies. In contrast, Fleiss and Gross (1991) believe that question addressed by the fixed effects model is less important than the one addressed by the random effects model. Consideration of the differences in the questions involved does not seem to resolve the question of which model to use.

12.3.3   Homogeneity

In all of the methods based on the assumption of fixed effects, the variance component of the meta-analytic estimate of the pooled effect size is composed only of terms for the within-study variance of each component study. The assumption of the random effects model that studies are a random sample from some population of studies makes it necessary to include a between-studies as well as a within-study component of variation in estimation of effect size and statistical significance. Because the random effects model incorporates a between-studies component of variance, it will be more 'conservative' than an analysis of the same data based on a method that assumes fixed effects. That is, an analysis based on a random effects model will generally yield a wider confidence interval and will be less likely to declare a difference significant than an analysis based on fixed effects.

As the between-studies variance becomes large (i.e. when there is heterogeneity), the between-studies variance term will dominate the weights assigned to the study using the random effects model and the large studies will tend to be weighted equally. In this situation, the results of the analysis based on a fixed effects model, which weights studies according to their sample size, and the random effects models may differ considerably. When there is not much heterogeneity, the fixed effects and the random effects models will both weight studies according to sample size and they will yield results that are essentially identical (Petitti, 1999).

12.3.4   Fixed effects model

Box 12.1 describes the fixed effects method for combining results across studies. Table 12.5 shows the computer output from using a fixed effects model to combine the QoL outcomes for the 15 RCTs comparing glucosamine and placebo for the treatment of osteoarthrtitis.

The overall estimated SMD is −0.33 (95% CI: −0.435 to −0.225), which appears to significantly favour glucosamine treatment (since it wholly excludes the null value of zero). However, both the test for heterogeneity and I^2 statistics suggest considerable between-studies heterogeneity and that a random effects statistical model may be more appropriate for these data.

Box 12.1 Fixed effects inverse variance based method for combining SMDs across studies

Suppose we have QoL outcomes in k studies which are to be combined.

1. Calculate the SMD effect size for each of the k studies, as described in Table 12.3. Let the SMD estimate for the ith study be denoted by $\hat{\theta}_i$.

2. Calculate the standard error for the SMD each of the k studies, as described in Table 12.3. Let the standard error of SMD estimate for the ith study be denoted by $SE\{\hat{\theta}_i\}$.

3. The individual study effect sizes are weighted according to the reciprocal of their variance using

$$w_i = \frac{1}{(SE\{\hat{\theta}_i\})^2}.$$

4. Calculate the pooled estimate of the effect size,

$$\hat{\theta}_{IV} = \frac{\sum_{i=1}^{k} w_i \hat{\theta}_i}{\sum_{i=1}^{k} w_i}.$$

5. Calculate the standard error of the pooled estimate of the effect size,

$$SE\{\hat{\theta}_{IV}\} = \frac{1}{\sqrt{\sum_{i=1}^{k} w_i}}.$$

6. The $100(1 - \alpha)\%$ confidence interval for $\hat{\theta}_{IV}$ is given by

$$\hat{\theta}_{IV} - z_{1-\frac{\alpha}{2}} SE\{\hat{\theta}_{IV}\} \text{ to } \hat{\theta}_{IV} + z_{1-\frac{\alpha}{2}} SE\{\hat{\theta}_{IV}\}.$$

where $z_{1-\alpha/2}$ are the appropriate values from the standard Normal distribution for the $100(1 - \alpha/2)$ percentiles (see Table B.1).

7. The heterogeneity statistic is given by

$$Q_{IV} = \sum_{i=1}^{k} w_i (\hat{\theta}_i - \hat{\theta}_{IV})^2.$$

Under the null hypothesis that there are no differences in intervention effect among studies, this follows a chi-squared distribution with $k - 1$ degrees of freedom (where k is the number of studies in the meta-analysis).

8. The I^2 statistic is calculated as

$$I^2 = \max\left\{100\% \times \frac{Q_{IV} - (k - 1)}{Q_{IV}}, 0\right\}.$$

This measures the extent of the inconsistency among the studies' results, and is interpreted as approximately the proportion of the total variation in study estimates that is due to heterogeneity rather than sampling error.

9. The test for the presence of an overall intervention effect is given by

$$Z = \frac{\hat{\theta}_{IV}}{SE\{\hat{\theta}_{IV}\}}.$$

Under the null hypothesis that there is no overall effect of the intervention, Z follows a standard Normal distribution (see Table B.1).

12.3.5 Forest plots

A forest plot is commonly used to display the quantitative results of studies included in systematic reviews and meta-analyses. The forest plot consists of a graph that shows the estimated effects and the corresponding confidence interval from each study. The forest plot can also be used for displaying the results from other studies or the results of different outcomes within the same study. Figure 12.2 is an example of a forest plot from a meta-analysis of 15 RCTs that compare glucosamine against placebo treatment for osteoarthritis. It shows the standardized mean difference in post-randomization pain score

Table 12.5 Fixed effects model estimates and confidence intervals for the SMD from 15 RCTs comparing glucosamine and placebo treatment for osteoarthritis (data from Towheed *et al.*, 2005).

Study	SMD_g	95% CI Lower	Upper	% Weight
Cibere 2004	0.001	−0.334	0.336	9.82
Crolle 1980	−1.281	−2.076	−0.485	1.74
D'ambrosio 1981	−5.327	−6.941	−3.713	0.42
Drovanti 1980	−1.4	−1.891	−0.908	4.57
Houpt 1999	−0.124	−0.522	0.274	6.98
Hughes 2002	0.032	−0.412	0.476	5.6
McAklindon 2004	0.053	−0.221	0.327	14.71
Pavelka 2002	−0.127	−0.403	0.149	14.48
Pujalte 1980	−1.814	−2.892	−0.736	0.95
Reginster 2001	−0.078	−0.348	0.191	15.21
Rindone 2000	−0.079	−0.476	0.317	7.03
Rovati 1997	−1.237	−1.58	−0.894	9.36
Usha 2004	−0.685	−1.216	−0.154	3.91
Vajaradul 1981	−0.775	−1.33	−0.22	3.58
Zenk 2002	0.067	−0.757	0.892	1.62
IV pooled SMD$_g$	**−0.33**	**−0.435**	**−0.225**	**100**

Heterogeneity chi-squared = 121.50 (df = 14), $P = 0.001$
I^2 (variation in SMD attributable to heterogeneity) = 88.5%
Test of SMD=0: $z = 6.16$, $P < 0.001$

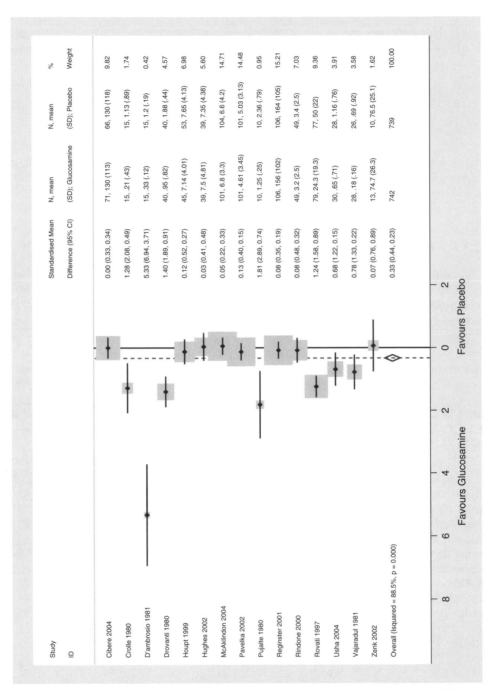

Figure 12.2 Forest plot of standardized mean differences in post-randomization pain score in 15 RCTs comparing glucosamine and placebo treatment for Osteoarthritis based on a fixed effects model. From Towheed, T.E., Maxwell, L., Anastassiades, *et al.*, Glucosamine therapy for treating osteoarthritis. *Cochrane Database of Systematic Reviews* 2005, Issue 2. Art. No.: CD002946. DOI: 10.1002/14651858.CD002946.pub2. © 2005 Cochrane Collaboration, reproduced with permission.

between the two groups (Towheed *et al.*, 2005). A negative SMD favours the glucosamine treated group.

The point estimates are sometimes marked using square shapes of size proportional to the size of the study represented. This counters a tendency for the viewers' eyes to be drawn to the studies which have the widest confidence interval estimates, and are therefore graphically more impressive, but are the least significant (Deeks and Everitt, 2005). Sometimes, too, the individual lines are ordered by date of study, by some index of study quality or by the point estimate of effect size.

Figure 12.2 contains both graphical and tabular elements. Data from each study are summarized in the rows of the diagram, with the name of the study's first author, the year of publication, summary measure of the treatment effect and confidence interval and the weight each study is given in the overall meta-analysis. The estimates of the treatment effect are marked by a block and the associated uncertainty shown by horizontal lines extending between the upper and lower confidence intervals. The size of the block varies between studies to reflect the weight given to each in the meta-analysis, more influential studies having the larger blocks. The overall estimate of effect is marked at the bottom of the plot as a diamond, the central point indicating the point estimate while the outer points mark the confidence limits. A vertical line is drawn across the diagram at the meta-analytical point estimate. The percentage weight that each study contributes to the meta-analysis is included. From the plots it is often possible to assess visually the degree of heterogeneity in study results by noting the overlap of confidence intervals of individual studies with the overall combined point estimate from the meta-analysis.

The forest plot and the heterogeneity statistic suggest considerable heterogeneity across the 15 studies. The I^2 statistic further suggests that 88% of the total variability in SMD estimates is due to heterogeneity rather than sampling error. This implies that a random effects model may be more appropriate to analyse the data.

12.3.6 Random effects

The DerSimonian and Laird (1986) random effects model is described in Box 12.2. Table 12.6 shows that the overall estimated SMD from the random effects model is larger −0.615 (95% CI: −0.946 to −0.283), with wider confidence limits than its fixed effects counterpart. However, the results still significantly favour glucosamine treatment (since it wholly excludes the null value of zero). The forest plot of Figure 12.3 shows the results graphically.

12.3.7 Funnel plots

Funnel plots are a particular type of scatter plot used to detect publication bias in systematic reviews and meta-analysis. For each study in a review the estimated treatment effect is plotted against a measure of trial precision such as the variance or standard error (SE) of the treatment effect as shown in Figure 12.4. In a change from the standard graphical practice for scatter plots where the outcome variable or treatment effect is plotted on the vertical axis (see Chapter 7), funnel plots depict precision (Variance of the treatment effect or sample size) on the vertical axis and the treatment effect on the horizontal axis. The overall combined summary from the meta-analysis may be marked by a vertical line. When all study results are published it is expected that the studies will have a symmetrical distribution around the average or overall effect line, the spread of studies

Box 12.2 DerSimoninan and Laird random effects inverse variance based method for combining SMD across studies

Suppose that we have QoL outcomes in k studies which are to be combined. Under the random effects model, the assumption of a common intervention effect is relaxed, and the effect sizes are assumed to have a Normal distribution, $\theta_i \sim N(\theta, \tau^2)$.

1. Calculate the SMD effect size for each of the k studies, as described in Table 12.3. Let the SMD estimate for the ith study be denoted by $\hat{\theta}_i$.

2. Calculate the standard error for the SMD for each of the k studies, as described in Table 12.3. Let the standard error of SMD estimate for the ith study be denoted by $SE\{\hat{\theta}_i\}$.

3. Calculate the inverse variance weights for each study.

$$w_i^{RE} = \frac{1}{\left(SE\{\hat{\theta}_i\}\right)^2}$$

4. Calculate the estimate of τ^2

$$\hat{\tau}^2 = \max\left\{\frac{Q_{IV} - (k-1)}{\sum w_i - (\sum w_i^2)/\sum w_i}, 0\right\}$$

5. Each study's effect size weight is given by

$$w_i^{RE} = \frac{1}{SE\{\hat{\theta}_i\}^2 + \hat{\tau}^2}$$

6. The pooled effect size is given by

$$\hat{\theta}_{RE} = \frac{\sum w_i^{RE}\hat{\theta}_i}{\sum w_i^{RE}}.$$

7. Calculate the standard error of the pooled estimate of the effect size,

$$SE\{\hat{\theta}_{RE}\} = \frac{1}{\sqrt{w_i^{RE}}}$$

8. The $100(1-\alpha)\%$ confidence interval for $\hat{\theta}_{RE}$ is given by

$$\hat{\theta}_{RE} - z_{1-\frac{\alpha}{2}} SE\{\hat{\theta}_{RE}\} \text{ to } \hat{\theta}_{RE} + z_{1-\frac{\alpha}{2}} SE\{\hat{\theta}_{RE}\}.$$

where $z_{1-\alpha/2}$ are the appropriate values from the standard Normal distribution for the $100(1-\alpha/2)$ percentiles (see Table B.1).

9. The heterogeneity statistic is given by

$$Q_{IV} = \sum_{i=1}^{k} w_i(\hat{\theta}_i - \hat{\theta}_{IV})^2.$$

Under the null hypothesis that there are no differences in intervention effect among studies, this follows a chi-squared distribution with $k - 1$ degrees of freedom (where k is the number of studies in the meta-analysis).

10. The I^2 statistic is calculated as

$$I^2 = \max\left\{100\% \times \frac{Q_{IV} - (k-1)}{Q_{IV}}, 0\right\}.$$

This measures the extent of the inconsistency among the studies' results, and is interpreted as approximately the proportion of the total variation in study estimates that is due to heterogeneity rather than sampling error.

11. The test for the presence of an overall intervention effect is given by

$$Z = \frac{\hat{\theta}_{IV}}{SE\{\hat{\theta}_{IV}\}}.$$

Under the null hypothesis that there is no overall effect of the intervention, Z, follows a standard Normal distribution (see Table B.1).

Table 12.6 Random effects model estimates and confidence intervals for the SMD from 15 RCTs comparing glucosamine and placebo treatment for osteoarthritis (data from Towheed *et al.*, 2005).

Study	SMD	95% CI Lower	Upper	% Weight
Cibere 2004	0.001	−0.334	0.336	7.67
Crolle 1980	−1.281	−2.076	−0.485	5.62
D'Ambrosio 1981	−5.327	−6.941	−3.713	2.8
Drovanti 1980	−1.4	−1.891	−0.908	7.03
Houpt 1999	−0.124	−0.522	0.274	7.43
Hughes 2002	0.032	−0.412	0.476	7.24
McAklindon 2004	0.053	−0.221	0.327	7.87
Pavelka 2002	−0.127	−0.403	0.149	7.86
Pujalte 1980	−1.814	−2.892	−0.736	4.43
Reginster 2001	−0.078	−0.348	0.191	7.88
Rindone 2000	−0.079	−0.476	0.317	7.43
Rovati 1997	−1.237	−1.58	−0.894	7.64
Usha 2004	−0.685	−1.216	−0.154	6.86
Vajaradul 1981	−0.775	−1.33	−0.22	6.75
Zenk 2002	0.067	−0.757	0.892	5.49
D+L pooled SMD	**−0.615**	**−0.946**	**−0.283**	**100**

Heterogeneity chi-squared $= 121.50$ (df $= 14$), $P < 0.001$ $I^2 = 88.5\%$
Estimate of between-studies variance $\tau^2 = 0.3441$
Test of SMD$=0$: $z = 3.63$, $P < 0.001$

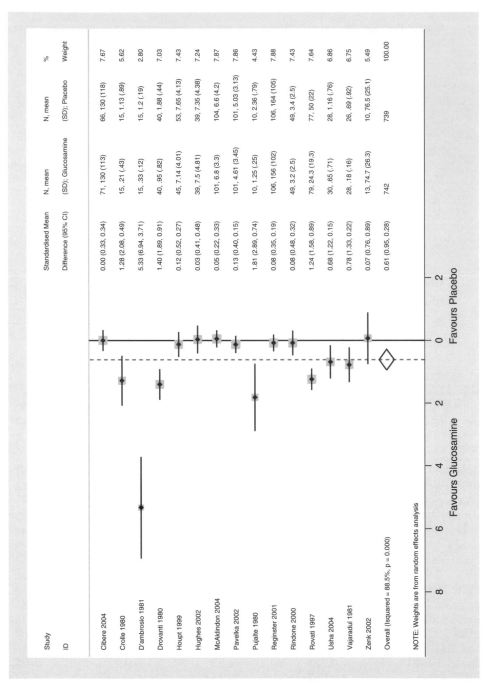

Figure 12.3 Forest plot of standardized mean differences in post-randomization pain score in 15 RCTs comparing glucosamine and placebo treatment for osteoarthritis based on a random effects model. From Towheed, T.E., Maxwell, L., Anastassiades, *et al.*, Glucosamine therapy for treating osteoarthritis. *Cochrane Database of Systematic Reviews* 2005, Issue 2. Art. No.: CD002946. DOI: 10.1002/14651858.CD002946.pub2. © 2005 Cochrane Collaboration, reproduced with permission.

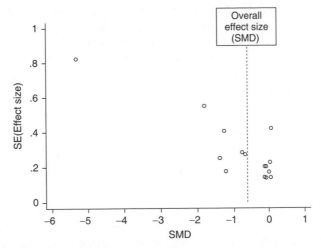

Figure 12.4   Funnel plot of standard error of the treatment effect against the standardized mean differences (SMD) in post-randomization pain score in 15 randomised controlled trials comparing Glucosamine vs. Placebo treatment for Osteoarthritis based on a random effects model (data from Towheed *et al.*, 2005).

with low precision being larger than that of studies with high precision, resulting in a funnel-like shape. Some graphs mark the funnel with lines within which 95% of studies would fall were there no between-studies heterogeneity. The choice of the measure of treatment effect and the measure of precision makes a difference to the shape of the plot. Plots of treatment effects against standard errors are usually to be preferred, as the funnel will have straight rather than curved sides (Deeks, 2005). Figure 12.4 shows a funnel plot with effect size data from the random effects model. The plot appears to have a reasonably symmetrical distribution around the overall effect line, but again there does appear to be an outlying study.

   Interpretation of funnel plots is often visually difficult due to there being inadequate numbers of studies. Assessing the causes of funnel plot asymmetry is also difficult as between-studies heterogeneity, relationships between study quality and sample size, as well as publication bias can all cause similar patterns in funnel plots (Egger *et al.*, 1997).

   The forest and funnel plots can be produced using the Cochrane Collaborations Review Manager software, commonly known as 'Rev Man'. Alternatively, they can be produced in more general statistical packages such as STATA. STATA does not have a meta-analysis command. STATA users, however, have developed an excellent suite of commands for performing meta-analyses, such as `metan` and `funnel`.

12.4   Presentation of results

The published report of the results of a meta-analysis is usually the only information about the study that is available to readers. So the description of the study methods and procedures must be comprehensive, and the presentation of study findings must be especially clear. Specific information that should be included in the published reports is as follows (Pettiti, 1999):

1. *Identification of eligible studies.* The details of the procedures that were used to identify studies eligible for the meta-analysis should be given. The report should describe the exact terms that were used to search MEDLINE etc. Methods for finding unpublished studies should be described. All of the studies with relevant material that were identified should be cited. For excluded studies, the reason for exclusion should be presented.

2. *Quality rating.* If the studies were rated on quality, the methods for obtaining the ratings should be described.

3. *Data abstraction.* The report should describe the procedures for abstracting data from the study reports. The procedures for handling missing data should be described.

4. *Statistical analysis.* The report should explain the reason for the choice of effect measure. The rationale for the choice of fixed or random effects model should be stated. The method for arriving at the summary estimate of effect and its confidence limits should be described. The statistical test for homogeneity should be described along with the results of the test. If the statistical test suggests the studies are heterogeneous then the effect of this heterogeneity on the conclusions and model choice should be discussed. If the quality of studies was rated, the method for taking it into account should be described.

5. *Discussion.* The possibility of publication bias should be addressed. Evidence for or against publication bias should be presented.

12.5   Conclusion

There is no empirical basis for preferring the fixed effects model over the random effects model (Petitti, 1999). Thompson and Pocock (1991) point out that the choice of a fixed or random effects model is secondary to the examination of the reasons for lack of homogeneity. If the studies are homogeneous, then the choice between the fixed effects model and the random effects model is unimportant as the models will yield results that are identical (Petitti, 1999).

Petitti (1999) states that use of the random effects model is not considered to be a defensible solution to the problem of heterogeneity and the random effects model is generally 'conservative'. In most situations the use of the random effects model will lead to wider confidence intervals and a lower chance of calling a difference 'statistically significant'. The desire to be conservative is a reason to use the random effects model, but only in the absence of heterogeneity.

Some of the concerns about meta-analysis are broad concerns based on philosophy. Meta-analysis has been subjected to formal evaluations, and the results of these formal evaluations are not all favourable. Although the use of meta-analysis is growing rapidly, enthusiasm about it is not universal. Eysenck (1978), in an often quoted letter titled 'an exercise in mega-silliness', said of meta-analysis: '"Garbage in garbage out" is a well known axiom of computer specialists; it applies here with equal force.'

The quality of meta-analysis, its reproducibility and its correlation with the results of 'definitive' studies have all been formally evaluated. The results of these evaluations give a mixed picture of meta-analysis.

12.6   Further reading

For up-to-date information about systematic reviews and meta-analysis the interested reader is referred to the Cochrane Collaboration website http://www.cochrane. org/. This includes the Cochrane Library which contains high-quality, independent evidence to inform health-care decision-making. It includes reliable evidence from Cochrane and other systematic reviews, clinical trials and more. The Cochrane Handbook for Systematic Reviews of Interventions is the official document that describes in detail the process of preparing and maintaining Cochrane systematic reviews on the effects of health-care interventions (Higgins and Green, 2008). The current version of the Handbook is 5.0.1 (updated September 2008). It is available to browse online (or to download) at www.cochrane-handbook.org. The browsable Handbook is also available from the help menu in Review Manager 5 (software for composing Cochrane Reviews) which is available to download at http://www.cc-ims.net/RevMan. There are also a number of useful books that cover meta-analysis; see Egger *et al.* (2001), Hedges and Olkin (1985), Petitti (1999) and Sutton *et al.* (2000).

Exercises

12.1 Towheed *et al.* (2005) reviewed the use of glucosamine for treating osteoarthritis and identified 20 RCTs, with 2750 patients overall, suitable for inclusion. Of these, eight trials were found to have adequate allocation concealment and be placebo controlled and reported pain QoL outcomes post randomization. Table 12.7 shows the results for these eight studies. Each study is listed with its sample size, mean pain scale score and its variability separately for the glucosamine and placebo groups.

   (a) Overall how many osteoarthritis patients were involved in the eight RCTs?

   (b) Calculate the standardized mean difference (SMD) for each study using Hedges' adjusted g.

Table 12.7   Summary statistics for post-randomization pain scores for the eight randomized controlled trials comparing glucosamine and placebo treatment for osteoarthritis (data from Towheed *et al* 2005).

Study	Author	Glucosamine			Placebo		
		n	Mean	SD	n	mean	SD
1	Cibere 2004	71	129.72	113.23	66	129.62	118.02
2	Houpt 1999	45	7.14	4.01	53	7.65	4.13
3	Hughes 2002	39	7.50	4.81	39	7.35	4.38
4	McAklindon 2004	101	6.80	3.30	104	6.60	4.20
5	Pavelka 2002	101	4.61	3.45	101	5.03	3.13
6	Reginster 2001	106	156.10	101.90	106	164.20	104.50
7	Rovati 1997	79	24.30	19.30	77	50.00	22.00
8	Zenk 2002	13	−74.70	26.30	10	−76.50	25.10

(c) Calculate the standard error of the SMD (from Hedges' adjusted g) for each study.

(d) Using the fixed effects inverse variance method, calculate the weights for each study. Which study or studies has the largest weight?

(e) Calculate 95% confidence intervals for each of the SMD estimates for the eight studies.

(f) Calculate the heterogeneity chi-squared statistic and comment on the results. Does the heterogeneity chi-squared statistic suggest that the results from the eight studies are homogenous and broadly similar?

(g) Calculate the I^2 statistic and comment on the results.

(h) Calculate the overall pooled SMD across the eight studies and its associated 95% confidence interval. Comment on the results. Do the pooled SMD and its confidence interval favour glucosamine treatment over placebo treatment?

(i) Plot the individual study SMDs and their associated 95% confidence intervals on a forest plot. Include the overall pooled SMD and its associated confidence interval in this forest plot.

12.2 Using the data from Table 12.6 (and some of the calculations from Exercise 12.1) repeat the meta-analysis but this time using a random effects model.

(a) Comment on the results of the random effects model meta-analysis. Do the pooled SMD and its confidence interval favour glucosamine treatment over placebo treatment?

(b) Do you think a fixed or random effects model is appropriate for the data?

(c) Using the results from the random effects meta-analysis, produce a funnel plot of the SMD against its standard error. Include in the plot a line with the overall pooled SMD. Comment on the shape of the funnel plot.

13

Practical issues

Summary

This chapter will look at some practical issues when analysing and reporting studies which have used QoL outcomes. It will describe the problems that arise through missing QoL data, and how missing QoL values may be estimated or imputed. When many hypothesis tests are performed in the analysis of one study, looking at many QoL variables, a number of spurious positive results can be expected to arise by chance alone. Clearly, the greater the number of tests carried out, the greater the likelihood of finding some significant results, but the expected number of false positive findings will increase too. The problem of multiple comparisons is particularly acute in QoL outcomes. This chapter will describe several ways of adjusting significance levels in order to allow for multiple testing. The chapter will end with a checklist of recommended guidelines for reporting QoL studies.

13.1   Missing data

Quality of life outcome measures are becoming increasingly used in research. QoL measures typically have several dimensions and use multiple questions or items to measure these dimensions. This section will provide a practical overview of methods for dealing with missing QoL data. It will also discuss the draft guidance of the US Food and Drug Administration (FDA) for using QoL outcomes (and dealing with missing data) in medicinal product development (FDA, 2006).

13.1.1   Why do missing data matter?

Missing data matter because, if there are missing data in a study then the results may be biased and not reflect the true state of affairs. If the proportion of missing data is small

Quality of Life Outcomes in Clinical Trials and Health-Care Evaluation   Stephen J. Walters
© 2009 John Wiley & Sons, Ltd

Box 13.1 Patterns of missing data

1. *Missing completely at random (MCAR).* when the probability of response at time t is independent of both the previously observed values and the unobserved values at time t.

2. *Not missing at random (NMAR).* when the probability of response at time t depends on the unobserved values at time t.

3. *Missing at random (MAR).* when the probability of response at time t depends on the previously observed values but not the unobserved values at time t.

---

then little bias will result. If the proportion of data missing is not small then a crucial question is: are the characteristics of patients with missing data different from those for whom complete data are available? If the answer is yes then the study results will be biased and will not reflect the truth.

There are essentially two main types of missing QoL data: item non-response and unit non-response. *Item non-response* arises when there are single missing item(s) from an otherwise complete questionnaire. *Unit non-response* is when the whole QoL questionnaire missing when one was anticipated from the patient. Box 13.1 also shows that there are essentially three patterns of missing data.

13.1.2 Methods for missing items within a form

When individual items from a multi-item scale are missing there are problems in calculating scores for the summated scale. Methods have been developed to impute the most likely value for these missing items.

13.1.2.1 Treat the score for the scale as missing

If any of the constituent items are missing, the scale score for that patient is excluded from all statistical analyses. When data are MCAR, this reduced data set represents a randomly drawn subsample of the full data set and inferences drawn can be considered reasonable.

13.1.2.2 Simple mean imputation

For instruments that use unweighted scores, the missing item can be estimated from the mean of the items that are available. The Role Physical (RP) scale of the SF-36v2 is formed by summing the raw responses to the four items and then transforming this sum onto a 0–100 scale. Figure 13.1 shows that question 4b is missing from the RP scale. The mean score of the three completed items is

$$(Q_{4a} + Q_{4c} + Q_{4d})/3 = (1 + 2 + 2)/3 = 1.67.$$

This mean score of 1.67 can then be substituted for the missing Q_{4b} and used to calculate the RP scale score.

4. During the <u>past 4 Weeks,</u> how much of the time have you had any of
    the following problems with your work or other regular daily
    activities as a result of your <u>physical health?</u>

(Please circle one number on each line)

	All of the time	Most of the time	Some of the time	A little of the time	None of the time
a. Cut down on the **amount of time** you spent on work or other activities	①	2	3	4	5
b. **Accomplished less** than you would like	1	2	3	4	5
c. Were limited in the **kind** of work or other activities	1	②	3	4	5
d. Had **difficulty** performing the work or other activities (for example, it took extra effort)	1	②	3	4	5

Figure 13.1   The Role Physical dimension of the SF-36v2.

	Not at all	A little	Quite a bit	Very Much
1. Do you have any trouble doing strenuous activities, like carrying a heavy shopping bag or a suitcase?	1	2✓	3	4
2. Do you have any trouble taking a <u>long</u> walk?	1	2	3	4
3. Do you have any trouble taking a <u>short</u> walk outside of the house?	1	2	3	4✓
4. Do you have to stay in a bed or chair during the day?	1	2✓	3	4
5. Do you need help with eating, dressing, washing yourself or using the toilet?	1✓	2	3	4

Figure 13.2   The Physical Functioning (PF) scale of the EORTC-C30 (V3.0).

13.1.2.3   Hierarchical scales

Figure 13.2 shows that the five items in the Physical Function (PF) scale of the EORTC QLQ-C30 are *hierarchical*. If a patient replies 'very much' to Q3 about troubles with a short walk, but does not answer Q2, it would not be sensible to base an imputed value for this missing response on the average of all answered items. Clearly those who have difficulties with short walks would have even greater problems with a long walk. It may be reasonable to impute a value of 4 (very much) for Q2 for troubles with a long walk.

13.1.2.4   Regression imputation

This technique replaces missing values by predicted values obtained from a regression of the missing item variable on the remaining items of the scale. The data used for this calculation are from all those subjects in the study with complete information on all variables within the scale. For example, suppose that the missing item is Q4b on the RP scale, but the patient completed Q4a, Q4c, and Q4d. Then a value for the missing Q4b item can be estimated from the following equation:

$$Q_{4b} = b_0 + b_1 Q_{4a} + b_2 Q_{4c} + b_3 Q_{4d}. \qquad (13.1)$$

13.1.3   Methods for missing forms

Missing forms tend to be a far more serious problem than missing items. Forms are more frequently missing, and if a form is missing, so are all the constituent items on the form. When a whole QoL assessment is missing the imputation procedure must use information from other 'similar' patients, values from previous and/or later assessments by the same patient, or a mixture of both. If items are used only as components of the scale, it may not be necessary to impute values for those items, only for the scale score itself. Table 13.1 shows some patterns of missing SF-36 Bodily Pain data from 10 randomly selected patients with low back pain from an RCT to compare the effectiveness of acupuncture vs. usual care for the treatment of low back pain (Thomas *et al.*, 2006). All 10 subjects had a valid baseline (0 months) SF-36 Bodily Pain score and three had valid SF-36 Bodily Pain scores at all four assessment points. The primary outcome for this study was the SF-36 Bodily Pain score at 12 months post randomization.

13.1.3.1   Last observation carried forward

A simple method of missing data imputation is the last observation carried forward (LOCF). The values that were recorded by the patient at the last previously completed QoL assessment are carried forward. For example, in Table 13.1 patient number 1 has three missing QoL assessments at 3, 12 and 24 months respectively. Using LOCF, the

Table 13.1   Patterns of missing SF-36 Bodily Pain data for 10 patients with low back pain from the acupuncture study (data from Thomas *et al.*, 2006).

Patient No.	Group	Age	Sex	0 months	3 months	12 months	24 months
1	Usual care	30	Female	33.3	.	.	.
2	Usual care	38	Female	0	11.1	.	.
3	Acupuncture care	36	Female	11.1	.	77.8	77.8
4	Acupuncture care	23	Male	33.3	44.4	.	.
5	Usual care	32	Male	11.1	22.2	22.2	.
6	Usual care	46	Male	44.4	.	100	.
7	Usual care	46	Male	11.1	44.4	44.4	100
8	Acupuncture care	50	Male	44.4	88.9	88.9	.
9	Usual care	41	Male	55.6	100	55.6	77.8
10	Usual care	34	Male	22.2	55.6	22.2	22.2
		Mean		26.7	52.4	58.7	69.5
		SD		18.3	32.5	31.3	33.2
		Valid *n*		10	7	7	4

baseline value of the pain score would be carried forward to give the following imputed scores (in italics).

Patient 1:   33.3   *33.3   33.3   33.3*

13.1.3.2   Simple mean imputation

This is usually the replacement of missing QoL scores by the mean score calculated for patients who *did* complete the assessment. For example, Table 13.1 shows that the mean SF-36 Bodily Pain score at 12 months was $\bar{x} = 58.7$ for those seven patients who were assessed. For those patients who are missing, their missing QoL score will be imputed as $x_i = \bar{x} = 58.7$. So patients would now have the following imputed Pain scores at 12 months.

Patient 1:	33.3		*58.7*
Patient 2:	0	11.1	*58.7*
Patient 4:	33.3	44.4	*58.7*

13.1.3.3   Reduced standard deviation

A feature of mean imputation is that the estimate of the mean of the augmented dataset remains the same as $\bar{x}$, the mean for the original data. For example, if we use mean imputation to calculate the three missing 12-month SF-36 Bodily Pain scores in Table 13.1 the mean is still 58.7. However, the estimate of the standard deviation will be reduced artificially. It has gone down from 31.3 to 25.5. This can lead to a reduced standard error and hence distorted significance tests and falsely narrow confidence intervals. The SD can be corrected or equivalently use the SD of the non-missing values, i.e. 31.3 in this example.

13.1.3.4   Horizontal mean imputation

Unlike LOCF, mean imputation takes no account of the longitudinal nature of the data. An alternative to simple mean imputation is to impute the missing value from the mean of the patient's own previous scores. This method is termed horizontal as it takes into account the longitudinal nature of the QoL data. It reduces to the LOCF method if there is only one previous assessment available or if there has been no change in QoL score over time.

For example, in Table 13.1, patients 2 and 4 have valid baseline and 3-month SF-36 Bodily Pain scores. The mean baseline and 3-month scores for patients 2 and 4 are 5.6 and 38.9, respectively. So patients 2 and 4 would now have the following imputed Pain scores at 12 months:

Patient 2:	0	11.1	*5.6*
Patient 4:	33.3	44.4	*38.9*

13.1.3.5   Regression imputation of missing forms

Multiple linear regression models are another way of imputing missing QoL values. The simplest regression method uses patients with valid QoL scores at the time point of interest to develop a regression model to predict this value. The regression equation is then applied to subjects with missing QoL values (but with valid values for the predictor variables in the regression model) to impute the missing QoL values. The regression models may contain baseline characteristics or other prognostic factors as covariates (such as age and sex) as well as previous or later QoL assessments.

For example, we could use the seven patients with valid baseline and 12-month SF-36 Bodily Pain score data (in Table 13.1) to develop a regression model to impute the missing 12-month SF-36 Bodily Pain score, using the baseline Pain score and covariates such as age and sex. A multiple linear regression imputation, based on the seven patients who completed both a baseline and 12-month SF-36 Bodily Pain score, produced the following model:

$$\text{Pain}_{12-\text{months}} = -90.20 + 0.68\text{Pain}_{\text{baseline}} + 3.00\text{Age} + 52.50\text{Sex} \qquad (13.2)$$

$$(\text{SE } 46.94) \quad (0.47) \qquad (1.24) \qquad (20.90) \qquad (R^2 = 0.84)$$

Sex was coded as $0 = $ male and $1 = $ female.

This model suggests that SF-36 Bodily Pain score increases with baseline Pain score, increasing age and being female. For example, patient 1, a woman aged 30 with a baseline Pain score of 33.3 (and a missing 12-month Pain score) would have a regression imputed 12-month Pain score of

$$-90.2 + (0.68 \times 33.3) + (3.00 \times 30) + (52.50 \times 1) = 74.8.$$

Similarly, patient 2, another woman aged 38 with a baseline Pain score of 0, would have an imputed 12-month SF-36 Bodily Pain score of 76.3. Patient 4, a man aged 23 with a baseline pain score of 33.3, would have an imputed 12-month SF-36 Bodily Pain score of 1.3. Of course, the regression model would use the available data from all low back patients in the acupuncture trial and not just this random sample of 10 subjects.

Example: The PONDER cRCT

The PONDER study was a cluster randomized controlled trial (cRCT) in primary care designed to evaluate the effectiveness of new health visitor (HV) led psychological intervention in detecting and treating new mothers with postnatal depression (PND) compared to usual care. The PONDER trial randomized 100 clusters (GP practices and their associated health visitors) and collected data on 2659 new mothers with an 18-month follow-up. The participants were 1745 women (in 63 clusters) allocated to intervention, and 914 (in 37 clusters) allocated to control. The main outcome measure was the 6-month Edinburgh Postnatal Depression Scale score, on a 0–30 scale, with a higher score indicating more depressive symptoms; a score greater than 12 is regarded as being 'at higher risk' of PND. Table 13.2 shows the mean EPDS score for the 'higher risk' mothers with a 6-week score of 12 or more for the two treatment groups: 595 women reported a 6-week EPDS score of 12 or more. At 6-month follow-up 418 women had both a 6-week and 6-month EPDS score and were available for the complete case based statistical analysis. A sensitivity analysis was performed to impute the missing 6-month EPDS data for the 177/595 (30%) of women who were lost to follow-up.

Two forms of missing data imputation were performed: LOCF and regression imputation. LOCF imputation is very conservative and represents the worst-case scenario,

Table 13.2 Comparison of mean 6-month EPDS scores between control and intervention groups with regression and LOCF imputation of missing 6-month EPDS data.

	Group Control			Intervention			95% CI			P-
	n	Mean	SD	n	Mean	SD	Difference	Lower	Upper	value
EPDS score (6 weeks)	191	15.4	(3.2)	404	15.4	(3.2)				
EPDS score (6 months)	147	11.3	(5.8)	271	9.2	(5.4)	−2.1	−3.4	−0.8	0.002
EPDS 6 month (with LOCF)	191	12.1	(5.5)	404	11.5	(5.9)	−0.7	−1.8	0.4	0.233
EPDS 6 month (Regression Imputed)	191	11.0	(5.2)	404	9.7	(4.6)	−1.3	−2.3	−0.3	0.009

EPDS = Edinburgh Postnatal Depression Scale.
LOCF (Last observation carried forward) imputation (i.e. 6-week EPDS score carried forward to 6 months).
Regression imputation, based on the following model, from $n = 2659$ women who completed both a 6-week and 6-month EPDS:

$$EPDS_{6\text{-months}} = 2.287 \text{ (SE } 0.135) + 0.526 \text{ (SE } 0.17) \text{ } EPDS_{6\text{-weeks}} \text{ } (R^2 = 0.269)$$

where the 6-week EPDS score is carried forward to 6 months. For example, a woman with a 6-week EPDS score of, say, 12 (and a missing 6-month EPDS score) would have an LOCF imputed 6-month EPDS score of 12. A more realistic form of imputation is regression imputation, which better reflects the natural aetiology and epidemiology of PND and PND symptoms which tend to decline over time after childbirth. Regression imputation, based on the $n = 2659$ women who completed both a 6-week and 6-month EPDS, produced the following model (see Figure 13.3):

$$EPDS_{6\text{-months}} = 2.287 \text{ (SE } 0.135) + 0.526 \text{ (SE } 0.17) \text{ } EPDS_{6\text{-weeks}} \text{ } (R^2 = 0.269) \quad (13.3)$$

For example, a woman with a 6-week EPDS score of 12 (and a missing 6-month EPDS score) would have a regression imputed 6-month EPDS score of $2.287 + (12 \times 0.526)$, i.e. 9.2. □

Table 13.2 shows the results of sensitivity analysis for the imputation of missing data and compares it with the complete-case analysis. Using LOCF imputation, the results change markedly and the observed treatment effect is now smaller and not statistically significant. Using regression imputation, the results are similar to the complete-case analysis, although the observed treatment effect is now smaller.

13.1.3.6 Markov chain imputation

In the methods described so far, the imputed values will be the same for any two patients with the same profile of successive non-missing values. Markov chain (MC) imputation allows these two patients to have different imputed QoL values. It assigns, for a patient

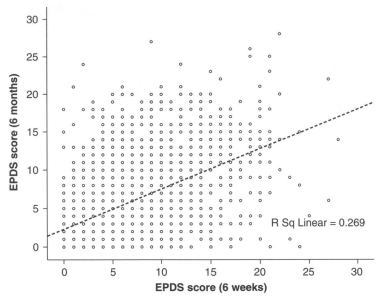

Figure 13.3   Scatter plot of the relationship between the 6-month and 6-week EPDS scores ($n = 2659$) with the regression line of best fit (data from Morrell *et al.*, 2009).

in a particular QoL state at one assessment, *transition* probabilities of being in each of the possible states, including the same at the next assessment. Table 13.3 shows an estimated matrix of transition probabilities between baseline and 12-month SF-36 Bodily Pain scores for 215 low back pain patients in the acupuncture trial.

Example: MC imputation

For patients 1 and 4 in Table 13.1 the 12-month QoL assessment was missing. For both patients the baseline SF-36 Bodily Pain score was 33.3. Table 13.4 shows a simplified version of the transition matrix of Table 13.3 with only the baseline SF-36 Bodily Pain score of 33.3 and the associated transition probabilities. Table 13.4 shows that the probability of having a 12-month Pain score of 22.2, given a baseline score of 33.3, is 0.02. The probability of having a 12-month Pain score of 33.3 (i.e. unchanged) is 0.10. To impute missing values we make use of these transition probabilities together with a table of random numbers from 0 to 100. Table 13.4 shows the correspondence between the random numbers and the imputed 12-month SF-36 Bodily Pain score. If the random number generated is between 0 and 2 we impute a score of 22.2 for the missing QoL score at 12 months. If the random number generated is greater than 2 and less than or equal to 12 we impute a score of 33.3 for the missing QoL score at 12 months. Suppose, for patient 1, the random number generated is 10; then a 12-month SF-36 Bodily Pain score of 33.3 is imputed. Suppose for patient 4 the random number generated is 50; then a 12-month SF-36 Bodily Pain score of 66.7 is imputed from Table 13.4.   □

This example clearly illustrates that MC imputation allows two patients, both with the same baseline pain scores to have different imputed pain scores at 12 months.

Table 13.3 Matrix of transition probabilities between baseline and 12-month SF-36 Bodily Pain scores for 215 low back pain patients in the acupuncture trial.

		SF-36 Bodily Pain (12 months)									
		0.0	11.1	22.2	33.3	44.4	55.6	66.7	77.8	88.9	100.0	Total
SF-36 Bodily Pain (baseline)	**0.0**	*0.10*	*0.00*	*0.10*	*0.00*	*0.20*	*0.30*	*0.00*	*0.20*	*0.00*	*0.10*	1.00
	11.1	*0.06*	*0.09*	*0.22*	*0.06*	*0.13*	*0.09*	*0.06*	*0.06*	*0.16*	*0.06*	*1.00*
	22.2	*0.00*	*0.00*	*0.10*	*0.06*	*0.27*	*0.08*	*0.11*	*0.10*	*0.16*	*0.13*	*1.00*
	33.3	*0.00*	*0.00*	*0.02*	*0.10*	*0.14*	*0.21*	*0.21*	*0.14*	*0.07*	*0.10*	*1.00*
	44.4	*0.00*	*0.00*	*0.03*	*0.00*	*0.13*	*0.25*	*0.13*	*0.20*	*0.15*	*0.13*	*1.00*
	55.6	*0.00*	*0.00*	*0.00*	*0.06*	*0.25*	*0.31*	*0.06*	*0.00*	*0.19*	*0.13*	*1.00*
	66.7	*0.00*	*0.00*	*0.00*	*0.00*	*0.10*	*0.10*	*0.20*	*0.30*	*0.10*	*0.20*	*1.00*
	77.8	*0.00*	*0.00*	*0.00*	*0.00*	*0.00*	*0.00*	*0.00*	*0.50*	*0.50*	*0.00*	*1.00*

Table 13.4 Transition probabilities and associated random number values between baseline and 12-month SF-36 Bodily Pain scores for patients with a baseline SF-36 Bodily Pain score of 33.2.

| | | SF-36 Bodily Pain (12 months) | | | | | | | |
		22.2	33.3	44.4	55.6	66.7	77.8	88.9	100.0
SF-36 Bodily Pain (baseline)	**33.3** *Probability*	0.02	0.10	0.14	0.21	0.21	0.14	0.07	0.10
	Random number (0 to 100)	0 to 2	>2 to 12	>12 to 26	>26 to 47	>47 to 68	>68 to 82	>82 to 90	>90 to 100

Of course for patient 4 who has a 3-month QoL assessment we could use a different matrix of transition probabilities based on the 3-month and 12-month SF-36 Bodily Pain scores and not the baseline and 12-months outcomes.

13.1.3.7   Hot deck imputation

This technique selects at random, from patients with observed QoL data, the QoL score from one of these and substitutes this as the imputed value for the patient with the missing QoL assessment. The *hot deck* refers to the deck of responses of patients with observed data from which the missing QoL score is selected. The particular deck chosen may be restricted to those patients who are similar to the patient (e.g. the same age or sex) with the missing QoL score.

For example, in Table 13.1, patient 4 is male and aged 23 and has a missing 12-month SF-36 Bodily Pain score. We could use a hot deck of male patients to impute the missing 12-month SF-36 Bodily Pain score. Restricting the hot deck to male subjects means we would use the six patients (numbered 5 to 10 in Table 13.1) with valid 12-month QoL scores to impute the missing Pain score for patient 4.

13.1.3.8   The expectation–maximization algorithm

Fayers and Machin (2007) describe another method for imputing missing values called the expectation–maximization (EM) algorithm. The EM method is particularly useful when many patients have missing forms at different time points, because there may be too few patients with complete data for whom we are able to derive hot decks or transition probabilities.

To use the EM algorithm we must first decide on the imputation method for estimating the missing items. For example, we could use multiple linear regression to estimate the missing QoL outcomes. The EM algorithm is as follows:

1. Replace all missing values with the estimates that are predicted from the regression.

2. With the new data set, recalculate the parameters of the regression equation.

3. Now repeat from (1), using the revised regression equation as just calculated in (2).

This iterative procedure is continued until the values 'put back' do not differ from those just 'taken out'.

13.1.3.9   Multiple imputation

If deterministic methods such as LOCF are used, then the augmented data set will be unique. If a random element is included in the choice of missing values, the augmented data set will be just a single random one out of many potential datasets. The idea of multiple imputation is that many alternative 'complete' datasets can be created. The analysis can be repeated for each data set and then combined into a final summary analysis (Rubin, 1987).

13.1.4   The regulator's view on statistical considerations for patient-level missing data

The FDA regulator recommends that the Statistical Analysis Plan (SAP) describes how the statistical analyses will handle missing QoL data when evaluating treatment efficacy and when considering patient success or patient response (FDA, 2006). At a specific patient visit, a QoL dimension measurement may be missing some, but not all, items. Defining rules that specify the number of items that can be missing and still consider the dimension to have been measured is one approach to handling this type of missing data. Rules for handling missing data should be specific to each QoL instrument and should usually be determined during the instrument development and validation process. The FDA recommends that all rules be specified in the SAP. For example, the SAP can specify that a domain will be treated as missing if more than 25% of the items are missing; if less than 25% of the items are missing, the domain score can be taken to be the average of the non-missing items.

When the amount of missing data becomes large, study results can be inconclusive. As described earlier, the FDA encourages pre-specified procedures in the study protocol, particularly when patients discontinue study treatment. Because missing data may be due to the treatment received or the underlying disease and can introduce bias in the analysis of treatment differences and conclusions about treatment impact, the FDA encourages investigators to obtain data on each patient at the time of withdrawal to determine the reason for withdrawal. When available, this information can be taken into account in the analysis.

A variety of statistical strategies have been proposed in the literature and in applications to the FDA to deal with missing data due to patient withdrawal from assigned treatment exposure prior to planned completion of the trial. The FDA (2006) draft guidance states that: 'No single method is generally accepted as preferred.' One strategy used in the past was to exclude subjects from the analyses if they did not complete the study (i.e. completers' analysis). The FDA states that this strategy is generally inadvisable because the reason for missing data can be treatment-related and these patients may not adequately represent the study population.

The FDA is equally sceptical of other methods of imputation such as LOCF. LOCF enables every patient randomized to contribute some observation to the analysis, but the FDA (2006) believes it can be problematic for the following reasons:

> 'If the objective of the trial is to detect a treatment effect after a certain duration of treatment (e.g. at 8 weeks), then a comparison that includes only measurements on patients at earlier times or visits is not addressing the original trial objective. The average of patient responses, many of which are at different times or visits, may be uninterpretable. LOCF makes an implicit assumption that the patient would sustain the same response seen at an early study visit for the entire duration of the trial. This assumption is untestable and potentially unrealistic.'

The FDA guidance on other imputation strategies, such as regression, hot deck and MC, for imputing missing QoL data is equally sceptical. These strategies try to predict missing outcomes for a patient who has withdrawn from the trial using data from subjects who stayed in the trial and for whom all data have been collected. 'All of these strategies are imperfect, as they involve strong or weak assumptions about what caused data to be missing, assumptions that usually cannot be verified from the data' (FDA, 2006). If missing data are associated with the treatment effect in ways that cannot be predicted from measurements on subjects with complete data, analyses using imputation procedures will be biased.

The FDA recommends use of several imputation methods. When there are few patients with missing measurements and the frequency of missing data or proportion of patients with missing data is comparable across treatment groups, most approaches will yield similar results. When a higher proportion of patients have missing data, the FDA recommends the use of several different imputation methods (including a worst-case scenario in which missing data are assumed to be unfavourable for those on the investigational treatment and favourable for those in the control group) and an assessment of the consistency of the study results using each method. These analyses will demonstrate the sensitivity of the conclusions to the assumptions made by the different methods.

Many investigators (and the FDA) are suspicious about using imputation techniques, because of the assumptions overtly involved. However, not imputing missing data makes the assumption that patients failing to respond are similar to those who do. Imputation tries to use the available information to make better allowances for patients with missing data. Markov chain and hot deck imputation are more efficient as they take additional patient information into account and preserve the magnitude of the standard deviations so standard errors, confidence intervals, and P-values can be correctly calculated. The best imputation method may be specific to the individual items or scales concerned as well as the assessment sequence. The key points are to decide the method(s) of imputation in advance. The QoL scales which are primary outcomes should be the focus for determining the imputation process. Sophisticated imputation methods are no substitute for the real data. The best way of dealing with missing data is not to have any!

13.1.5   Conclusions and further reading on missing QoL data

Throughout this book I have assumed that any missing QoL values in the datasets are MCAR. This means that the probability of the QoL response being missing is independent of the scores on the previous observed questionnaires and independent of the current and future scores had they been observed. I have assumed that the reduced data set represents a randomly drawn subsample of the full data set and the inferences drawn can be considered reasonable. This is a strong assumption and needs to be checked. However, there is an extensive literature on the issue of missing values and QoL outcomes. The imputation of missing QoL scores and the analysis of QoL data with missing values is discussed in Curran et al., (1998a, 1998b), Fayers et al., (1998), Troxel et al., (1998), Fairclough (2002) and Fayers and Machin (2007).

This section has provided a practical overview of methods for dealing with missing QoL data, including methods for dealing with:

(i) missing items within dimensions;

(ii) missing entire dimensions or measurements.

The US regulator the FDA regards most imputation methods as 'imperfect'. However, the FDA recommends:

(i) specifying imputation methods in advance in the SAP;

(ii) imputing missing QoL items according to instrument developer's guidelines;

(iii) using several imputation methods with a sensitivity analysis of the results.

Pragmatically, I think the FDA recommendations on missing data imputation methods are valid for most studies with QoL outcomes, not just pharmaceutical trials, and I would recommend their use.

13.2   Multiplicity, multi-dimensionality and multiple quality of life outcomes

The SF-36 is an example of a profile measure of QoL with eight different dimensions, plus two further summary components. This is a common feature of many other QoL instruments such as the NHP and EORTC QLQ-C30 that can have a number of dimensions. For example, in an RCT with three treatment groups (A, B, C) using the SF-36 measure, with repeated QoL assessments at baseline and 1, 2 and 3 months post randomization, there is a multiplicity of QoL outcomes. We have three groups with three post-randomization QoL assessments using a QoL instrument with eight dimensions. This leads to $3 \times 3 \times 8 = 72$ possible outcomes. When several QoL outcomes are collected on the same people, it is always possible to test each variable separately. However, this will lead to potential problem of multiple comparisons or multiple hypothesis testing.

Throughout this book I have taken a simpler *univariate* approach where each individual QoL dimension is analysed separately (although in some cases the test statistic is derived from a multiple-variable longitudinal marginal analysis). For example, in an RCT, if two groups are compared using the SF-36 then a difference between the means for the two groups can be tested separately for each of the eight dimensions of the SF-36. Unfortunately, there is a drawback to this approach because of the repeated use of significance tests means the probability of falsely finding at least one significant difference accumulates with the number of tests carried out. That is, univariate tests of each QoL dimension and time point can seriously inflate the Type I (false positive) α error rate for the overall trial such that the analyst is unable to distinguish between true and false positive differences. Multiple comparisons arise from three main sources (Pocock, 1983; Fairclough, 2002):

1. multiple QoL measures;

2. repeated post randomization assessments;

3. multiple (three or more) treatment arms.

Three strategies to reduce the problem of multiple comparisons and multiple outcomes (Pocock, 1983; Fairclough, 2002) are:

1. a priori specification of a limited number of *confirmatory* tests;

2. the use of summary measures or statistics (e.g. AUC);

3. multiple comparison procedures including α adjustments (e.g. Bonferroni).

In practice, a combination of all three strategies, that is, focused hypotheses, summary measures, and multiple comparison procedures are necessary.

One recommended solution (Fayers and Machin, 2007) to the multiple comparison problem is to specify a limited number of a priori endpoints in the design of the trial (say, no more than three). While theoretically improving the overall Type I error rate for a study, in practice investigators are reluctant to ignore the remaining data and still present CI and even formal hypothesis test results for the remaining scales/outcomes. A more important critique of this approach is an ethical question about the collection of data that will not be used in the primary analysis (Fairclough, 2002).

Well-chosen summary measures or statistics often have a greater power to detect patterns of consistent QoL differences across time or measures (Fairclough, 2002). The use of summary measures such as the AUC (as described in Chapter 9) is a good strategy that both simplifies the presentation of the results and reduces the multiplicity of the repeated assessments over time. For example, the use of summary measures such as the AUC in the acupuncture study can reduce the number of hypothesis tests from three (the number of follow-up QoL assessments) to one for each dimension of the SF-36.

Another way of reducing the number of comparisons is to use a *single global multivariate test* that uses the information from all the variables simultaneously. A global test generates a single statistic for testing the overall treatment effect and results in the acceptance or rejection of a set of K hypotheses $\mathbf{H}_0$: $H_{0(1)}$, $H_{0(2)}$, ...,$H_{0(K)}$. For example, in a two-group RCT design using the SF-36 outcome, a null hypothesis would be that the vector of all eight mean QoL dimension scores of the SF-36 in the intervention group is the same as the vector for all eight mean scores for the control group. One global multivariate test is Hotelling's T^2 test for the two-group situation or Multivariate Analysis of Variance (MANOVA) for more than two groups (Manly, 1994). However, the problem with such multivariate methods is that they test very general hypotheses (e.g. whether one group differs in some non-specified way in their QoL from another) and so consequently have very poor power to detect any real difference. Thus, more often than not they will give a non-significant result (Walters et al., 2001c). When the overall test of $\mathbf{H}_0$ has been rejected, the question still remains as to which of the individual hypotheses can be rejected. Unfortunately, a global test does not allow inferences to be made about individual QoL outcomes and a series of univariate tests must be performed for these comparisons.

Tandon (1990) suggested a parametric method that was more specific. For example, to compare two groups, calculate t-tests for each dimension and then find

$$z = \frac{\mathbf{J}' S^{-1} \mathbf{t}}{(\mathbf{J}' S^{-1} \mathbf{J})^{1/2}}, \tag{13.4}$$

where $\mathbf{J}' = (1, \ldots, 1, 1)$, S is the estimated correlation matrix and $\mathbf{t}$ is the vector of t-statistics from the separate univariate t-tests. The test statistic z has an asymptotic standard Normal distribution. The main drawback of this method is that it does not give an estimate of the treatment effect; it just provides a test statistic.

A second way of allowing for multiple comparisons is to adjust the significance level from each univariate test or make what is called an *alpha* adjustment for the K univariate tests, to control the overall Type I error rate. Fairclough (2002) comprehensively describes a number of procedures that can be used to control the Type I error rate for K multiple comparisons using the following notation. Let $H_{0(1)}$, $H_{0(2)}$, ...,$H_{0(K)}$ denote the K null hypotheses that are to be tested and $T_{0(1)}$, $T_{0(2)}$, ... , $T_{0(K)}$ the corresponding K test statistics. The observed P-value, $P_{(k)}$, denotes the *unadjusted* probability of observing the test statistic, $T_{(k)}$, or a more extreme value if the null hypothesis $H_{0(k)}$ is true. The K ordered P-values from smallest to largest can be written as $P_{[1]} \leqslant P_{[2]} \leqslant \cdots \leqslant P_{[K]}$.

Most of the alpha adjustments for K univariate tests described in Fairclough (2002) are a variation of the simple Bonferroni correction described in Chapter 4. The Bonferroni correction adjusts the test statistics on K outcomes. The *global test* is based on the smallest P-value, $P_{[1]}$, for the K QoL outcomes. The global null hypothesis $\mathbf{H}_0$: $H_{0(1)}$, $H_{0(2)}$, ...,$H_{0(K)}$ is rejected when

$$P_{[1]} \leq \alpha/K. \tag{13.5}$$

For individual QoL outcomes the Bonferroni procedure is to accept as statistically significant only those tests with P-values that are less than α/K.

The Bonferroni procedure controls the *experiment-wise error rate* well but is well known to be quite conservative. (The experiment-wise error rate is the probability of incorrectly rejecting at least one true null hypothesis, regardless of which (if any) null hypotheses are true.) If the K outcomes are uncorrelated (the tests are independent) and the null hypotheses are all true, then the probability of rejecting at least one of the K hypotheses is approximately[1] αK when α is small. The Bonferroni approach focuses on the detection of large differences in one or more outcomes and is insensitive to a pattern of smaller differences that are all in the same direction.

The major limitation of all the global tests is that they were developed to control the Type I error rate under the most conservative condition, K independent tests. However, in most studies of QoL, the K outcomes, in this case the various dimensions of the QoL outcomes, are likely to be moderately correlated. As a result, these procedures are very conservative and the power to detect meaningful differences is severely reduced. Fairclough describes a bootstrap algorithm for global hypothesis tests (Box 13.2, from Fairclough, 2002) to address this problem.

The general idea is to obtain an estimate of the distribution of the cut-off test statistic (T_{COT}) for the multiple comparison procedure for outcomes with unknown correlation structure. For example, the simple Bonferroni cut-off test statistic and its associated P-value are $T_{[1]}$ and $P_{[1]}$, respectively (the largest test statistic or the corresponding smallest P-value from the K univariate tests). The bootstrap procedure was first proposed by Westfall and Young (1989) and adapted by Reitmeir and Wasser (1999) for multiple comparisons of K outcomes between two treatment groups.

13.2.1   Which multiple comparison procedure to use?

Pragmatically, I do not like to use multivariate global hypothesis tests, since the interpretation of the results of such tests is difficult. So throughout this book I have tended to use univariate methods and analyse each dimension of the QoL dimension separately,

---

[1] Pr $[\min(P\text{-value}) \leq \alpha] = 1 - (1 - \alpha)^K \approx \alpha K$.

one at a time. Indeed, Fairclough (2002) advocates the use of multiple comparison procedures using a *set of univariate test statistics* rather than those using a single multivariate statistic.

I have not used the bootstrap resampling method (Box 13.2), since there is no general consensus on what procedure to adopt to allow for multiple comparisons (Altman *et al.*, 2000). I believe in following Altman's recommendation of reporting unadjusted *P*-values (to three decimal places or significant figures) and confidence limits with a suitable note of caution with respect to interpretation. As Perneger (1998) concludes: 'Simply describing

---

Box 13.2 Algorithm for computation of the bootstrap global test statistic for K outcomes for a two-group study

Suppose we have two groups of subjects $\mathbf{Z} = (\mathbf{Z}_1, \mathbf{Z}_2, \ldots, \mathbf{Z}_n)$ and $\mathbf{Y} = (\mathbf{Y}_1, \mathbf{Y}_2, \ldots, \mathbf{Y}_m)$, where the $\mathbf{Z}_i$ (and $\mathbf{Y}_i$) consists of a row vector of K QoL responses for subject i, that is, $\mathbf{Z}_i = (z_{i1}, z_{i2}, \ldots, z_{iK})$. If we let the combined sample of QoL responses for $\mathbf{Z}$ and $\mathbf{Y}$ be denoted by $\mathbf{X}$.

1. Identify the statistic for the global test T_{COT} or P_{COT} and calculate it from the observed data. For example, the simple Bonferroni cut-off test statistic and its associated *P*-value are $T_{[1]}$ and $P_{[1]}$ respectively (the largest test statistic or the corresponding smallest *P*-value from the K univariate tests).

2. Draw a random sample of subjects with replacement (bootstrap sample) from the pooled sample $\mathbf{X}$ of the same size as the original sample, call the first n observations $\mathbf{Z}^*$ and the remaining m observations $\mathbf{Y}^*$.

3. Evaluate the global test T_{COT}^* or P_{COT}^* statistic from the data associated with the subjects drawn from the bootstrap sample, b.

4. Repeat the previous two steps B times; $B = 10\,000$ is recommended (Reitmeir and Wassmer, 1999). We now have a bootstrap distribution of B values of T_{COT}^* and P_{COT}^* respectively, that is,

$$(T_{\text{COT}}^{*1}, T_{\text{COT}}^{*2}, \ldots, T_{\text{COT}}^{*B}) \text{ and } (P_{\text{COT}}^{*1}, P_{\text{COT}}^{*2}, \ldots, P_{\text{COT}}^{*B}). \tag{13.6}$$

5. Since the bootstrap statistics were calculated under the null hypothesis by generating the bootstrap samples from the pooled sample, $\mathbf{X}$, the distribution of the global test statistic is approximated by the distribution of the P_{COT}^{*b}.

6. The *P*-value, achieved significance level (ASL^{boot}), for the global test is the proportion of the B bootstrap statistics that are equal to or more extreme than the observed data statistic:

$$\hat{\text{ASL}}_{\text{boot}} = \frac{\#\{P_{\text{COT}}^{*b} \leq P_{\text{COT}}\}}{B} \text{ or } \hat{\text{ASL}}_{\text{boot}} = \frac{\#\{T_{\text{COT}}^{*b} \geq T_{\text{COT}}\}}{B} \tag{13.7}$$

7. If this proportion is less than α, the global test is rejected.

what tests of significance have been performed, and why, is generally the best way of dealing with multiple comparisons.'

Throughout this book, I have favoured a combination of Fayers and Machin's (2007) and Altman *et al.* (2000) approaches to multiple comparisons or endpoints. My favoured approach is to identify the main study QoL endpoints in advance, limit the number of confirmatory hypothesis tests to these outcomes, and report unadjusted *P*-values and confidence limits with a suitable note of caution with respect to interpretation.

13.3   Guidelines for reporting quality of life studies

Quality of life outcome measures are becoming increasing used in clinical trials. Fayers and Machin have produced some general guidelines for the reporting of studies that include a QoL measurement. Table 13.5 shows a checklist of items to include when reporting a study which has used QoL outcomes.

Table 13.5   Checklist of items to include when reporting studies which have used QoL outcomes. Adapted with permission from Fayers, P.M., Machin, D., *Quality of Life: The Assessment, Analysis and Interpretation of Patient-reported Outcomes*. 2nd edition. John Wiley & Sons Ltd, Chichester. © 2007.

	Descriptor
Abstract	Describe the purpose of the study, the methods, the main results and conclusions.
Introduction	
Background	Describe the objective of the study.
	Briefly describe the epidemiology and aetiology of the disease and why QoL is being assessed in this study.
	The study hypotheses for QoL assessment should be stated.
	The definition of QoL should be described.
Methods	
Participants	Eligibility criteria for participants and the settings and locations where the data were collected.
QoL instrument selection	Rationale for choice of QoL instrument, including details of validation and psychometric properties of the instrument.
Sample size	How sample size was determined, on which QoL outcome, and the definition of the minimum important difference.
Outcomes/endpoints	State the dimension(s) of the QoL instrument that are the main outcomes.
Timing and administration of QoL assessments	The scheduled times of instrument administration should be reported.
	Describe the method of administration (e.g. self-completion; interview or proxy assessment; at home or at hospital; by post or at a clinic).

Table 13.5 *(Continued)*

	Descriptor
Data	The procedure for evaluating the quality of the QoL data collected should be described. Methods for imputing missing item and/or form QoL data should be specified.
Statistical methods	Definition of *P*-value level for statistical significance. Statistical methods used to compare groups for primary outcome(s) should be described. As should methods for additional analyses, such as sub-group analyses and adjusted analyses. Any allowance for multiple comparisons should be stated.
Results	
Participant flow	Flow of participants through each stage (a diagram is strongly recommended). Specifically, for each group report the numbers of participants randomly assigned, receiving intended treatment, completing the study pro-tocol, and analysed for the primary outcome. Describe protocol deviations from study as planned, together with reasons.
Recruitment	Dates defining the periods of recruitment and follow-up.
Baseline data	Baseline demographic, clinical and QoL characteristics of each group should be reported.
Numbers analysed	Number of participants (denominator) in each group included in each analysis and whether the analysis was by 'intention to treat'. State the results as absolute numbers when feasible (e.g. 10/20, not 50%).
Outcomes and estimation	For each primary and secondary QoL outcome, give a summary of results for each group, and the estimated effect size and its precision (e.g. 95% confidence interval).
Ancillary analyses	Address multiplicity by reporting any other analyses per-formed, including subgroup analyses and adjusted analy-ses, indicating those pre-specified and those exploratory.
Discussion	
Interpretation	Interpretation of QoL results, taking into account study hypotheses, sources of potential bias or imprecision and the dangers associated with multiplicity of analyses and outcomes. A summary of the clinical results should be reported alongside the QoL results so that a balanced interpretation of the results can be made.
Generalizability	Generalizability (external validity) of the trial findings.
Overall evidence	General interpretation of the results in the context of cur-rent evidence.

Exercises

13.1 Table 13.6 shows the available EQ-5D Visual Analogue Scale (VAS) data for a random sample of 10 patients, with low back pain, from an RCT to compare the effectiveness of acupuncture and usual care for the treatment of low back pain (Thomas *et al.*, 2006). The EQ-5D VAS is scored on a 0 to 100 (good health) scale. Only five of the 10 patients had valid 12-month EQ-5D data.

(a) Use the LOCF method to impute the missing 12-month EQ-5D VAS data.

(b) Use the simple mean method to impute the missing 12-month EQ-5D VAS data.

(c) Use the horizontal mean imputation method to estimate the missing 12-month EQ-5D VAS scores.

(d) Use a multiple regression method with baseline EQ-5D score, age and sex as covariates to impute the missing 12-month EQ-5D VAS scores.

(e) Use a simple hot deck procedure, using all patients with valid 12-month EQ-5D data, to estimate the missing 12-month EQ-5D VAS scores.

13.2 Table 7.2 shows a comparison of the mean scores on the eight dimensions of the SF-36 between a group of IBS patients and control group. The P-values reported in the table have not been adjusted for multiple hypothesis testing.

(a) Use a Bonferroni correction to adjust the P-values in Table 7.2. Compare the Bonferroni corrected P-values with the original unadjusted P-values.

Table 13.6 Patterns of missing EQ-5D VAS data for 10 patients with low back pain, from the acupuncture study (data from Thomas *et al.*, 2006).

Patient No.	Group	Age	Sex	EQ-5D Visual Analogue Scale score 0 months	3 months	12 months
1	Usual care	36	Female	80	80	
2	Acupuncture care	53	Female	60	75	58
3	Usual care	51	Female	44		
4	Acupuncture care	29	Female	90	100	
5	Usual care	44	Male	85	75	60
6	Acupuncture care	39	Male	85		
7	Usual care	26	Male	60	70	
8	Usual care	35	Male	80	88	75
9	Usual care	31	Female	40	58	68
10	Usual care	41	Male	95	95	74
	Mean			71.9	80.1	67.0
	SD			19.5	13.7	7.8
	Valid *n*			10	8	5

What do you now conclude? Is there any evidence of difference in QoL between the IBS group and the control group?

(b) Use Fairclough's method to carry out a global hypothesis test to compare the eight SF-36 dimension scores between the IBS and control groups. Is there any evidence of difference in QoL between the IBS group and the control group? Comment on the results.

13.3 Table 8.6 shows a comparison of the mean scores for 10 QoL outcomes at 6 weeks after childbirth between a group of new mothers randomized to receive additional postnatal support (intervention) and usual care (control). The P-values reported in the Table 8.6 have not been adjusted for multiple hypothesis testing.

(a) Use a Bonferroni correction to adjust the P-values in Table 8.6. Compare the Bonferroni corrected P-values with the original unadjusted P-values. What do you now conclude? Is there any evidence of difference in QoL between the intervention group and the control group?

(b) Use Fairclough's method to carry out a global hypothesis test to compare the 10 QoL outcome scores between the Intervention and control groups. Is there any evidence of difference in QoL between the intervention group and the control group? Comment on the results.

Solutions to exercises

Chapter 4

4.1 (a) 76 per group (152 in total)

   (b) 102 per group (204 in total)

4.2 (a) SD = 8.2

   (b) 158 per group (316 in total)

   (c) 198 per group (396 in total)

4.3 (a) 85 per group (170 in total)

   (b) 192 in total (64 and 128 per group)

   (c) 240 in total (80 and 160 per group)

4.4 (a) 124 per group (248 in total)

   (b) 199 per group (398 in total)

   (c) $OR_{Int/Con} = 0.444$

   (d) 93 per group (186 in total)

   (e) 179 women per group (358 in total). This is the same as 18 HV per group (36 HV in total)

   (f) 285 women per group (570 in total). This is the same as 29 HV per group (58 HV in total)

   (g) 196 per group (392). This is the same as 20 HV per group (40 HV in total)

4.5 (a) 85

    (b) 170

4.6 (a) 173 case–control pairs

    (b) $s_{Difference} = 0.208$

    (c) 138 case–control pairs

4.7 (a) SD $= 22.2$

    (b) 1936 per group (3872 in total)

    (c) 2420 per group (4840 in total)

Chapter 5

5.1 (a) The graph below plots the difference between baseline and 2-week postnatal family scale scores against average family score from ($n = 9$) cancer patients; it also shows the observed mean difference and 95% limits of agreement.

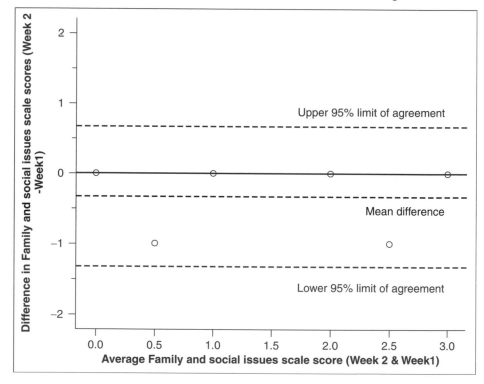

    (b) 95% limits of agreement -1.33 to 0.67

(c) No relationship

(d) ICC $= 0.88$ (good test–retest reliability).

5.2 (a) All nine patients responded 'not at all' to question 3 about lack of support from family.

(b) Item 3 can be removed from the calculations, $\alpha_{\text{Cronbach}} = 0.19$, which is very low indicating poor correlations between the items and scale.

5.3 (a) Cohen's kappa is 0.52 which suggests moderate agreement between the items.

(b) Weighted kappa (using quadratic weights) is 0.84 which suggests very high agreement between the items.

(c) The weighted kappa value is higher than the unweighted kappa. The overall agreement is 6/9 (67%) and the remaining three patients only disagree by one category, so weighted kappa is preferred.

Chapter 6

6.1

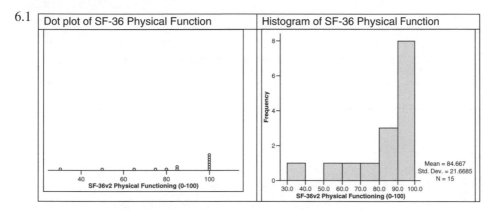

(a) The SF-36 Physical Function data are negatively skewed.

(b) Mean $= 84.7$, median $= 100.0$, mode $= 100.0$. The median is best summary as the data are skewed.

(c) Range 30.0 to 100.0, IQR $= 75.0$ to 100.0, SD $= 21.7$. The IQR is the best summary as the data ares skewed.

6.2 (a) A scatter plot of total body fat mass versus SF36v2 Physical Function dimension score in 15 young male cancer survivors is shown below.

(b) Yes, there appears to be a positive linear relationship between the two variables.

6.3 (a) A scatter plot of SF36v2 Physical Function score versus SF36v2 PCS score in 15 young male cancer survivors is given below.

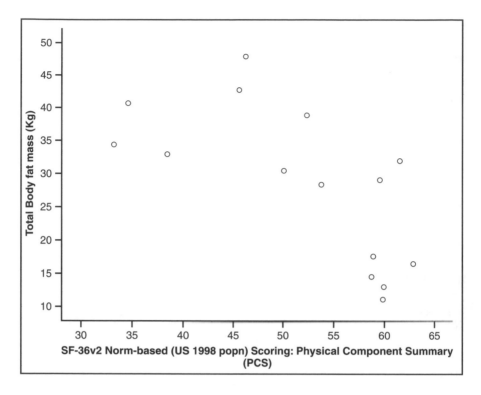

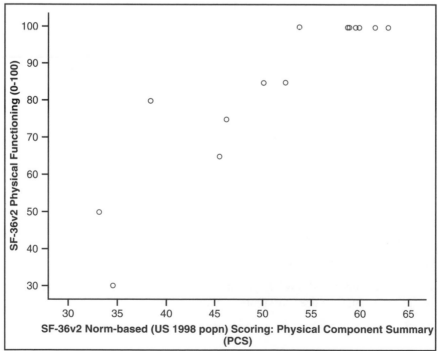

(b) Yes there appears to be a very strong positive linear relationship between the two variables.

6.4 (a) A radar plot of the median scores for the eight dimensions of the SF-36 by gender from a general population survey of 7213 Sheffield residents (Walters *et al.*, 2001) is given below.

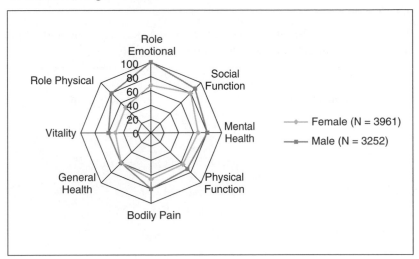

(b) Yes, there does appear to be a difference in the median QoL scores between the males and females.

Chapter 7

7.1 (a) H_0: No difference in population mean SF-36 Physical Function scores between male cancer survivors with normal and low levels of testosterone, that is, $\mu_{Normal} - \mu_{Low} = 0$.
H_A: There is a difference in population SF-36 Physical Function scores between male cancer survivors with normal and low levels of testosterone, that is, $\mu_{Normal} - \mu_{Low} \neq 0$.

(b) The assumptions for a two independent samples *t*-test are: the groups are independent; the variables of interest are continuous; the data in both groups have similar standard deviations; the data are Normally distributed in both groups.
T Test for comparing the means of two independent groups

| | Normal Testosterone | | | Low Testosterone | | | Mean | Pooled | | | | | 95% CI | |
	N_1	MEAN$_1$	SD$_1$	N_2	MEAN$_2$	SD$_2$	Difference	SD	SE	df	t	p	Lower	Upper
Physical Function	10	89	17.1	10	49.5	36.9	39.5		28.76	12.86	18	3.07	0.007	12.5	66.5

The *P*-value is 0.007, which is less than 0.05 and so is statistically significant. Therefore there is sufficient evidence to reject the null hypothesis of no difference in population mean SF-36 Physical Function scores between male cancer survivors with normal and low levels of testosterone. We conclude that there is a difference in population SF-36 Physical Function scores between male cancer survivors with normal and low levels of testosterone

(c) The mean difference is 39.5 (95% CI: 12.5 to 66.5). The CI excludes zero, suggesting that male cancer survivors with normal levels of testosterone have better SF-36 Physical Function scores than cancer survivors with low levels of testosterone.

7.2 (a) From the dot plot below, the data appear to be skewed in the normal group and symmetric in the low testosterone group.

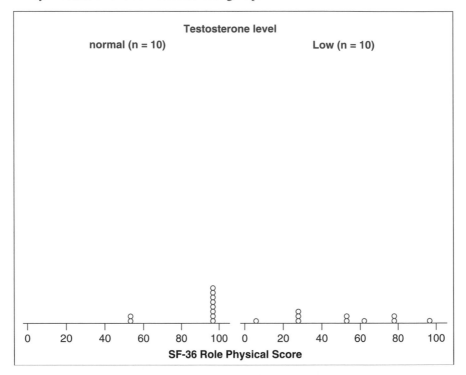

(b) The assumptions for a two independent samples t-test are: the groups are independent; the variables of interest are continuous; the data in both groups have similar standard deviations; the data are Normally distributed in both groups.

T Test for comparing the means of two independent groups

	Normal Testosterone			Low Testosterone			Mean	Pooled						95% CI	
	N_1	$MEAN_1$	SD_1	N_2	$MEAN_2$	SD_2	Difference	SD	SE	df	t	p	Lower	Upper
Role Physical	10	88.1	20.3	10	51.3	29.4	36.8	25.26	11.30	18	3.26	0.004	13.1	60.5

The P-value is 0.004, which is less than 0.05 and so is statistically significant. Therefore there is sufficient evidence to reject the null hypothesis of no difference in population mean SF-36 Role Physical scores between male cancer survivors with normal and low levels of testosterone. We conclude that there is a difference in population SF-36 Role Physical scores between male cancer survivors with normal and low levels of testosterone

(c) The mean difference is 36.8 (95%CI 13.1 to 60.5). The CI excludes zero, suggesting that male cancer survivors with normal levels of testosterone have better SF-36 Role Physical scores than cancer survivors with low levels of testosterone.

7.3 (a) The assumptions for the paired t-test are: the paired individual differences in outcomes are plausibly Normally distributed and independent of each other. The paired t-test gives $t = 4.252$ on 9 degrees of freedom. The P-value from this test is 0.002, which is less than 0.05 and so is statistically significant. Therefore there is sufficient evidence to reject the null hypothesis of no difference in population mean HAD anxiety scores between Gypsies/Travellers and their age- and sex-matched controls. We conclude that there is a difference in population mean HAD anxiety scores between Gypsies/Travellers and their age- and sex-matched controls.

(b) The Gypsies/Travellers have higher levels of anxiety than their age- and sex-matched controls. On average the mean HAD anxiety score of Gypsies/Travellers is 9.6 (95% CI: 4.5 to 14.7) points higher than the control group.

(c) The Wilcoxon test statistic $Z = -2.549$. The P-value is 0.011, which is less than 0.05 and statistically significant. Therefore we can reject the null hypothesis and accept the alternative that there is a difference in HAD depression scores between the Gypsies/Travellers and their age- and sex-matched controls.

7.4 (a) There is no obvious pattern in the scatter plot, although there is a slight suggestion that lower Physical Function scores are associated with increasing age.

(b) The negative value for the correlation coefficient suggests that high Physical Function scores are associated with younger ages. The P-value is the probability of observing the data, and the correlation coefficient, or more extreme values if the null hypothesis that the population correlation coefficient between age and SF-36 Physical Function score is zero. Since this P-value is less than 0.05, it is statistically significant and we can reject the null hypothesis and accept the alternative that the population correlation coefficient between age and SF-36 Physical Function score is non-zero. Table 7.10 suggests a 'moderate relationship' between age and SF-36 Physical Function score.

7.5 (a) $A = 47.980$; $B = 6.60$

(b) Both age and sex are significant predictors of Physical Function.

(c) 79.8

(d) 93.6

(e) The adjusted R^2 is 0.26, that is, 26% of the variability in SF-36 Physical Function scores is explained by age and sex. The model is likely to be a poor fit to the data, as 74% of the variability in the outcome, SF-36 Physical Function score, cannot be explained by the variables in the model.

7.6 The null hypothesis for the one-way ANOVA is that the four population mean SF-36 Physical Function scores for the young male cancer survivor groups are the same, $H_0 : \mu_{Germcell} = \mu_{Lymphoma} = \mu_{Leukaemia} = \mu_{Other} = \mu$. The alternative hypothesis that they are not the same.

The P-value is 0.604, which is greater than 0.05 and not statistically significant. Therefore there is insufficient evidence to reject the null hypothesis. That is, the four population mean SF-36 Physical Function scores for the young male cancer survivor groups are the same.

Chapter 8

8.1 (a) H_0: No difference in population mean 3-month WOMAC pain scores between the W. *somnifera* and placebo treated OA knee patients, that is, $\mu_{Withania} - \mu_{Placebo} = 0$

H_A: There is a difference in population mean 3-month WOMAC pain scores between the W. *somnifera* and placebo treated OA knee patients, that is, $\mu_{Withania} - \mu_{Placebo} \neq 0$

(b) The assumptions for a two independent samples t-test are: the groups are independent; the variables of interest are continuous; the data in both groups have similar standard deviations; the data are Normally distributed in both groups.

T Test for comparing the means of two independent groups

		Placebo			Withania Somnifera		Mean	Pooled						95%	CI
	N_1	$MEAN_1$	SD_1	N_2	$MEAN_2$	SD_2	Difference	SD		SE	df	t	p	Upper	Lower
WOMAC Pain	10	7.2	5	10	8	4.2	−0.80		4.62	2.06	18	0.39	0.7030	3.54	−5.14

The P-value is 0.70, which is greater than 0.05 and is not statistically significant. Therefore there is insufficient evidence to reject the null hypothesis of no difference in 3-month WOMAC Pain scores between the W. *somnifera* and placebo treated OA knee patients.

(c) The mean difference is 0.80 (95%CI −3.5 to 5.1). The CI includes zero, which is consistent with there being no difference in 3-month WOMAC pain scores between the groups.

8.2 (a) Mean difference in $HAMD_{17}$ scores = 0.21.

(b) 95% CI for the mean difference in $HAMD_{17}$ scores is −1.01 to 0.58. The 95% CI is within the pre-defined non-inferiority margin of 2.2 points on the $HAMD_{17}$. It appears that duloxetine is non-inferior to paroxetine in patients with non-psychotic MDD with respect to the $HAMD_{17}$ outcome.

(c) Mean difference in HAMA scores = −0.08.

(d) 95% CI for the mean difference in HAMA scores is −0.88 to 0.72. The 95% CI is within the non-inferiority margin of 2.2 points on the HAMA. It appears that duloxetine is non-inferior to paroxetine in patients with non-psychotic MDD with respect to the HAMA outcome.

8.3 (a) The possibility of a period effect is tested by a two independent samples t-test to compare the difference between the periods in the two groups of patients. The assumptions for a two independent samples t-test are: the groups are independent;

the variables of interest are continuous; the data in both groups have similar standard deviations; the data are Normally distributed in both groups. If there was no general tendency for patients do better in one period than in the other period we would expect the mean differences between the periods in the two groups to be of the same size but having opposite signs. Therefore the test for a period effect is a two independent samples t-test comparing $\bar{d}_{AB}$ with $-\bar{d}_{BA}$. The test gives $t = 1.851$ on 18 df, $P = 0.081$, mean difference 19.8, 95% CI: -2.7 to 42.3. This is not statistically significant and implies no tendency for asthma patients to do better in one of the two periods, that is, no period effect.

(b) We can investigate the possibility of a carry-over effect by noticing that in the absence of a carry-over effect, a patient's average response to the two treatments would be the same regardless of the order in which they were received. The test for a carry-over effect is therefore a two independent samples t-test comparing $\bar{a}_{AB}$ with $\bar{a}_{BA}$. The assumptions for a two independent samples t-test are: the groups are independent; the variables of interest are continuous; the data in both groups have similar standard deviations; the data are Normally distributed in both groups. The test gives $t = 0.621$ on 18 df, $P = 0.542$, mean difference 6.9, 95% CI: -16.4 to 30.2. This is not statistically significant and implies no tendency for the treatment effect to carry over from one period to the next.

(c) The patients report on average a 23.2 point higher score whilst on active treatment compared to placebo (95% CI: 0.7 to 45.7, $P = 0.044$). This result is statistically significant and suggests that asthma patients on the active treatment have a better QoL than when on placebo treatment. The 95% CI excludes zero, again suggesting that when on active treatment asthma patients have better QoL than when on placebo treatment.

8.4 (a) The P-value is 0.78, which is greater than 0.05 and is not statistically significant. Therefore there is insufficient evidence to reject the null hypothesis of no difference in baseline Barthel scores between the supplementation and placebo treated patients.

(b) The P-value is 0.41, which is greater than 0.05 and is not statistically significant. Therefore there is insufficient evidence to reject the null hypothesis of no difference in 6-month Barthel scores between the supplementation and placebo treated patients.

(c) The 95% CI for POST is -0.44 to 1.07. The CI includes zero, which is consistent with their being no difference in 6-month Barthel scores between the groups.

(d) ANCOVA is to be preferred. This method has the narrowest confidence interval, from 0.40 to 0.94, compared to POST and CHANGE.

(e) The observed difference, between the placebo and supplementation groups, in Barthel scores at 6 months is 0.32 (95% CI: -0.44 to 1.07). Both the difference and CI are less than the MCID of 1.85 points. Therefore the difference is not statistically significant and not clinically important. The change in Barthel scores from baseline to 6 months is 2.1 and 1.9 points for the placebo and supplementation groups, respectively. These changes over time are bigger than the MCID of 1.85 points. Therefore the changes over time in Barthel scores are potentially clinically important.

Chapter 9

9.1 (a) The SF-36 Pain QoL outcome appears to increase (i.e. improve) post randomisation (baseline) till about week 16 and then flatten out.

   (b) A suitable summary measure would be the AUC or mean of the follow-up QoL assessments.

9.2 (a) Yes, the P-value is 0.742, which is greater than 0.05 and is not statistically significant. Therefore there is insufficient evidence to reject the null hypothesis of no difference in baseline SF-36 Pain scores between the Neoral and placebo treated patients.

   (b) The P-value is 0.238, which is greater than 0.05 and is not statistically significant. Therefore there is insufficient evidence to reject the null hypothesis of no difference in 8-week SF-36 Pain scores between the Neoral and placebo treated patients.

   (c) The P-value is 0.016, which is less than 0.05 and is statistically significant. Therefore there is sufficient evidence to reject the null hypothesis (of no difference in 16-week SF-36 Pain scores between the Neoral and placebo treated patients) and accept the alternative hypothesis. That is, there is a difference in mean 16-week SF-36 Pain scores between the Neoral and placebo treated patients)

   (d) The 95% CI for the difference in mean follow-up SF-36 Pain scores is 1.5 to 9.9. The CI excludes zero, which is consistent with there being a difference in average follow-up Pain scores between the Neoral and placebo groups, with the Neoral treated patients having the better outcome (i.e. improved pain scores).

   (e) Given the pattern of how the QoL data changes over time, the analysis with the mean follow-up SF-36 Pain score as the outcome is to be preferred as this uses all the available data.

   (f) The observed difference, between the placebo and Neoral group, in Pain AUC scores is 5.0 (95% CI: 0.6 to 9.3, $P = 0.026$). The mean difference is 5.0 which equals the MCID of 5.0 points. The CI excludes zero, and includes the MCID, therefore the difference in AUC, between the groups, is statistically significant and potentially clinically important.

9.3 (a) Equal correlations between the follow-up QoL scores.

   (b) No, the analysis suggests that Neoral and placebo treated groups have different SF-36 Pain scores at follow-up. The estimated mean follow-up SF-36 Pain score is 5.01 (95% CI: 1.45 to 8.56, $P = 0.006$) points higher (better) in Neoral treated patients, after allowing for other covariates. The CI excludes zero and the P-value is less than 0.05 and is statistically significant.

   (c) Yes, the analysis suggests that the SF-36 Pain scores change over time. The estimated regression coefficient for time is 0.15 (95% CI: 0.09 to 0.22, $P =$

0.001) after allowing for other covariates The CI excludes zero and the P-value is less than 0.05 and statistically significant. This implies that for every one-unit (week) increase in follow-up, SF-36 Pain scores increase (improve) by 0.15 points.

(d) The estimated mean difference between the Neoral and placebo groups in follow-up SF-36 Pain scores is 5.01 (95% CI: 1.45 to 8.56, $P = 0.006$) points. The difference is just bigger than the MCID of 5, but the lower limit of the CI, although non-zero, is less than 5 points. Therefore the difference is statistically significant and potentially of clinical and practical importance.

(e) Follow-up SF-36 Pain score is significantly associated with baseline Pain score but not age and sex after allowing for other covariates (time and group). The regression coefficient for baseline SF-36 Pain suggests that for every one-unit increase in baseline Pain score, follow-up SF-36 Pain score will increase by 0.49 points (95% CI: 0.38 to 0.59, $P = 0.001$).

9.4 (a) The ICC of 0.016 is low, suggesting little correlation or clustering by health visit with respect to 6-month MCS outcome.

(b) Yes, the analysis suggests that mothers in the intervention and control groups have different 6-month MCS scores. The estimated mean 6-month MCS score is 1.4 (95% CI: 0.46 to 2.28, $P = 0.003$) points higher (better) in intervention group mothers, after allowing for other covariates. The CI excludes zero and the P-value is less than 0.05 and is statistically significant.

(c) The estimated mean difference between the intervention and control groups in 6-month MCS scores is 1.4 (95% CI: 0.5 to 2.3, $P = 0.003$) points. The difference is less than the MCID of 5, and the upper limit of the CI is less than five points. The CI clearly excludes zero. Therefore the difference is statistically significant but not of clinical and practical importance.

(d) Six-month MCS score is significantly associated with 6-week MCS score, History of PND and life events but not living alone after allowing for other covariates (group). The regression coefficient for 6-week MCS score suggests that for every one-unit increase in 6-week MCS score, 6-month MCS score will increase by 0.4 points (95% CI: 0.4 to 0.5, $P = 0.001$).
The regression coefficient for history of PND (0 = no, 1 = yes) suggests that mothers with a previous history of PND will have their 6-month MCS score reduced (made worse) by -3.1 points (95% CI: -4.5 to -1.7, $P = 0.001$) compared to mothers without a previous history of PND. The regression coefficient for life vents (0 = no, 1 = yes) suggests that mothers who have experienced a life event will have their 6-month MCS score reduced (made worse) by -1.4 points (95% CI: -2.1 to -0.7, $P = 0.001$) compared to mothers without a previous experience of a life event.

Chapter 11

11.1 (a) 1.300

(b) 1.300

(c) Patients A and B have the same QALY but different utility scores at the four assessment points.

(d)

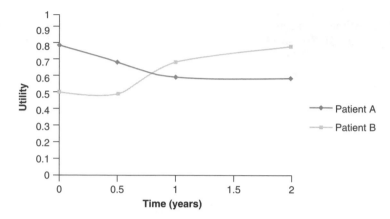

Patient A's QoL declines over time, whereas patient B's increases over time.

11.2 (a) 0.113 QALYs; 95% CI: 0.023 to 0.203

(b) £14.51; 95% CI: −£185 to £214

(c) ICER = £128/QALY

(d) NE quadrant

(e) A probability of about 0.99

(f) Yes

Chapter 12

12.1 (a) $N = 1111$

Fixed effects model estimates and confidence intervals for the SMD from eight RCTs comparing glucosamine and placebo treatment for osteoarthritis (data from Towheed *et al.*, 2005)

Study	SMD$_{Hedgesg}$	SE$_{SMD}$	95% CI Lower	Upper	% Weight
Cibere 2004	0.001	0.171	−0.334	0.336	12.6
Houpt 1999	−0.124	0.203	−0.522	0.274	9.0
Hughes 2002	0.032	0.227	−0.412	0.476	7.2
McAklindon 2004	0.053	0.140	−0.221	0.327	18.9
Pavelka 2002	−0.127	0.141	−0.403	0.149	18.6
Reginster 2001	−0.078	0.137	−0.348	0.191	19.6
Rovati 1997	−1.237	0.175	−1.58	−0.894	12.0
Zenk 2002	0.067	0.421	−0.757	0.892	2.1
I-V pooled SMD	−0.185		−0.304	−0.066	100.0

Heterogeneity $\chi^2 = 42.29$ (df = 7), $P = 0.001$ I^2 (variation in SMD attributable to heterogeneity) = 83.4%

Test of SMD = 0: $z = 3.05$, $P = 0.002$

(d) The Reginster 2001 study has the largest weight.

(f) Heterogeneity chi-squared = 42.29 (df = 7), $P = 0.001$. Significant evidence of heterogeneity across the eight studies.

(g) $I^2 = 83.4\%$ of the variation in SMD attributable to heterogeneity across the eight studies.

(h) Pooled SMD = -0.185 (95% CI: -0.034 to -0.066). The CI excludes zero, favouring glucosamine treatment over placebo.

Forest plot of standardized mean differences in post-randomization pain score in eight RCTs comparing glucosamine and placebo treatment for osteoarthritis based on a fixed effects model (data from Towheed et al., 2005)

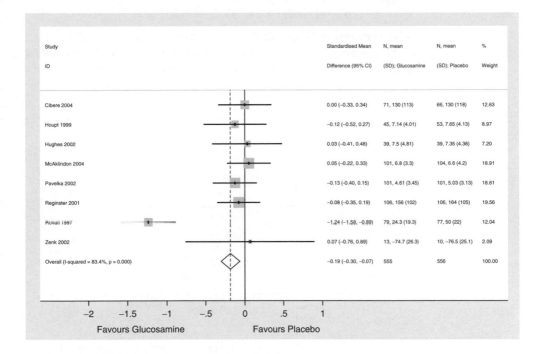

12.2 (a) The random effects model estimate of the pooled SMD is -0.191 (95% CI: -0.496 to $+0.115$). This is less than the fixed effects model of -0.185 and the CI is much wider. The CI includes zero and suggests no difference between glucosamine treatment and placebo.

Random effects model estimates and confidence intervals for the SMD from eight RCTs comparing glucosamine and placebo treatment for osteoarthritis (data from Towheed et al., 2005)

Study	SMD	95% CI Lower	Upper	% Weight
Cibere 2004	0.001	−0.334	0.336	13.25
Houpt 1999	−0.124	−0.522	0.274	12.44
Hughes 2002	0.032	−0.412	0.476	11.83
McAklindon 2004	0.053	−0.221	0.327	13.99
Pavelka 2002	−0.127	−0.403	0.149	13.97
Reginster 2001	−0.078	−0.348	0.191	14.05
Rovati 1997	−1.237	−1.58	−0.894	13.15
Zenk 2002	0.067	−0.757	0.892	7.33
D+L pooled SMD	−0.191	−0.496	0.115	100

Heterogeneity chi-squared $= 42.29$ (df $= 7$), $P = 0.000$
I^2 (variation in SMD attributable to heterogeneity) $= 83.4\%$
Estimate of between-study variance Tau-squared $\tau^2 = 0.1538$

Test of SMD $= 0 : z = 1.22$, $P = 0.221$

Forest plot of standardized mean differences in post-randomization Pain score in eight RCTs comparing glucosamine and placebo treatment for Osteoarthritis based on a random effects model (data from Towheed et al., 2005)

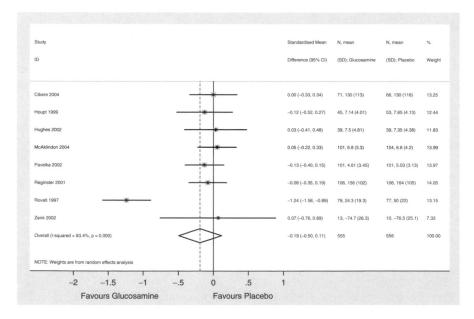

(b) A random effects model is more appropriate because of the heterogeneity across the eight studies.

(c) Funnel plot of standard error of the treatment effect against the standardized mean differences in post-randomization Pain score in eight RCTs comparing glucosamine and placebo treatment for osteoarthritis based on a random effects model (data from Towheed *et al.*, 2005)

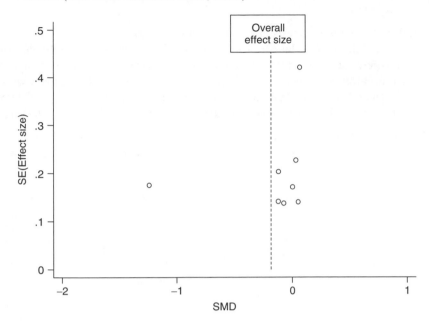

No obvious pattern in the funnel plot.

Chapter 13

13.1 (a) LOCF patient 1 = 80; patient 3 = 44; patient 4 = 100; patient 6 = 85; patient 7 = 70.

(b) Simple mean imputation = 67.0 for all five patients.

(c) Patient 1 = 80; patient 2 = 44; patient 4 = 95; patient 6 = 85; patient 7 = 65.

(d) The regression equation is:
$$\text{EQ-5D VAS}_{12\text{months}} = 53.13 + 0.80\text{VAS}_{\text{baseline}} - 1.32\text{Age} + 25.33\text{Sex}$$
Sex coded as (0 = male, 1 = female).
The regression imputed values are patient 1 = 94.9; patient 3 = 46.3; patient 4 = 112.2 (rounded down to 100 the maximum possible VAS score); patient 6 = 69.7; patient 7 = 66.8.

(e) The hot deck is 58, 60, 75, 68 and 74. So the imputed missing scores are randomly sampled from this hot deck.

13.2 (a) With eight hypothesis tests at $\alpha = 0.05$; $\alpha/K = 0.05/8 = 0.00625$.
All eight P-values are less than this value, so there is still reliable evidence of difference in QoL on all eight dimensions of the SF-36 between the IBS and control groups after adjustment for multiple hypothesis testing.

(b) The smallest P-value is 0.001. This is less than 0.00625, so the global null hypothesis (of equality of QoL scores across all eight dimensions of the SF-36) is rejected.

13.3 (a) With 10 hypothesis tests at $\alpha = 0.05$; $\alpha/K = 0.05/10 = 0.005$.
None of the 10 P-values are less than this value, so there is no reliable evidence of difference in QoL on all 10 dimensions between the intervention and control groups after adjustment for multiple hypothesis testing. This contrast with three P-values being less than 0.05 (and statistically significant with $\alpha = 0.05$) and a fourth equal to 0.05 without adjustment for multiple hypothesis testing.

(b) The smallest P-value is 0.008. This is clearly more than 0.005, so the global null hypothesis (of equality of QoL scores across the 10 outcomes) cannot be rejected.

Appendix A

Examples of questionnaires

Health status questionnaire (SF-36)

The following questions ask you about your health, how you feel and how well you are able to do your usual activities.
If you are unsure how to answer a question, please give the best answer you can.

1. In general, would you say your health is:

(tick one)

Excellent . . . . ○
Very good . . . . ○
Good. . . . . ○
Fair . . . . ○
Poor . . . . ○

2. Compared to one year ago, how would you rate your health in general now?

(tick one)

Much better than one year ago . . . . ○
Somewhat better than one year ago . . . . ○
About the same . . . . ○
Somewhat worse now than one year ago . . . . ○
Much worse now than one year ago . . . . ○

Quality of Life Outcomes in Clinical Trials and Health-Care Evaluation   Stephen J. Walters
© 2009 John Wiley & Sons, Ltd

Health and daily activities

3. The following questions are about activities that you might do during a typical day. Does your health limit you in these activities? If so, how much?

(circle one number on each line)

Activities	Yes, limited a lot	Yes, limited a little	No, not limited at all
a. **Vigorous activities**, such as running, lifting heavy objects, participating in strenuous sports	1	2	3
b. **Moderate activities**, such as moving a table, pushing a vacuum cleaner, bowling or playing golf	1	2	3
c. Lifting or carrying groceries	1	2	3
d. Climbing **several** flights of stairs	1	2	3
e. Climbing **one** flight of stairs	1	2	3
f. Bending, kneeling or stooping	1	2	3
g. Walking **more than a mile**	1	2	3
h. Walking **half a mile**	1	2	3
i. Walking **100 yards**	1	2	3
j. Bathing and dressing yourself	1	2	3

4. During the <u>past 4 weeks</u>, have you had any of the following problems with your work or other regular daily activities <u>as a result of your physical health</u>?

(circle one number on each line)

	YES	NO
a. Cut down on the **amount of time** you spent on work or other activities	1	2
b. **Accomplished less** than you would like	1	2
c. Were limited in the **kind** of work or other activities	1	2
d. Had **difficulty** in performing the work or other activities (e.g. it took extra effort)	1	2

5. During the <u>past 4 weeks</u>, have you had any of the following problems with your work or other regular daily activities <u>as a result of any emotional problems</u> (such as feeling depressed or anxious)?

(circle one number on each line)

	YES	NO
a. Cut down on the **amount of time** you spent on work or other activities	1	2
b. **Accomplished less** than you would like	1	2
c. Didn't do work or other activities as **carefully** as usual	1	2

6. During the <u>past 4 weeks</u>, to what extent have your physical health or emotional problems interfered with your normal social activities with family, friends, neighbours or groups?

(circle one number)

Not at all...................... 1
Slightly 2
Moderately 3
Quite a bit.................... 4
Extremely 5

7. How much <u>bodily</u> pain have you had during <u>the past 4 weeks</u>?

(circle one number)

None.......................... 1
Very mild 2
Mild.......................... 3
Moderate 4
Severe 5
Very severe.................. 6

8. During the <u>past 4 weeks</u>, how much did pain interfere with your normal work (including work both outside the home and housework)?

(circle one number)

Not at all..................... 1
A little bit................... 2
Moderately 3
Quite a bit................... 4
Extremely 5

Your feelings

9. These questions are about how you feel and how things have been with you during <u>the past 4 weeks</u>. (For each question, please indicate the <u>one</u> answer that comes closest to the way you have been feeling.)

(circle one number on each line)

How much of the time during the past 4 weeks:	All of the time	Most of the time	A good bit of time	Some of the time	A little of the time	None of the time
a. Did you feel full of life?	1	2	3	4	5	6
b. Have you been a very nervous person?	1	2	3	4	5	6
c. Have you felt so down in the dumps that nothing could cheer you up?	1	2	3	4	5	6
d. Have you felt calm and peaceful?	1	2	3	4	5	6
e. Did you have a lot of energy?	1	2	3	4	5	6
f. Have you felt down-hearted and low?	1	2	3	4	5	6
g. Did you feel worn-out?	1	2	3	4	5	6
h. Have you been a happy person?	1	2	3	4	5	6
i. Did you feel tired?	1	2	3	4	5	6
j. Has your health limited your social activities (like visiting friends or close relatives)	1	2	3	4	5	6

Health in general

1. Please choose the answer that best describes how <u>true</u> or <u>false</u> each of the following statements is for you.

(circle one number on each line)

	Definitely true	Mostly true	Not sure	Mostly false	Definitely false
a. I seem to get ill more easily than other people	1	2	3	4	5
b. I am as healthy as anybody I know	1	2	3	4	5
c. I expect my health to get worse	1	2	3	4	5
d. My health is excellent	1	2	3	4	5

Hospital Anxiety and Depression (HAD) scale

Instructions: Using the scale provided as a guide, indicate how much you agree or disagree with each of the following statements. Read each question and <u>circle the number</u> in the box opposite the reply that comes closest to how you have been feeling in the **past week**. Please choose <u>one response</u> from the four given for each question. Please give an immediate response and don't think too long about your answers.

1A	**I feel tense or 'wound up':**	
	Most of the time	3
	A lot of the time	2
	From time to time, occasionally	1
	Not at all	0
2D	**I still enjoy the things I used to enjoy:**	
	Definitely as much	0
	Not quite so much	1
	Only a little	2
	Hardly at all	3
3A	**I get a sort of frightened feeling as if something awful is about to happen:**	
	Very definitely and quite badly	3
	Yes, but not too badly	2
	A little, but it doesn't worry me	1
	Not at all	0
4D	**I can laugh and see the funny side of things:**	
	As much as I always could	0
	Not quite so much now	1

	Definitely not so much now	2
	Not at all	3
5A	**Worrying thoughts go through my mind:**	
	A great deal of the time	3
	A lot of the time	2
	From time to time, but not too often	1
	Only occasionally	0
6D	**I feel cheerful:**	
	Not at all	3
	Not often	2
	Sometimes	1
	Most of the time	0
7A	**I can sit at ease and feel relaxed:**	
	Definitely	0
	Usually	1
	Not often	2
	Not at all	3
8D	**I feel as if I am slowed down:**	
	Nearly all the time	3
	Very often	2
	Sometimes	1
	Not at all	0
9A	**I get a sort of frightened feeling like 'butterflies' in the stomach:**	
	Not at all	0
	Occasionally	1
	Quite often	2
	Very often	3
10D	**I have lost interest in my appearance:**	
	Definitely	3
	I don't take as much care as I should	2
	I may not take quite as much care	1
	I take just as much care as ever	0
11A	**I feel restlessas I have to be on the move:**	
	Very much indeed	3
	Quite a lot	2
	Not very much	1
	Not at all	0
12D	**I look forward with enjoyment to things:**	
	As much as I ever did	0
	Rather less than I used to	1
	Definitely less than I used to	2
	Hardly at all	3

13A	I get sudden feelings of panic:	
	Very often indeed	3
	Quite often	2
	Not very often	1
	Not at all	0
14D	I can enjoy a good book or radio or TV program:	
	Often	0
	Sometimes	1
	Not often	2
	Very seldom	3
	Total 'A' =	
	Total 'D' =	

Euroqol© health questionnaire

Here are some simple questions about your health in general. By ticking one answer in each group below, please indicate which statements best describe your own health state TODAY.

Please tick one

1. **Mobility**
   I have no problems in walking about ○
   I have some problems in walking about ○
   I am confined to bed ○
2. **Self-care**
   I have no problems with self-care ○
   I have some problems washing or dressing myself ○
   I am unable to wash or dress myself ○
3. **Usual Activities**
   I have no problems with performing my usual activities ○
   (*e.g. work, study, housework, family or leisure activities*)
   I have some problems with performing my usual activities ○
   I am unable to perform my usual activities ○
4. **Pain/Discomfort**
   I have no pain or discomfort ○
   I have moderate pain or discomfort ○
   I have extreme pain or discomfort ○
5. **Anxiety/Depression**
   I am not anxious or depressed ○
   I am moderately anxious or depressed ○
   I am extremely anxious or depressed ○

6.   To help people say how good or bad their health is, we have
     drawn a scale (rather like a thermometer) on which the best
     state you can imagine is marked by 100 and the worst state
     you can imagine is marked by 0.
   We would like you to indicate on this scale how good or bad
     your own health is today, in your opinion. Please do this by
     drawing a line from the box below to whichever point on the
     scale indicates how good or bad your current health state is.

Your own health state today

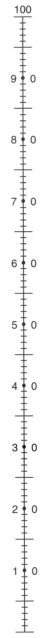

**Best imaginable
health state**

100

9 0

8 0

7 0

6 0

5 0

4 0

3 0

2 0

1 0

**Worst
imaginable
health state**

Measure Yourself Medical Outcome Profile (MYMOP)

```
The MYMOP follow up questionnaire
--------------------------------------------------------------------
PLEASE FILL THIS IN ON ........................... MYMOP. Follow up

Please circle the number to show how severe your problem has been IN THE LAST WEEK.
- this should be YOUR opinion, no-one else's!

SYMPTOM 1: ....................    as good as it    1 2 3 4 5 6 7    as bad as it
...........................        could be                          could be
...........................

SYMPTOM 2: ....................    as good as it    1 2 3 4 5 6 7    as bad as it
...........................        could be                          could be
...........................

ACTIVITY: 1 cannot ...........     able to do it    1 2 3 4 5 6 7    not able to
...........................        normally                          do it at all
...........................


WELLBEING: How would               as good as it    1 2 3 4 5 6 7    as bad as it
you rate your general feeling      could be                          could be
of wellbeing

If an important new symptom has appeared you may describe it and mark how bad it is
below. Otherwise do not use this line.

SYMPTOM 3:.....................    as good as it    1 2 3 4 5 6 7    as bad as it
...........................        could be                          could be
...........................
--------------------------------------------------------------------
```

```
The MYMOP follow up questionnaire
--------------------------------------------------------------------
How would you rate your condition now compared to the last time you measured it?
please tick one only)
                              Much better      ()
...............               A little better ()
                              About the same   ()
                              A little worse   ()
                              Much worse       ()

Present treatment for this problem is............................................
and is given by..................................................................

Who else have you sought help from, for this problem, since you last completed a
MYMOP form? (please tick the boxes)

At Warwick House                          Not at Warwick House
   GP                                        Doctor at hospital
   Complementary practitioner or             Complementary  practitioner or
   therapist (please specify)                therapist (please specify)
   Nurse/health vistor/midwife               Physiotherapist
   Counsellor                                Counsellor
                                             Chemist/pharmacist (talked to)
                                             Family
                                             Friends
                                             Magazine or book
   Other (please specify) ........           Other (please specify).......
...........................               ...........................

THANK YOU!
Please return this in the envelope (no stamp required)
Or if you are due to see your doctor /practitioner on or near this date
please bring it with you to the surgery.
```

From Paterson (1996).

Appendix B

Statistical tables

Quality of Life Outcomes in Clinical Trials and Health-Care Evaluation   Stephen J. Walters
© 2009 John Wiley & Sons, Ltd

Table B.1   The standard Normal distribution. The value tabulated is the probability, xα, that a random variable, Normally distributed with mean 0 and standard deviation 1, will be greater than z_α or less than $-z_\alpha$

z	0.00	0.01	0.02	0.03	0.04	0.05	0.06	0.07	0.08	0.09
0.00	1.0000	0.9920	0.9840	0.9761	0.9681	0.9601	0.9522	0.9442	0.9362	0.9283
0.10	0.9203	0.9124	0.9045	0.8966	0.8887	0.8808	0.8729	0.8650	0.8572	0.8493
0.20	0.8415	0.8337	0.8259	0.8181	0.8103	0.8026	0.7949	0.7872	0.7795	0.7718
0.30	0.7642	0.7566	0.7490	0.7414	0.7339	0.7263	0.7188	0.7114	0.7039	0.6965
0.40	0.6892	0.6818	0.6745	0.6672	0.6599	0.6527	0.6455	0.6384	0.6312	0.6241
0.50	0.6171	0.6101	0.6031	0.5961	0.5892	0.5823	0.5755	0.5687	0.5619	0.5552
0.60	0.5485	0.5419	0.5353	0.5287	0.5222	0.5157	0.5093	0.5029	0.4965	0.4902
0.70	0.4839	0.4777	0.4715	0.4654	0.4593	0.4533	0.4473	0.4413	0.4354	0.4295
0.80	0.4237	0.4179	0.4122	0.4065	0.4009	0.3953	0.3898	0.3843	0.3789	0.3735
0.90	0.3681	0.3628	0.3576	0.3524	0.3472	0.3421	0.3371	0.3320	0.3271	0.3222
1.00	0.3173	0.3125	0.3077	0.3030	0.2983	0.2937	0.2891	0.2846	0.2801	0.2757
1.10	0.2713	0.2670	0.2627	0.2585	0.2543	0.2501	0.2460	0.2420	0.2380	0.2340
1.20	0.2301	0.2263	0.2225	0.2187	0.2150	0.2113	0.2077	0.2041	0.2005	0.1971
1.30	0.1936	0.1902	0.1868	0.1835	0.1802	0.1770	0.1738	0.1707	0.1676	0.1645
1.40	0.1615	0.1585	0.1556	0.1527	0.1499	0.1471	0.1443	0.1416	0.1389	0.1362
1.50	0.1336	0.1310	0.1285	0.1260	0.1236	0.1211	0.1188	0.1164	0.1141	0.1118
1.60	0.1096	0.1074	0.1052	0.1031	0.1010	0.0989	0.0969	0.0949	0.0930	0.0910
1.70	0.0891	0.0873	0.0854	0.0836	0.0819	0.0801	0.0784	0.0767	0.0751	0.0735
1.80	0.0719	0.0703	0.0688	0.0672	0.0658	0.0643	0.0629	0.0615	0.0601	0.0588
1.90	0.0574	0.0561	0.0549	0.0536	0.0524	0.0512	0.0500	0.0488	0.0477	0.0466
2.00	0.0455	0.0444	0.0434	0.0424	0.0414	0.0404	0.0394	0.0385	0.0375	0.0366
2.10	0.0357	0.0349	0.0340	0.0332	0.0324	0.0316	0.0308	0.0300	0.0293	0.0285
2.20	0.0278	0.0271	0.0264	0.0257	0.0251	0.0244	0.0238	0.0232	0.0226	0.0220
2.30	0.0214	0.0209	0.0203	0.0198	0.0193	0.0188	0.0183	0.0178	0.0173	0.0168
2.40	0.0164	0.0160	0.0155	0.0151	0.0147	0.0143	0.0139	0.0135	0.0131	0.0128
2.50	0.0124	0.0121	0.0117	0.0114	0.0111	0.0108	0.0105	0.0102	0.0099	0.0096
2.60	0.0093	0.0091	0.0088	0.0085	0.0083	0.0080	0.0078	0.0076	0.0074	0.0071
2.70	0.0069	0.0067	0.0065	0.0063	0.0061	0.0060	0.0058	0.0056	0.0054	0.0053
2.80	0.0051	0.0050	0.0048	0.0047	0.0045	0.0044	0.0042	0.0041	0.0040	0.0039
2.90	0.0037	0.0036	0.0035	0.0034	0.0033	0.0032	0.0031	0.0030	0.0029	0.0028
3.00	0.0027	0.0026	0.0025	0.0024	0.0024	0.0023	0.0022	0.0021	0.0021	0.0020
3.10	0.0019	0.0019	0.0018	0.0017	0.0017	0.0016	0.0016	0.0015	0.0015	0.0014
3.20	0.0014	0.0013	0.0013	0.0012	0.0012	0.0012	0.0011	0.0011	0.0010	0.0010
3.30	0.0010	0.0009	0.0009	0.0009	0.0008	0.0008	0.0008	0.0008	0.0007	0.0007
3.40	0.0007	0.0006	0.0006	0.0006	0.0006	0.0006	0.0005	0.0005	0.0005	0.0005
3.50	0.0005	0.0004	0.0004	0.0004	0.0004	0.0004	0.0004	0.0004	0.0003	0.0003

Table B.2 Student t distribution. The value tabulated is t_α such that if X is distributed as Student's t with df degrees of freedom, then α is the probability that $X \leq -t_\alpha$ or $X \geq t_\alpha$

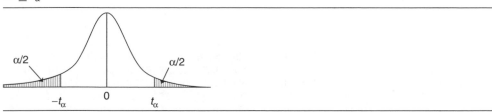

df	α 0.20	0.10	0.05	0.04	0.03	0.02	0.01	0.001
1	3.078	6.314	12.706	15.895	21.205	31.821	63.657	636.619
2	1.886	2.920	4.303	4.849	5.643	6.965	9.925	31.599
3	1.638	2.353	3.182	3.482	3.896	4.541	5.841	12.924
4	1.533	2.132	2.776	2.999	3.298	3.747	4.604	8.610
5	1.476	2.015	2.571	2.757	3.003	3.365	4.032	6.869
6	1.440	1.943	2.447	2.612	2.829	3.143	3.707	5.959
7	1.415	1.895	2.365	2.517	2.715	2.998	3.499	5.408
8	1.397	1.860	2.306	2.449	2.634	2.896	3.355	5.041
9	1.383	1.833	2.262	2.398	2.574	2.821	3.250	4.781
10	1.372	1.812	2.228	2.359	2.527	2.764	3.169	4.587
11	1.363	1.796	2.201	2.328	2.491	2.718	3.106	4.437
12	1.356	1.782	2.179	2.303	2.461	2.681	3.055	4.318
13	1.350	1.771	2.160	2.282	2.436	2.650	3.012	4.221
14	1.345	1.761	2.145	2.264	2.415	2.624	2.977	4.140
15	1.341	1.753	2.131	2.249	2.397	2.602	2.947	4.073
16	1.337	1.746	2.120	2.235	2.382	2.583	2.921	4.015
17	1.333	1.740	2.110	2.224	2.368	2.567	2.898	3.965
18	1.330	1.734	2.101	2.214	2.356	2.552	2.878	3.922
19	1.328	1.729	2.093	2.205	2.346	2.539	2.861	3.883
20	1.325	1.725	2.086	2.197	2.336	2.528	2.845	3.850
21	1.323	1.721	2.080	2.189	2.328	2.518	2.831	3.819
22	1.321	1.717	2.074	2.183	2.320	2.508	2.819	3.792
23	1.319	1.714	2.069	2.177	2.313	2.500	2.807	3.768
24	1.318	1.711	2.064	2.172	2.307	2.492	2.797	3.745
25	1.316	1.708	2.060	2.167	2.301	2.485	2.787	3.725
26	1.315	1.706	2.056	2.162	2.296	2.479	2.779	3.707
27	1.314	1.703	2.052	2.158	2.291	2.473	2.771	3.690
28	1.313	1.701	2.048	2.154	2.286	2.467	2.763	3.674
29	1.311	1.699	2.045	2.150	2.282	2.462	2.756	3.659
30	1.310	1.697	2.042	2.147	2.278	2.457	2.750	3.646
50	1.299	1.676	2.009	2.109	2.234	2.403	2.678	3.496
100	1.290	1.660	1.984	2.081	2.201	2.364	2.626	3.390
150	1.287	1.655	1.976	2.072	2.191	2.351	2.609	3.357
200	1.286	1.653	1.972	2.067	2.186	2.345	2.601	3.340
500	1.283	1.648	1.965	2.059	2.176	2.334	2.586	3.310
∞	1.282	1.645	1.960	2.054	2.170	2.326	2.576	3.291

Table B.3 F distribution. The value tabulated is $F(\alpha, \nu_1, \nu_2)$ such that if X has F distribution with ν_1 and ν_2 degrees of freedom, then α is the probability that $X \geq F(\alpha, \nu_1, \nu_2)$

ν_2	α	ν_1 1	2	3	4	5	6	7	8	9	10	20	∞
1	0.10	39.86	49.50	53.59	55.83	57.24	58.20	58.91	59.44	59.86	60.19	61.74	63.33
1	0.05	161.45	199.50	215.71	224.58	230.16	233.99	236.77	238.88	240.54	241.88	248.01	254.31
1	0.01	4052.18	4999.50	5403.35	5624.58	5763.65	5858.99	5928.36	5981.07	6022.47	6055.85	6208.73	6365.68
2	0.10	8.53	9.00	9.16	9.24	9.29	9.33	9.35	9.37	9.38	9.39	9.44	9.49
2	0.05	18.51	19.00	19.16	19.25	19.30	19.33	19.35	19.37	19.38	19.40	19.45	19.50
2	0.01	98.50	99.00	99.17	99.25	99.30	99.33	99.36	99.37	99.39	99.40	99.45	99.50
3	0.10	5.54	5.46	5.39	5.34	5.31	5.28	5.27	5.25	5.24	5.23	5.18	5.13
3	0.05	10.13	9.55	9.28	9.12	9.01	8.94	8.89	8.85	8.81	8.79	8.66	8.53
3	0.01	34.12	30.82	29.46	28.71	28.24	27.91	27.67	27.49	27.35	27.23	26.69	26.13
4	0.10	4.54	4.32	4.19	4.11	4.05	4.01	3.98	3.95	3.94	3.92	3.84	3.76
4	0.05	7.71	6.94	6.59	6.39	6.26	6.16	6.09	6.04	6.00	5.96	5.80	5.63
4	0.01	21.20	18.00	16.69	15.98	15.52	15.21	14.98	14.80	14.66	14.55	14.02	13.46
5	0.10	4.06	3.78	3.62	3.52	3.45	3.40	3.37	3.34	3.32	3.30	3.21	3.10
5	0.05	6.61	5.79	5.41	5.19	5.05	4.95	4.88	4.82	4.77	4.74	4.56	4.36
5	0.01	16.26	13.27	12.06	11.39	10.97	10.67	10.46	10.29	10.16	10.05	9.55	9.02
6	0.10	3.78	3.46	3.29	3.18	3.11	3.05	3.01	2.98	2.96	2.94	2.84	2.72
6	0.05	5.99	5.14	4.76	4.53	4.39	4.28	4.21	4.15	4.10	4.06	3.87	3.67
6	0.01	13.75	10.92	9.78	9.15	8.75	8.47	8.26	8.10	7.98	7.87	7.40	6.88
7	0.10	3.59	3.26	3.07	2.96	2.88	2.83	2.78	2.75	2.72	2.70	2.59	2.47
7	0.05	5.59	4.74	4.35	4.12	3.97	3.87	3.79	3.73	3.68	3.64	3.44	3.23
7	0.01	12.25	9.55	8.45	7.85	7.46	7.19	6.99	6.84	6.72	6.62	6.16	5.65
8	0.10	3.46	3.11	2.92	2.81	2.73	2.67	2.62	2.59	2.56	2.54	2.42	2.29
8	0.05	5.32	4.46	4.07	3.84	3.69	3.58	3.50	3.44	3.39	3.35	3.15	2.93
8	0.01	11.26	8.65	7.59	7.01	6.63	6.37	6.18	6.03	5.91	5.81	5.36	4.86
9	0.10	3.36	3.01	2.81	2.69	2.61	2.55	2.51	2.47	2.44	2.42	2.30	2.16
9	0.05	5.12	4.26	3.86	3.63	3.48	3.37	3.29	3.23	3.18	3.14	2.94	2.71
9	0.01	10.56	8.02	6.99	6.42	6.06	5.80	5.61	5.47	5.35	5.26	4.81	4.31
10	0.10	3.29	2.92	2.73	2.61	2.52	2.46	2.41	2.38	2.35	2.32	2.20	2.06
10	0.05	4.96	4.10	3.71	3.48	3.33	3.22	3.14	3.07	3.02	2.98	2.77	2.54
10	0.01	10.04	7.56	6.55	5.99	5.64	5.39	5.20	5.06	4.94	4.85	4.41	3.91
20	0.10	2.97	2.59	2.38	2.25	2.16	2.09	2.04	2.00	1.96	1.94	1.79	1.61
20	0.05	4.35	3.49	3.10	2.87	2.71	2.60	2.51	2.45	2.39	2.35	2.12	1.84
20	0.01	8.10	5.85	4.94	4.43	4.10	3.87	3.70	3.56	3.46	3.37	2.94	2.42
30	0.10	2.88	2.49	2.28	2.14	2.05	1.98	1.93	1.88	1.85	1.82	1.67	1.46
30	0.05	4.17	3.32	2.92	2.69	2.53	2.42	2.33	2.27	2.21	2.16	1.93	1.62
30	0.01	7.56	5.39	4.51	4.02	3.70	3.47	3.30	3.17	3.07	2.98	2.55	2.01
40	0.10	2.84	2.44	2.23	2.09	2.00	1.93	1.87	1.83	1.79	1.76	1.61	1.38
40	0.05	4.08	3.23	2.84	2.61	2.45	2.34	2.25	2.18	2.12	2.08	1.84	1.51
40	0.01	7.31	5.18	4.31	3.83	3.51	3.29	3.12	2.99	2.89	2.80	2.37	1.80
50	0.10	2.81	2.41	2.20	2.06	1.97	1.90	1.84	1.80	1.76	1.73	1.57	1.33
50	0.05	4.03	3.18	2.79	2.56	2.40	2.29	2.20	2.13	2.07	2.03	1.78	1.44
50	0.01	7.17	5.06	4.20	3.72	3.41	3.19	3.02	2.89	2.78	2.70	2.27	1.68
100	0.10	2.76	2.36	2.14	2.00	1.91	1.83	1.78	1.73	1.69	1.66	1.49	1.21
100	0.05	3.94	3.09	2.70	2.46	2.31	2.19	2.10	2.03	1.97	1.93	1.68	1.28
100	0.01	6.90	4.82	3.98	3.51	3.21	2.99	2.82	2.69	2.59	2.50	2.07	1.43
∞	0.10	2.71	2.30	2.08	1.94	1.85	1.77	1.72	1.67	1.63	1.60	1.42	1.01
∞	0.05	3.84	3.00	2.60	2.37	2.21	2.10	2.01	1.94	1.88	1.83	1.57	1.01
∞	0.01	6.64	4.61	3.78	3.32	3.02	2.80	2.64	2.51	2.41	2.32	1.88	1.01

Table B.4 The χ^2 distribution. The value tabulated is $\chi^2(\alpha)$, such that if X is distributed as χ^2 with df degrees of freedom, then α is the probability that $X \geq \chi^2$

df	α 0.20	0.10	0.05	0.04	0.03	0.02	0.01	0.001
1	1.64	2.71	3.84	4.22	4.71	5.41	6.63	10.83
2	3.22	4.61	5.99	6.44	7.01	7.82	9.21	13.82
3	4.64	6.25	7.81	8.31	8.95	9.84	11.34	16.27
4	5.99	7.78	9.49	10.03	10.71	11.67	13.28	18.47
5	7.29	9.24	11.07	11.64	12.37	13.39	15.09	20.52
6	8.56	10.64	12.59	13.20	13.97	15.03	16.81	22.46
7	9.80	12.02	14.07	14.70	15.51	16.62	18.48	24.32
8	11.03	13.36	15.51	16.17	17.01	18.17	20.09	26.12
9	12.24	14.68	16.92	17.61	18.48	19.68	21.67	27.88
10	13.44	15.99	18.31	19.02	19.92	21.16	23.21	29.59
11	14.63	17.28	19.68	20.41	21.34	22.62	24.72	31.26
12	15.81	18.55	21.03	21.79	22.74	24.05	26.22	32.91
13	16.98	19.81	22.36	23.14	24.12	25.47	27.69	34.53
14	18.15	21.06	23.68	24.49	25.49	26.87	29.14	36.12
15	19.31	22.31	25.00	25.82	26.85	28.26	30.58	37.70
16	20.47	23.54	26.30	27.14	28.19	29.63	32.00	39.25
17	21.61	24.77	27.59	28.44	29.52	31.00	33.41	40.79
18	22.76	25.99	28.87	29.75	30.84	32.35	34.81	42.31
19	23.90	27.20	30.14	31.04	32.16	33.69	36.19	43.82
20	25.04	28.41	31.41	32.32	33.46	35.02	37.57	45.31
21	26.17	29.62	32.67	33.60	34.76	36.34	38.93	46.80
22	27.30	30.81	33.92	34.87	36.05	37.66	40.29	48.27
23	28.43	32.01	35.17	36.13	37.33	38.97	41.64	49.73
24	29.55	33.20	36.42	37.39	38.61	40.27	42.98	51.18
25	30.68	34.38	37.65	38.64	39.88	41.57	44.31	52.62
26	31.79	35.56	38.89	39.89	41.15	42.86	45.64	54.05
27	32.91	36.74	40.11	41.13	42.41	44.14	46.96	55.48
28	34.03	37.92	41.34	42.37	43.66	45.42	48.28	56.89
29	35.14	39.09	42.56	43.60	44.91	46.69	49.59	58.30
30	36.25	40.26	43.77	44.83	46.16	47.96	50.89	59.70
50	58.16	63.17	67.50	68.80	70.42	72.61	76.15	86.66
200	216.61	226.02	233.99	236.35	239.27	243.19	249.45	267.54
500	526.40	540.93	553.13	556.71	561.14	567.07	576.49	603.45

References

Aaronson, N. K., Ahmedzai, S., Bergman, B. *et al*. (1993) The European Organization for Research and Treatment of Cancer QLQ-C30: A quality-of-life instrument for use in international clinical trials in oncology. *Journal of the National Cancer Institute*, 85, 365–376.

Agresti, A. (1984) *Analysis of Ordinal Categorical Data*. New York: John Wiley & Sons, Inc.

Agresti, A. (2002) *Categorical Data Analysis*, 2nd edition. New York: John Wiley & Sons, Inc.

Agresti, A. (2007) *An Introduction to Categorical Data Analysis*, 2nd edition. Hoboken, NJ: John Wiley & Sons, Inc.

Akehurst, R. L., Brazier, J. E., Mathers, N., O'Keefe, C., Kaltenthaler, E., Morgan, A., Platts, M., Walters, S. J. (2002) Health-related quality of life and cost impact of irritable bowel syndrome in a UK primary care setting. *Pharmacoeconomics*, 20(7), 455–462.

Allard, S., and the NAME IT Study Group. (2000) *Phase IIIB.IV Clinical Study Report of a Double-Blind, Randomised, Controlled Study to Compare Methotrexate plus Neoral® versus Methotrexate plus Placebo in Subjects with Early Severe Rheumatoid Arthritis*. Basel, Switzerland, Novartis Pharma AG.

Altman, D. G. (1991) *Practical Statistics for Medical Research*. London: Chapman & Hall.

Altman, D. G., Machin, D., Bryant, T. N., and Gardner, M. J. (2000) *Statistics with Confidence: Confidence Intervals and Statistical Guidelines*, 2nd edition. London: British Medical Journal.

Ananth, C. and Kleinbaum, D. (1997) Regression models for ordinal responses: a review of methods and applications. *International Journal of Epidemiology*, 26(6), 1323–1333.

Anderson, J. A. (1984) Regression and ordered categorical variables (with discussion). *Journal of Royal Statistical Society Series B*, 46, 1–30.

Apgar, V. (1953) A proposal for a new method of evaluation of the newborn infant. *Current Researches in Anesthesia and Analgesia*, 32(4), 260–267.

Armitage, P., Berry, G., and Matthews, J. N. S. (2002) *Statistical Methods in Medical Research*, 4th edition. Oxford: Blackwell Science.

Armstrong, B. G. and Sloan, M. (1989) Ordinal regression models for epidemiologic data. *American Journal of Epidemiology*, 129, 191–204.

Bailey K. R. (1987) Inter-study differences: how should they influence the interpretation and analysis of results? *Statistics in Medicine*, 6, 351–358.

Beck, A. T., Ward, C. H., Mendelson, M., Mock, J. and Erbaugh, J. (1961) An inventory for measuring depression. *Archives of General Psychiatry*, 4, 53–63.

Bellamy, N., Buchanan, W. W., Goldsmith, C. H., Campbell, J., Stitt, L. W. (1988) Validation study of WOMAC: a health status instrument for measuring clinically important patient relevant outcomes to antirheumatic drug therapy in patients with osteoarthritis of the hip or knee. *Journal of Rheumatology* 15(12), 1833–1840.

Bjordal, K., Ahlner-Elmqvist, M., Tollesson, E., Jensen, A. B., Razavi, D., Maher, E. J. and Kaasa, S. (1994) Development of a European Organization for Research and Treatment of Cancer (EORTC) questionnaire module to be used in quality of life assessments in head and neck cancer patients. EORTC Quality of Life Study Group. *Acta Oncologica*, 33(8), 879–885.

Bland, J. M. and Altman, D. G. (1986) Statistical methods for assessing agreement between two methods of clinical measurement. *Lancet*, 1, 307–310.

Blazeby, J., Sprangers, M., Cull, A., Groenvold, M. and Bottomley, A. (2002). *Guidelines for Developing Questionnaire Modules*, 3rd edition revised. EORTC Quality of Life Group.

Bowling, A. (2001) *Measuring Disease: A Review of Disease-Specific Quality of Life Measurement Scales*, 2nd edition. Buckingham: Open University Press.

Bowling, A. (2004) *Measuring Health: A Review of Quality of Life Measurement Scales*, 2nd edition. Buckingham: Open University Press.

Brant, R. (1990) Assessing proportionality in the proportional odds model for ordinal logistic regression. *Biometrics*, 46, 1171–1178.

Brazier, J. E., Harper, R., Jones, N. M. B., O'Cathain, A., Thomas, K. J., Usherwood, T. and Westlake, L. (1992) Validating the SF-36 health survey questionnaire: new outcome measure for primary care. *British Medical Journal*, 305, 160–164.

Brazier, J. E., Walters, S. J., Nicholl, J. P. and Kohler, B. (1996) Using the SF-36 and Euroqol on an elderly population. *Quality of Life Research*, 5, 195–204.

Brazier, J. E., Harper, R., Munro, J. F., Walters, S. J. and Snaith, M. L. (1999) Generic and condition-specific outcome measures for people with osteoarthritis of the knee. *Rheumatology*, 38, 870–877.

Brazier, J. E., Roberts, J. F. and Deverill, M. D. (2002) The estimation of a preference based measure of health for the SF-36. *Journal of Health Economics*, 21, 271–292.

Brazier J., Ratcliffe J., Salomon J. A. and Tsuchiya A. (2007) *Measuring and Valuing Health Benefits for Economic Evaluation*. Oxford: Oxford University Press.

Briggs, A. H. (2001) Handling uncertainty in economic evaluation. In M. Drummond and A. McGuire (eds), *Economic Evaluation in Health Care: Merging Theory with Practice*, pp. 172–214. Oxford: Oxford University Press.

Briggs, A. H. and Gray, A. M. (1999) Handling uncertainty when performing economic evaluation of healthcare interventions. *Health Technology Assessment*, 3(2), 1–134.

Briggs, AH, Mooney, C. Z. and Wondering, D. E. (1999) Constructing confidence intervals for cost-effectiveness ratios: an evaluation of parametric and non-parametric techniques using Monte Carlo simulation. *Statistics in Medicine*, 18, 3245–3262.

Brown, C. T., Yap, T., Cromwell, D. A., Rixon, L., Steed, L., Mulligan, K., Mundy, A., Newman, S. P., van der Meulen, J. and Emberton, E. (2007) Self management for men with lower urinary tract symptoms: randomised controlled trial. *British Medical Journal*; 334, 25–28.

Campbell, M. J. (2006) *Statistics at Square Two: Understanding Modern Statistical Applications in Medicine*, 2nd edition. London: BMJ.

Campbell, M. J., Machin, D. and Walters, S. J. (2007) *Medical Statistics: A Text Book for the Health Sciences*, 4th edition. Chichester: John Wiley & Sons, Ltd.

Carpenter, J. and Bithell, J. (2000) Bootstrap confidence intervals: when, which, what? A practical guide for medical statisticians. *Statistics in Medicine*, 19, 1141–1164.

Cohen, J. (1988) *Statistical Power Analysis for the Behavioral Sciences*, 2nd edition. Hillsdale, NJ: Lawrence Earlbaum.

Cronbach, L. J. (1951) Coefficient alpha and the internal structure of tests. *Psychometrika*, 16, 297–334.

Curran, D., Molenberghs, G., Fayers, P. M. and Machin, D. (1998a). Analysis of incomplete quality of life data in clinical trials. In M. J. Staquet, R. D. Hays and P. M. Fayers (eds) *Quality of Life Assessment in Clinical Trials*. Oxford: Oxford University Press.

Curran, D., Molenberghs, G., Fayers, P. M. and Machin, D. (1998b) Incomplete quality of life data in randomised trials: missing forms. *Statistics in Medicine*, 17, 697–709.

Davison, A. C. and Hinkley, D. V. (1997) *Bootstrap Methods and their Applications*. Cambridge: Cambridge University Press.

Day, S. J. and Graham, D. F. (1989) Sample size and power for comparing two or more treatment groups in clinical trials. *British Medical Journal*, 299, 663–665.

de Haes, J. C. J. M., van Knippenberg, F. C. E. and Neijt, J. P. (1990) Measuring psychological and physical distress in cancer patients: structure and application of the Rotterdam Symptom Checklist. *British Journal of Cancer*, 62, 1034–1038.

Deeks, J. (2005) Funnel plots. In B. Everitt and C. Palmer (eds), *The Encyclopaedic Companion to Medical Statistics*. London: Arnold.

Deeks J. and Everitt B. S. (2005) Forest plot. In B. Everitt and C. Palmer (eds), *The Encyclopaedic Companion to Medical Statistics*. London: Arnold.

DerSimonian, R. and Laird, N. (1986) Meta-analysis in clinical trials. *Controlled Clinical Trials*, 7, 177–188.

Deyo, R. A., Inui, T. S., Leininger, J. and Overman, S. (1982) Physical and psychosocial function in rheumatoid arthritis. Clinical use of a self-administered health status instrument. *Archives of Internal Medicine*, 142(5), 879–882.

Diggle, P. J., Heagerty, P., Liang, K-Y. and Zeger, S. L. (2002) *Analysis of Longitudinal Data*, 2nd edition. Oxford: Oxford University Press.

Dolan, P., Gudex, C., Kind, P. and Williams, A. (1995) *A Social Tariff for the EuroQol: Results from a UK General Population Survey*. Centre for Health Economics discussion paper no. 138. York: University of York.

Donner, A. and Klar, N. (2000) *Design and Analysis of Cluster Randomization Trials in Health Research*. London: Arnold.

Drummond, M. and McGuire, A (eds). (2001) *Economic Evaluation in Health Care. Merging Theory with Practice*. Oxford: Oxford University Press.

Drummond, M. F., Sculpher, M., O'Brien, B., Stoddart, G. L. and Torrance, G. W. (2005) *Methods for the Economic Evaluation of Health Care Programmes*. Oxford: Oxford Medical Publications.

Efron, B. and Tibshirani, R. J. (1993) *An Introduction to the Bootstrap*. New York: Chapman & Hall.

Egger M., Davey-Smith, G., Schneider, M. and Minder, C. (1997) Bias in meta-analysis detected by a simple graphical test. *British Medical Journal*, 315(7109), 629–634.

Egger, M., Davey-Smith, G. and Altman, D. (eds) (2001) *Systematic Reviews in Health Care: Meta-analysis in Context*, 2nd edition. London: BMJ Books.

Elashoff, J. D. (1999) *nQuery Advisor Version 3.0 User's Guide*. Los Angeles: Statistical Solutions.

EuroQol Group (1990) EuroQol – a new facility for the measurement of health related quality of life. *Health Policy* 16, 199–208.

Everitt, B. S. (1995) *The Cambridge Dictionary of Statistics in the Medical Sciences*. Cambridge: Cambridge University Press.

Everitt, B. S. (2001) *Statistics for Psychologists*. Mahwah, NJ: Lawrence Erlbaum Associates.

Everitt, B. S. (2002) *A Handbook of Statistical Analyses using S-Plus*, 2nd edition. Boca Raton, FL: Chapman & Hall/CRC.

Eysenck, H. J. (1978) An exercise in mega-silliness. *American Psychologist*, 33: 517.

Fairclough, D. L. (2002) *Design and Analysis of Quality of Life Studies in Clinical Trials*. New York: Chapman & Hall.

Fayers, P. M. and Hays, R. D. (eds) (2005) *Assessing Quality of Life in Clinical Trials: Methods and Practice*, 2nd edition. Oxford: Oxford University Press.

Fayers, P. M. and Machin, D. (2007) *Quality of Life: The Assessment, Analysis and Interpretation of Patient-Reported Outcomes*, 2nd edition. Chichester: John Wiley & Sons, Ltd.

Fayers, P. M., Curran, D. and Machin, D. (1998) Incomplete quality of life data in randomised trials: missing items. *Statistics in Medicine*, 17, 679–696.

Fitzpatrick, R., Davey, C., Buxton, M. J., Jones, D. R. (1998) Evaluating patient-based outcome measures for use in clinical trials. *Health Technology Assessment*, 2(14), 1–74.

Fleiss, J. L. and Gross, A. J. (1991) Meta-analysis in epidemiology, with special reference to studies of the association between exposure to environmental tobacco smoke and lung cancer: a critique. *Journal of Clinical Epidemiology*, 44, 127–139.

Food and Drug Administration (2006) *Guidance for Industry: Patient-Reported Outcome Measures: Use in Medical Product Development to Support Labeling Claims* (draft). New York, Food and Drug Administration.

Freeman, J. V., Walters, S. J. and Campbell, M. J. (2008) *How to Display Data*. Oxford: Blackwell.

Frihagen, F., Nordsletten, L. and Madsen, J. E. (2007) Hemiarthroplasty or internal fixation for intracapsular displaced femoral neck fractures: randomised controlled trial. *British Medical Journal*, 335, 1251–1254.

Frison, L. and Pocock, S. J. (1992) Repeated measures in clinical trials: analysis using mean summary statistics and its implications for design. *Statistics in Medicine*, 11, 1685–1704.

Gariballa, S., Foster, S., Walters, S. and Power, H. (2006) A randomised, double-blind, placebo-controlled trial of nutritional supplementation during acute illness. *American Journal of Medicine*, 119, 693–699.

Goldstein, H., Rasbash, J., Plewis, I., Draper, D., Browne, W., Yang, M., Woodhouse, G. and Healy, M. (1998) *A User's Guide to MLwiN. Version 1.0*. Multilevel Models Project, Institute of Education, University of London, London.

Greenfield, D. M., Walters, S. J., Coleman, R. E., Hancock, B. W., Eastell, R., Davies, H. A., Snowden, J. A., Derogatis, L., Shalet, S. M. and Ross, RJ. (2007) Prevalence and consequences of androgen deficiency in young male cancer survivors in a controlled cross-sectional study. *Journal of Clinical Endocrinology & Metabolism*, 92(9), 3476–3482.

Greenland, S. (1994) Alternative models for ordinal logistic regression. *Statistics in Medicine*, 13, 1665–1677.

Guyatt, G. H., Feeny, D. H. and Patrick, D. L. (1993) Measuring health-related quality of life. *Annals of Internal Medicine*, 118(8), 622–629.

Harper, R., Brazier, J. E., Waterhouse, J. C., Walters, S. J., Jones, N. M. B. and Howard, P. (1997) Comparison of outcome measures for patients with chronic obstructive pulmonary disease (COPD) in an outpatient setting. *Thorax*, 52, 879–887.

Hedges, L. V. and Olkin, I (1985) *Statistical Method for Meta-analysis*. Orlando FL: Academic Press.

Heeren, T. and D'Agostino, R. (1987) Robustness of the two independent samples t-test when applied to ordinal scaled data. *Statistics in Medicine*, 6, 79–90.

Hendrickx, J. (2000) Special restrictions in multinomial logistic regression. *Stata Technical Bulletin*, STB-56, 18–26.

Higgins, J. P. T. and Green S. (eds) (2008) *Cochrane Handbook for Systematic Reviews of Interventions Version 5.0.1 [updated September 2008]*. The Cochrane Collaboration. Available from http://www.cochrane-handbook.org.

Hogg, R. V. and Tanis, E. A. (1988) *Probability and Statistical Inference*. New York: Macmillan.

Hsieh, Y.-W., Wang, C.-H., Wu, S.-C., Chen, P.-C., Sheu, C.-F., Hsieh, C.-L. (2007) Establishing the minimal clinically important difference of the Barthel index in stroke patients. *Neurorehabilitation and Neural Repair*, 21(3), 233–238.

Hunt, S. M., McKenna, S. P., McEwen, J., Backett, E. M., Williams, J. and Papp, E. (1980) A quantitative approach to perceived health status: a validation study. *Journal of Epidemiology & Community Health*, 34(4), 281–286.

Hunt, S. M., McKenna, S. P., McEwen, J., Williams, J. and Papp, E. (1981) The Nottingham health profile: subjective health status and medical consultations. *Social Science & Medicine Part A, Medical Sociology*, 15(3Pt 1), 221–229.

Jenkinson, C., Coulter, A. and Wright, L. (1993) Short form 36 (SF 36) health survey questionnaire: normative data for adults of working age. *British Medical Journal*, 306, 1437–1440.

Julious, S. A. and Campbell, M. J. (1996) Sample sizes calculations for ordered categorical data. *Statistics in Medicine*, 15, 1065–1066.

Julious, S. A., George, S. and Campbell, M. J. (1995) Sample sizes for studies using the short form 36 (SF-36). *Journal of Epidemiology & Community Health*, 49, 642–644.

Karnofsky, D. A. and Burchenal, J. H. (1949) The clinical evaluation of chemotherapeutic agents in cancer. In C. M. MacLeod (ed.) *Evaluation of Chemotherapeutic Agents*. New York: Columbia University Press.

Kazis, L. E., Anderson, J. J. and Meenan, R. F. (1989) Effect sizes for interpreting changes in health status. *Medical Care*, 27(3), S178–S189.

Lacey, E. A. and Walters, S. J. (2003) Continuing inequality: gender and social class influences on self-perceived health after a heart attack. *Journal of Epidemiology and Community Health*, 57, 622–627.

Lall, R., Campbell, M. J., Walters, S. J., Morgan, K., and MRC CFAS (2002) A review of ordinal regression models applied on health related quality of life assessments. *Statistical Methods in Medical Research*, 11(1), 49–67.

Lauti, M., Scott, D. and Thompson-Fawcett, M. W. (2008) Fibre supplementation in addition to loperamide for faecal incontinence in adults: a randomized trial. *Colorectal Disease*, 10(6): 553–562.

Lee, P., Shu, L., Xu, X., Wang, C. Y., Lee, M. S., Liu, C.-Y., Hong, J. P., Ruschel, S., Raskin, J., Colman, S. and Harrison, G. A. (2007) Once-daily duloxetine 60mg in the treatment of major depressive disorder: multicenter, double-blind, randomized, paroxetine-controlled, non-inferiority trial in China, Korea, Taiwan and Brazil. *Psychiatry & Clinical Neurosciences*, 61(3), 295–307.

Lee, Y. and Nelder, J. A. (2004) Conditional and marginal models: another view. *Statistical Science*, 19(2), 219–238.

Liang, K-Y. and Zeger, S. L. (1986) Longitudinal data analysis using generalized linear models. *Biometrika*, 73, 13–22.

Lovell, K., Cox, D., Haddock, G., Jones, C., Raines, D., Garvey, R. and Hadley, S. (2006) Telephone administered cognitive behaviour therapy for treatment of obsessive compulsive disorder: randomised controlled non-inferiority trial. *British Medical Journal*, 333(7574), 883–887.

Machin, D. and Campbell, M. J. (2005) *Design of Studies for Medical Research*. Chichester: John Wiley & Sons, Ltd.

Machin, D., Campbell, M. J., Fayers, P. M. and Pinol, A. P. Y. (1997) *Sample Size Tables for Clinical Studies*, 2nd edition. Oxford: Blackwell.

Machin, D., Campbell, M. J., Julious, S. A., Say Beng, T. and Sze Huey, T. (2008) *Statistical Tables for the Design of Clinical Studies*, 3rd edition. Oxford: Blackwell.

Mahoney, F. I. and Barthel, DW. (1965) Functional evaluation: the Barthel index. *Maryland State Medical Journal*, 14, 61–65.

Manly, B. F. J. (1994) *Multivariate Statistical Methods: A Primer*, 2nd edition. London: Chapman & Hall.

Manor, O., Matthews, S. and Power, C. (2000) Dichotomous or categorical response? Analysing self-rated health and lifetime social class. *International Journal of Epidemiology*, 29, 149–157.

Matthews, J. N. S., Altman, D. G., Campbell, M. J. and Royston, P. (1990) Analysis of serial measurements in medical research. *British Medical Journal*, 300, 230–235.

McCullagh, P. and Nelder, J. A. (1989) *Generalized Linear Models*, 2nd edition. London, Chapman & Hall/CRC.

McDowell, I. and Newell, C. (1996). *Measuring Health: A Guide to Rating Scales and Questionnaires*, 2nd edition. New York: Oxford University Press.

Meier, P. (1987) Commentary on 'Why do we need systematic overviews of randomised trials?' *Statistics in Medicine*, 6, 329–331.

Melzack, R. (1975) The McGill Pain Questionnaire: major properties and scoring methods. *Pain*, 1, 277–299.

Mitchell, C., Walker, J., Walters, S., Morgan, A., Binns, T. and Mathers, N. (2005) Costs and effectiveness of pre- and post-operative home physiotherapy for total knee replacement: randomised controlled trial. *Journal of Evaluation in Clinical Practice*, 11(3), 283–292.

Moher, D., Schulz, K. F. and Altman, D. G. for the CONSORT Group (2001) The CONSORT statement: revised recommendations for improving the quality of reports of parallel group randomised trials. *Lancet*, 357, 1191–1194.

Montgomery, A. A., Peters, T. J. and Little, P. (2003) Design, analysis and presentation of factorial randomised controlled trials. *BMC Medical Research Methodology*, 3, 26.

Morrell, C. J., Walters, S. J., Dixon, S., Collins, K. A., Brereton, L. M. L., Peters, J. and Brooker, C. G. D. (1998) Cost-effectiveness of community leg ulcer clinics: randomised controlled trial. *British Medical Journal*, 316, 1487–1491.

Morrell, C. J., Spiby, H., Stewart, P., Walters, S. and Morgan, A. (2000) Costs and effectiveness of community postnatal support workers: randomised controlled trial. *British Medical Journal*, 321, 593–598.

Morrell, C. J., Slade, P., Warner, R., Paley, G., Dixon, S., Walters, S. J., Brugha, T., Barkham, M., Parry, G. and Nicholl, J. P. (2009) Clinical effectiveness of health visitor training in psychologically informed approaches for depression in postnatal women: pragmatic cluster randomised trial in primary care. *British Medical Journal*, 338, 1–12.

Murray D. M. (1998) *Design and Analysis of Group Randomized Trials*. Oxford: Oxford University Press.

National Institute for Clinical Excellence (2004) *Guide to the Methods of Technology Appraisal*. London: NICE.

Noether, G. E. (1987) Sample size determination for some common non-parametric tests. *Journal of the American Statistical Association*, 82(398), 645–647.

Norman, G. R., Sloan, J. A. and Wyrwich, K. W. (2003) Interpretation of changes in health-related quality of life: the remarkable universality of half a standard deviation. *Medical Care*, 41(5), 582–592.

Nunnally, J. C. (1978) *Psychometric Theory*. New York: McGraw Hill.

Parry, G., Van Cleemput, P., Peters J., Walters, S. Thomas, K. and Cooper, C. (2007) Health status of Gypsies and Travellers in England. *Journal of Epidemiology and Community Health*, 61(3), 198–204. Erratum: 61(6), 559.

Paterson, C. (1996) Measuring outcomes in primary care: a patient generated measure, MYMOP, compared with the SF-36 health survey. *British Medical Journal*, 312(7037), 1016–1020.

Perneger, T. V. (1998) What's wrong with Bonferroni adjustments? *British Medical Journal*, 316, 1236–1238.

Peterson, B. and Harrell, F. (1990) Partial proportional odds model for ordinal response variables. *Applied Statistics*, 39(2), 205–217.

Petitti, D.-B. (1999) *Meta-analysis, Decision Analysis and Cost-Effectiveness Analysis: Methods for Quantitative Synthesis in Medicine*, 2nd edition. Oxford: Oxford University Press.

Peto, R. (1987) Why do we need systematic overviews of randomised trials? *Statistics in Medicine*, 6, 233–240.

Pocock, S. J. (1983) *Clinical Trials: A Practical Approach*. Chichester: John Wiley & Sons, Ltd.

Ratcliffe, J., Thomas, K. J. MacPherson, H. and Brazier, J. (2006) A randomised controlled trial of acupuncture care for persistent low back pain: cost effectiveness analysis. *British Medical Journal*, 333, 623.

Reitmeir, J., and Wassmer, G. (1999) Resampling-based methods for the analysis of multiple endpoints in clinical trials. *Statistics in Medicine*, 18, 3455–3462.

Rubin, D. B. (1987). *Multiple Imputation for Nonresponse in Surveys*. New York: John Wiley & Sons, Inc.

Ruta, D. A., Hurst, N. P., Kind, P., Hunter, M. and Stubbings, A. (1998) Measuring health status in British patients with rheumatoid arthritis: reliability, validity and responsiveness of the short form 36-item health survey (SF-36). *British Journal of Rheumatology*, 37, 425–436.

Senn, S. J. (1992) *The Design and Analysis of Cross-Over Trials*. Chichester: John Wiley & Sons, Ltd.

Simonoff, J. S., Hochberg, Y. and Reiser, B. (1986) Alternative estimation procedures for $Pr(X < Y)$ in categorised data. *Biometrics*, 42, 895–907.

Smets, E. M. A., Garssen, B., Bonke, B. and De Haes, J. C. J. M. (1995) The multidimensional fatigue inventory (MFI) psychometric qualities of an instrument to assess fatigue. *Journal of Psychosomatic Research*, 39(5), 315–25.

Spector, T. D. and Thompson, S. G. (1991) The potential and limitations of meta-analysis. *Journal of Epidemiology and Community Health*, 45, 89–92.

StataCorp. (2008) *Stata Statistical Software: Release 10.0*. College Station, TX: Stata Corporation.

Streiner, D. L. and Norman, G. R. (2003) *Health Measurement Scales: A Practical Guide to Their Development and Use*, 3rd edition. Oxford: Oxford University Press.

Sullivan, l. M. and D'Agostino, R. B. (2003) Robustness and power of analysis of covariance applied to ordinal scaled data as arising in randomized controlled trials. *Statistics in Medicine*, 22, 1317–1334.

Sutton, A. J., Jones, D. R., Abrams, K. R., Sheldon, T. A. and Song, F. (2000). *Methods for Meta-analysis in Medical Research*. New York: John Wiley & Sons, Inc..

Tandon, P. K. (1990) Applications of global statistics in analysing quality of life data. *Statistics in Medicine*, 9, 749–763.

Teasdale, G. and Jennett, B. (1974) Assessment of coma and impaired consciousness. A practical scale. *Lancet*, 2, 81–84.

Thomas, K. J., MacPherson, H., Thorpe, L., Brazier, J., Fitter, M., Campbell, M. J., Roman, M., Walters, S. J. and Nicholl, J. (2006) Randomised controlled trial of a short course of traditional acupuncture compared with usual care for persistent non-specific low back pain. *British Medical Journal*, 333(7569), 623.

Thompson, S. G. and Barber, J. A. (2000) How should cost data in pragmatic randomised trials be analysed? *British Medical Journal*, 320, 1197–1200.

Thompson, S. G. and Pocock, S. J. (1991) Can meta-analyses be trusted? *Lancet*; 338, 1127–1130.

Towheed, T. E., Maxwell, L., Anastassiades, T. P., Shea, B., Houpt, J., Robinson, V., Hochberg, M. C. amd Wells, G. (2005) Glucosamine therapy for treating osteoarthritis. *Cochrane Database of Systematic Reviews* 2005, Issue 2. Art. No.: CD002946. doi: 10.1002/14651858.CD002946.pub2.

Troxel, A. B., Fairclough, D. L., Curran, D. and Hahn, E. A. (1998) Statistical analysis of quality of life with missing data in cancer clinical trials. *Statistics in Medicine*, 17, 653–666.

Tufte, E. R. (1983) *The Visual Display of Quantitative Information*. Cheshire, CT: Graphics Press.

Ukoumunne, O. C., Gulliford, M. C., Chinn, S., Sterne, J. A. C. and Burney, P. G. J. (1999) Methods for evaluating area-wide and organisation-based interventions in health and health-care: a systematic review. *Health Technology Assessment*, 3(5), 1–99.

Underwood, M., Ashby, D., Cross, P., Hennessy, E., Letley, L., Martin, J., Mt-Isa, S., Parsons, S., Vickers, M., Whyte, K. and the TOIB Study Team (2008) Advice to use topical or oral ibuprofen for chronic knee pain in older people: randomised controlled trial and patient preference study. *British Medical Journal*, 336(7636), 138–142.

Van der Linden, W. J. and Hambleton, R. K. (eds) (1997). *Handbook of Modern Item Response Theory*. New York: Springer.

Walter, S. D., Eliasziw, M. amd Donner, A. (1998) Sample size and optimal designs for reliability studies. *Statistics in Medicine*, 17, 101–110.

Walters, S. J. (2003) The use of bootstrap methods for estimating sample size and analysing health-related quality of life outcomes. PhD thesis, University of Sheffield.

Walters S. J. (2004) Sample size and power estimation for studies with health related quality of life outcomes: a comparison of four methods using the SF-36. *Health & Quality of Life Outcomes*, 2(26), 1–17.

Walters S. J. (2009) Consultants' forum: Should post hoc sample size calculations be done? *Pharmaceutical Statistics*. 8(2): 163–169

Walters, S. J. and Brazier, J. E. (2005) Comparison of the minimally important difference for two health state utility measures: EQ-5D and SF-6D. *Quality of Life Research*, 14, 1523–1532.

Walters, S. J. and Campbell M. J. (2004) The use of bootstrap methods for analysing health-related quality of life outcomes (particularly the SF-36). *Health & Quality of Life Outcomes*, 2(70), 1–19.

Walters, S. J. and Campbell M. J. (2005) The use of bootstrap simulation methods for determining sample sizes for studies involving health-related quality of life measures. *Statistics in Medicine*, 24, 1075–1102.

Walters, S. J., Morrell, C. J. and Dixon, S. (1999) Measuring health-related quality of life in patients with venous leg ulcers. *Quality of Life Research*, 8(4), 327–336.

Walters, S. J., Campbell, M. J. and Paisley, S. (2000) Systematic review of literature on methods for determining sample sizes for studies involving health-related quality of life measures. Sheffield Health Economics Group Discussion Paper Series 00/3. Sheffield: ScHARR, University of Sheffield. Available from: http://www.shef.ac.uk/~sheg/discussion/00_3FT.pdf.

Walters, S. J., Munro, J. F. and Brazier, J. E. (2001a) Using the SF-36 with older adults: a cross-sectional community based survey. *Age & Ageing*; 30, 337–343.

Walters, S. J., Campbell, M. J. and Paisley, S. (2001b) Methods for determining sample sizes for studies involving health-related quality of life measures: a tutorial. *Health Services & Outcomes Research Methodology*, 2, 83–99.

Walters, S. J., Campbell, M. J. and Lall, R. (2001c) Design and analysis of trials with quality of life as an outcome: a practical guide. *Journal of Biopharmaceutical Statistics*, 11(3), 155–176.

Ware, J. E. Jr. and Sherbourne, C. D. (1992) The MOS 36-item short-form health survey (SF-36). I. Conceptual framework and item selection. *Medical Care*, 30, 473–483.

Ware, J. E., Snow, K. K., Kosinski, M. and Gandek, B. (1993) *SF-36 Health Survey Manual and Interpretation Guide*. Boston: Health Institute, New England Medical Centre.

Ware, J. Jr., Kosinski, M. and Keller, S. D. (1996) A 12-Item short-form health survey: construction of scales and preliminary tests of reliability and validity. *Medical Care*, 34(3), 220–233.

Waterhouse, J. C., Walters, S. J., Oluboyede, Y. and Lawson, R. A. (2009) The CoHoRT study: a randomised 2 × 2 trial of community versus hospital pulmonary rehabilitation, followed by telephone or conventional follow-up; impact on quality of life, exercise capacity and use of health care resources. *Health Technology Assessment*, to appear.

Wedderburn, R. W. M. (1974) Quasi-likelihood functions, generalised linear models and the Gaussian method. *Biometrika*, 61, 439–447.

Westfall, P. H. and Young, S. S. (1989) P-value adjustment for multiple testing in multivariate binomial model. *Journal of the American Statistical Association*, 84, 780–786.

Whitehead, J. (1993) Sample size calculations for ordered categorical data. *Statistics in Medicine*, 12, 2257–2271. Erratum: 13(8): 871.

Willan, A. R. and Briggs, A. H. (2006) *Statistical Analysis of Cost-Effectiveness Data*. Chichester: John Wiley & Sons, Ltd.

World Health Organisation (1948) *Constitution of the World Health Organisation*. Geneva: WHO.

Zigmond, A. S. and Snaith, R. P. (1983) The hospital anxiety and depression scale. *Acta Psychiatrica Scandinavica*, 67, 361–370.

Index

Quality of Life Outcomes in Clinical Trials and Health-Care Evaluation   Stephen J. Walters
© 2009 John Wiley & Sons, Ltd

STATISTICS IN PRACTICE

Human and Biological Sciences

Berger – Selection Bias and Covariate Imbalances in Randomized Clinical Trials
Berger and Wong – An Introduction to Optimal Designs for Social and Biomedical Research
Brown and Prescott – Applied Mixed Models in Medicine, Second Edition
Chevret (Ed) – Statistical Methods for Dose-Finding Experiments
Ellenberg, Fleming and DeMets – Data Monitoring Committees in Clinical Trials: A Practical Perspective
Hauschke, Steinijans & Pigeot – Bioequivalence Studies in Drug Development: Methods and Applications
Lawson, Browne and Vidal Rodeiro – Disease Mapping with WinBUGS and MLwiN
Lesaffre, Feine, Leroux & Declerck – Statistical and Methodological Aspects of Oral Health Research
Lui – Statistical Estimation of Epidemiological Risk
Marubini and Valsecchi – Analysing Survival Data from Clinical Trials and Observation Studies
Molenberghs and Kenward – Missing Data in Clinical Studies
O'Hagan, Buck, Daneshkhah, Eiser, Garthwaite, Jenkinson, Oakley & Rakow – Uncertain Judgements: Eliciting Expert's Probabilities
Parmigiani – Modeling in Medical Decision Making: A Bayesian Approach
Pintilie – Competing Risks: A Practical Perspective
Senn – Cross-over Trials in Clinical Research, Second Edition
Senn – Statistical Issues in Drug Development, Second Edition
Spiegelhalter, Abrams and Myles – Bayesian Approaches to Clinical Trials and Health-Care Evaluation
Walters – Quality of Life Outcomes in Clinical Trials and Health-Care Evaluation
Whitehead – Design and Analysis of Sequential Clinical Trials, Revised Second Edition
Whitehead – Meta-Analysis of Controlled Clinical Trials
Willan and Briggs – Statistical Analysis of Cost Effectiveness Data
Winkel and Zhang – Statistical Development of Quality in Medicine

Earth and Environmental Sciences

Buck, Cavanagh and Litton – Bayesian Approach to Interpreting Archaeological Data
Glasbey and Horgan – Image Analysis in the Biological Sciences
Helsel – Nondetects and Data Analysis: Statistics for Censored Environmental Data
Illian, Penttinen, Stoyan, H and Stoyan D–Statistical Analysis and Modelling of Spatial Point Patterns
McBride – Using Statistical Methods for Water Quality Management
Webster and Oliver – Geostatistics for Environmental Scientists, Second Edition
Wymer (Ed) – Statistical Framework for Recreational Water Quality Criteria and Monitoring

Industry, Commerce and Finance

Aitken – Statistics and the Evaluation of Evidence for Forensic Scientists, Second Edition
Balding – Weight-of-evidence for Forensic DNA Profiles
Brandimarte – Numerical Methods in Finance and Economics: A MATLAB-Based Introduction, Second Edition
Brandimarte and Zotteri – Introduction to Distribution Logistics
Chan – Simulation Techniques in Financial Risk Management
Coleman, Greenfield, Stewardson and Montgomery (Eds) – Statistical Practice in Business and Industry
Frisen (Ed) – Financial Surveillance
Fung and Hu – Statistical DNA Forensics
Gusti Ngurah Agung – Time Series Data Analysis Using EViews
Jank and Shmueli (Ed.) – Statistical Methods in e-Commerce Research
Lehtonen and Pahkinen – Practical Methods for Design and Analysis of Complex Surveys, Second Edition
Ohser and Mücklich – Statistical Analysis of Microstructures in Materials Science
Pourret, Naim & Marcot (Eds) – Bayesian Networks: A Practical Guide to Applications
Taroni, Aitken, Garbolino and Biedermann – Bayesian Networks and Probabilistic Inference in Forensic Science